T0249736

Orthobiologics

Editors

MICHAEL KHADAVI
LUGA PODESTA

PHYSICAL MEDICINE AND REHABILITATION CLINICS OF NORTH AMERICA

www.pmr.theclinics.com

Consulting Editor
SANTOS F. MARTINEZ

February 2023 • Volume 34 • Number 1

ELSEVIER

1600 John F. Kennedy Boulevard • Suite 1800 • Philadelphia, Pennsylvania, 19103-2899

http://www.theclinics.com

PHYSICAL MEDICINE AND REHABILITATION CLINICS OF NORTH AMERICA Volume 34, Number 1 February 2023 ISSN 1047-9651, 978-0-323-91989-0

Editor: Megan Ashdown
Developmental Editor: Diana Grace Ang

Reprints. For copies of 100 or more of articles in this publication, please contact the Commercial Reprints Department, Elsevier Inc., 360 Park Avenue South, New York, NY 10010-1710. Tel.: 212-633-3874; Fax: 212-633-3820; E-mail: reprints@elsevier.com.

Physical Medicine and Rehabilitation Clinics of North America (ISSN 1047-9651) is published quarterly by Elsevier Inc., 360 Park Avenue South, New York, NY 10010-1710. Months of issue are February, May, August, and November. Business and Editorial Offices: 1600 John F. Kennedy Blvd., Suite 1800, Philadelphia, PA 19103-2899. Customer Service Office: 3251 Riverport Lane, Maryland Heights, MO 63043. Periodicals postage paid at New York, NY and additional mailing offices. Subscription price per year is $342.00 (US individuals), $722.00 (US institutions), $100.00 (US students), $388.00 (Canadian individuals), $950.00 (Canadian institutions), $100.00 (Canadian students), $491.00 (foreign individuals), $950.00 (foreign institutions), and $210.00 (foreign students). Foreign air speed delivery is included in all *Clinics* subscription prices. All prices are subject to change without notice. **POSTMASTER:** Send address changes to *Physical Medicine and Rehabilitation Clinics of North America*, Customer Service Office: Elsevier Health Sciences Division, Subscription Customer Service, 3251 Riverport Lane, Maryland Heights, MO 63043. **Customer Service: 1-800-654-2452 (US). From outside of the United States, call 314-447-8871. Fax: 314-447-8029. E-mail: JournalsCustomerService-usa@elsevier.com (for print support); JournalsOnlineSupport-usa@elsevier.com (for online support).**

Physical Medicine and Rehabilitation Clinics of North America is indexed in *Excerpta Medica, MEDLINE/PubMed (Index Medicus), Cinahl, and Cumulative Index to Nursing and Allied Health Literature.*

Contributors

CONSULTING EDITOR

SANTOS F. MARTINEZ, MD, MS
Physical Medicine and Rehabilitation, Assistant Professor, Department of Orthopaedic Surgery and Biomedical Engineering, University of Tennessee College of Medicine, Campbell Clinic Orthopaedics, Memphis, Tennessee, USA

EDITORS

MICHAEL KHADAVI, MD, RMSK
Kansas City Orthopedic Alliance, Team Physician, Kansas City Ballet, Sporting Kansas City, Leawood, Kansas, USA

LUGA PODESTA, MD, FAAPMR
Director, Regenerative Sports Medicine, Bluetail Medical Group, Podesta Orthopedic & Sports Medicine Institute, Team Physician, Florida Everblades, Clinical Assistant Professor, Orlando College of Osteopathic Medicine, Naples, Florida, USA

AUTHORS

ANDRE ARMANDO ABADIN, DO
Department of Sports, Spine and Musculoskeletal Medicine, Swedish Medical Center, Seattle, Washington, USA

RAN ATZMON, MD
Sports Medicine Service, Department of Orthopedic Surgery, Stanford University, Stanford, California, USA

WILLIAM A. BERRIGAN, MD
Department of Orthopaedics, University of California, San Francisco, San Francisco, California, USA

JOANNE BORG-STEIN, MD
Department of Physical Medicine and Rehabilitation, Spaulding Rehabilitation Hospital, Harvard Medical School, Boston, Massachusetts, USA

ARTHUR JASON DE LUIGI, DO, MHSA
Chair, Department of Physical Medicine and Rehabilitation, Medical Director, Sports Medicine, Mayo Clinic, Scottsdale, Arizona, USA

PETER A. EVERTS, PhD, FRSM
Director, Gulf Coast Biologics, Research and Scientific Division, Fellow, Royal Society of Medicine London, England, Fort Myers, Florida, USA

RYAN FLOWERS, DO
University of Texas Southwestern, Dallas, Texas, USA

CHRISTOPHER S. FREY, MD
Sports Medicine Service, Department of Orthopedic Surgery, Stanford University, Stanford, California, USA

ALBERTO GOBBI, MD
O.A.S.I. Bioresearch Foundation Gobbi N.P.O, Milan, Italy

ANDREW H. GORDON, MD, PhD
US Physiatry, Reston, Virginia, USA

PHILLIP TROY HENNING, DO
Department of Sports, Spine and Musculoskeletal Medicine, Swedish Medical Center, Seattle, Washington, USA

KATARZYNA HERMAN, MD
O.A.S.I. Bioresearch Foundation Gobbi N.P.O, Milan, Italy; Department of Orthopedics and Traumatology, Brothers Hospitallers Hospital, Department of Medical Rehabilitation, Medical University of Silesia, Katowice, Poland

ERIC S. HONBO, PT, DPT, OCS, CERTDN
Diplomate, American Board of Physical Therapy Specialists; Regional Director, Advanced Physical Therapy and Sports Medicine - Spine and Sport PT, Adjunct Clinical Faculty, USC Department of Biokinesiology and Physical Therapy, Consultant, Chinese Olympic Committee/Team, Thousand Oaks, California, USA

CONNIE HSU, MD
Department of Physical Medicine and Rehabilitation, Spaulding Rehabilitation Hospital, Boston, Massachusetts, USA

KUDO JANG, MD
Department of Physical Medicine and Rehabilitation, Emory University School of Medicine, Atlanta, Georgia, USA

PRATHAP JAYARAM, MD
Associate Professor, Director of Regenerative Medicine, Department of Orthopedics, Emory University, Atlanta, Georgia, USA; Department of Rehabilitation Medicine, Emory University, Emory Sports Medicine Complex, Brookhaven, Georgia, USA

MICHAEL KHADAVI, MD, RMSK
Kansas City Orthopedic Alliance, Team Physician, Kansas City Ballet, Sporting Kansas City, Leawood, Kansas, USA

KENNETH M. LIN, MD
Sports Medicine Service, Department of Orthopedic Surgery, Stanford University, Stanford, California, USA

ALEXANDER RAPHAEL LLOYD, MD
Department of Sports, Spine and Musculoskeletal Medicine, Swedish Medical Center, Seattle, Washington, USA

GREGORY E. LUTZ, MD
Physiatrist-in-Chief Emeritus, Hospital for Special Surgery, Professor of Clinical Rehabilitation Medicine, Weill Medical College of Cornell University, Chief Medical Officer, Regenerative SportsCare Institute, New York, New York, USA

GERARD MALANGA, MD
Clinical Professor, Department of Physical Medicine and Rehabilitation, Rutgers School of Medicine, Partner, New Jersey Regenerative Institute, Cedar Knolls, New Jersey, USA

JOSHUA MARTIN, MD
Attending Physician at Regenerative Orthopedics and Sports Medicine, Washington, DC, USA

RAYMOND MATTFELD, PT, DPT, OCS, ATC
Director, Sports Rehab Consultants and Bright Bay Physical Therapy, Adjunct Professor of Physical Therapy, Touro College School of Health Sciences, Post-Professional DPT Program, Brightwaters, New York, USA

KEN MAUTNER, MD
Departments of Physical Medicine and Rehabilitation, and Orthopedics, Emory University School of Medicine, Atlanta, Georgia, USA

HIROTAKA NAKAGAWA, MD
Department of Orthopedics and Rehabilitation, Tufts Medical Center, Boston, Massachusetts, USA

RYAN P. NUSSBAUM, DO
Sports Medicine Fellow, Physical Medicine and Rehabilitation, University of Pittsburgh Medical Center, Pittsburgh, Pennsylvania, USA

KENTARO ONISHI, DO
Attending Physician, Physical Medicine and Rehabilitation, Orthopedic Surgery, University of Pittsburgh School of Medicine, University of Pittsburgh Medical Center, Pittsburgh, Pennsylvania, USA

JORDAN PEARL ORR, MD
Department of Sports, Spine and Musculoskeletal Medicine, Swedish Medical Center, Seattle, Washington, USA

ALBERTO J. PANERO, DO
Director, The BIOS Orthopedic Institute, Sacramento, California, USA

KINSLEY PIERRE, BS
Sports Medicine Service, Department of Orthopedic Surgery, Stanford University, Stanford, California, USA

LUGA PODESTA, MD, FAAPMR
Director, Regenerative Sports Medicine, Bluetail Medical Group, Podesta Orthopedic & Sports Medicine Institute, Team Physician, Florida Everblades, Clinical Assistant Professor, Orlando College of Osteopathic Medicine, Naples, Florida, USA

ADAM POURCHO, DO, RMSK
Elite Sports Performance Medicine, Seattle, Washington, USA

XIAOFEI QIN, PhD
Chief Scientist, Lifenet Health, Virginia Beach, Viginia, USA

DANIELLE REHOR, BS
Medical Student, University of Kansas School of Medicine, Kansas City, Kansas, USA

ALEX RONEY, BS
Medical Student, Liberty University College of Osteopathic Medicine, Lynchburg, Virginia, USA

PAYMAN SADEGHI, MD
Clinical Director, National Headache Institute and National Stem Cell Clinic, Miami, Florida, USA

SETH L. SHERMAN, MD
Associate Professor, Sports Medicine Service, Department of Orthopedic Surgery, Stanford University, Stanford, California, USA

DAVID R. SMITH, MD
Division of Anaesthesia, Adjunct Professor, Queens University, Astra Fellow in Regional Anesthesia, Virginia Mason Clinic, Staff Physician, Interventional Pain Medicine, Specialist in Orthobiologic Treatments, Kingston Orthopaedic Pain Institute, Kingston, Ontario, Canada

PHILIP M. STEPHENS, DO, MBA
Resident Physician, Physical Medicine and Rehabilitation, University of Pittsburgh Medical Center, Pittsburgh, Pennsylvania, USA

WALTER SUSSMAN, DO
Boston Sports & Biologics, Assistant Clinical Professor, Department of Orthopedics and Rehabilitation, Tufts Medical Center, Wellesley, Massachusetts, USA

STEPHANIE TOW, MD
University of Texas Southwestern, Scottish Rite for Children Orthopedic and Sports Medicine Center, Dallas, Texas, USA

MONICA S. VEL, BS
Sports Medicine Service, Department of Orthopedic Surgery, Stanford University, Stanford, California, USA

KEVIN VU, MD
Department of Physical Medicine and Rehabilitation, Spaulding Rehabilitation Hospital, Boston, Massachusetts, USA

PETER C. YEH, MD
Clinical Instructor, Department of Physical Medicine and Rehabilitation, Vanderbilt University, Vanderbilt Stallworth Rehabilitation Hospital, Nashville, Tennessee, USA

Contents

Foreword: Insights with Friends xiii

Santos F. Martinez

Preface: Expanding our Knowledge of Orthobiologic Therapies xv

Michael Khadavi and Luga Podesta

Basic Science of Autologous Orthobiologics Part 1. Platelet-Rich Plasma 1

Peter A. Everts, Payman Sadeghi, and David Smith

In recent years, autologous biological preparations have emerged as a growing area of medical innovation in interventional orthopedical procedures and surgical interventions. These cellular therapies are often referred to as orthobiologics and are derived from patient's own tissues, such as blood, bone marrow, and adipose tissue to prepare platelet-rich plasma (PRP), bone marrow concentrate, and adipose tissue concentrate, respectively. In this article, we will emphasize and discuss the physiological variability of autologous PRP bioformulations regarding their effectivity in tissue repair. Furthermore, recent developments concerning platelet dosing, potentially effecting immunomodulation, and pain killing will be described.

Basic Science of Autologous Orthobiologics: Part 2. Mesenchymal Stem Cells 25

Peter A. Everts and Alberto Panero

In recent years, autologous biological preparations have emerged as a growing area of medical innovation in interventional orthopedical procedures and surgical interventions. These cellular therapies are often referred to as orthobiologics and are derived from patient's own tissues, like blood, bone marrow, and adipose tissue to prepare platelet-rich plasma (PRP), bone marrow concentrate (BMC), and adipose tissue concentrate (ATC), respectively. In this article, we emphasize and discuss the physiologic variability of autologous prepared BMC and ATC for the delivery of mesenchymal stem cells to support tissue repair processes.

Basic Science of Allograft Orthobiologics 49

Alberto J. Panero, Peter A. Everts, Hirotaka Nakagawa, Walter Sussman, and Xiaofei Qin

Orthobiologic procedures are based on altering the microenvironment of musculoskeletal tissues to induce an anti-inflammatory effect and reduce pain, promote healing of these tissues, or provide mechanical support. Allograft tissues have these inherent qualities and can be used as such. This could provide patients whose own autologous tissues may be compromised or have contraindications to harvesting an alternative to treat their orthopedic conditions. Although these allograft therapies are promising, they lack high-quality clinical studies and regulatory guidelines currently limit their use.

Medical Concerns in Orthobiologics Procedures 63

Peter C. Yeh and Prathap Jayaram

Orthobiologics have shown immense treatment potential in many medical fields including sports medicine, musculoskeletal disorders, and pain management. As with the case of any medical procedures and treatments, there are potential side effects or caveats that physicians and patients should be cognizant of. Nevertheless, the use of orthobiologics does not seem to have consistent severe side effects and do not have increased risks with transmissible disease, immune-modulated reactions, or oncologic processes.

Evidence-Based Approach to Orthobiologics for Osteoarthritis and Other Joint Disorders 71

Katarzyna Herman and Alberto Gobbi

Osteoarthritis and cartilage lesions are a major cause of functional limitations which is why the goal of biological treatment is to preserve the native joint to delay the onset of OA. As a result of improvements in surgical techniques and technology, treatment options are more and more available, allowing the treatment of a whole range of injuries, from minor to extensive lesions both acute and chronic. In chondral lesion treatment, restoring hyaline-like cartilage provides improved durability of repaired tissue and desirable wear characteristics. Biological cell-based cartilage restoration treatment was developed to address the need for the long-term viability of repaired tissue. These procedures provide a reliable source of chondrocytes, whether directly or through the differentiation of multipotent precursor cells, capable of producing hyaline-like cartilage, with the minimal formation of fibrocartilage tissue. However, if arthritic changes begin biological therapies offer possibilities to delay. This chapter aims to discuss and give insights into these regenerative, joint preservation techniques for cartilage treatment and possible biological treatment in OA.

An Evidence-Based Approach to Orthobiologics for Tendon Disorders 83

Andre Armando Abadin, Jordan Pearl Orr, Alexander Raphael Lloyd, Phillip Troy Henning, and Adam Pourcho

Tendinopathy is a chronic injury that affects both the athletic and general population. Recalcitrant tendinopathy is both frustrating for patients and providers once typical conservative treatments have been exhausted. Current research in orthobiologics shows that they are safe and could improve pain and function in recalcitrant cases. Unfortunately, many studies show inconsistency in the content of the orthobiologic injectate and approach in treatment protocols. There are robust data to support the use of platelet-rich plasma for the treatment of recalcitrant common extensor tendinopathy and plantar fasciopathy, but high-quality random control trials are needed before drawing definitive conclusions for other tendinopathies.

Protocols and Techniques for Orthobiologic Procedures 105

Michael Khadavi, Adam Pourcho, and Luga Podesta

Many procedural techniques have been described and used for orthobiologics procedures with little research on the ideal technique. This section

outlines the commonly used materials and techniques from start to finish for these procedures. Post-procedure pain is common during and after many of these injections, and local and regional anesthesia during these procedures is discussed. Accuracy and safety of tendon, ligament, cartilage, intra-osseous, and spinal orthobiologic procedures are improved with the utilization of image guidance.

Intradiscal Leukocyte Rich Platelet Rich Plasma for Degenerative Disc Disease **117**

Gregory E. Lutz

If we could choose a single non-fatal medical condition to find a better solution that would make the greatest impact on global health it would be a solution for degenerative disc disease (DDD) - the number one cause of chronic low back pain (CLBP).

Orthobiologic Treatment of Ligament Injuries **135**

Luga Podesta, Eric S. Honbo, Raymond Mattfeld, and Michael Khadavi

Ligament injuries are common causes of joint pain, dysfunction, and disability resulting in disruption of joint homeostasis. Ligament injuries have historically been treated surgically. The autologous orthobiologic preparation used for treatment can influence the varying results reported. Therefore, to truly understand and compare results of these powerful therapies, reporting standardization, such as harvesting techniques, concentration techniques, quantification of the delivered product (platelets, progenitor cells), formulations (leukocyte content), number of injections performed, activation, injection technique (guided vs unguided), in addition to the post treatment rehabilitation process, are all important and necessary to evaluate and compare efficacy of future studies.

Prolotherapy: A Narrative Review of Mechanisms, Techniques, and Protocols, and Evidence for Common Musculoskeletal Conditions **165**

Connie Hsu, Kevin Vu, and Joanne Borg-Stein

Prolotherapy is a nonsurgical regenerative technique that allows small amounts of irritant solution to be injected into the site of painful tendon and ligament insertions to promote the growth of healthy cells and tissues. The goal of prolotherapy is to stimulate growth factors that may strengthen attachments and reduce pain. Prolotherapy injection technique is centered around a focused physical examination and strong anatomic knowledge for maximized results. Prolotherapy is beneficial in a variety of different musculoskeletal conditions, including, but not limited to, lateral epicondylosis, rotator cuff tendinopathy, plantar fasciitis, Achilles tendinopathy, osteoarthritis, low back pain, sacroiliac joint pain, and TMJ laxity.

Orthobiologic Interventions for Muscle Injuries **181**

Philip M. Stephens, Ryan P. Nussbaum, and Kentaro Onishi

Muscle injuries represent a common problem in active populations. Orthobiologics continue to be studied for their ability to improve muscle healing. To date, the basic science research for treating muscle injuries with platelet-rich plasma or stem cell remains novel. Furthermore, there are even fewer clinical studies on these topics, and their findings are inconclusive. Reviewing the literature, muscle injuries treated with ultrasound-

for safety and efficacy. These regulations are frequently updated and federally enforced. As the regulatory landscape changes, clinicians using biologic products must stay informed to remain within the purview of the FDA. This article describes the current regulations of the most common products: platelet-rich plasma, bone marrow aspirate concentrate, adipose-derived products, and birth tissue products.

Orthobiologic Standardization and Clinical Outcome Measurement **285**

Joshua Martin and Gerard Malanga

There is a pressing need for the standardization of orthobiologics, considering the cellular components, concentrations, and methods of injections may vary wildly, currently without significant standards of care. There is a growing body of evidence that these factors matter significantly for patient outcomes, so it is imperative that orthobiologic constituents are measured and standardized. Cell counts may be performed for platelet-rich plasma and bone marrow aspirate-based injections, whereas adipose should have standardized processing techniques as cellular quantification is more difficult.

Regional Anesthesia for Orthobiologic Procedures **291**

Michael Khadavi, Danielle Rehor, Alex Roney, Luga Podesta, and David R. Smith

Peripheral nerve blocks (PNB) can lessen procedural pain and eliminate the known detrimental effects of our local anesthetics on our orthobiologic target tissues. Local nerve damage and local anesthetic systemic toxicity are risks of PNBs that can be minimized with meticulous injection technique and an understanding of why these complications can occur. Herein, several PNB techniques are described in an effort to enhance procedural safety, efficacy, and comfort.

PHYSICAL MEDICINE AND REHABILITATION CLINICS OF NORTH AMERICA

Foreword

Insights with Friends

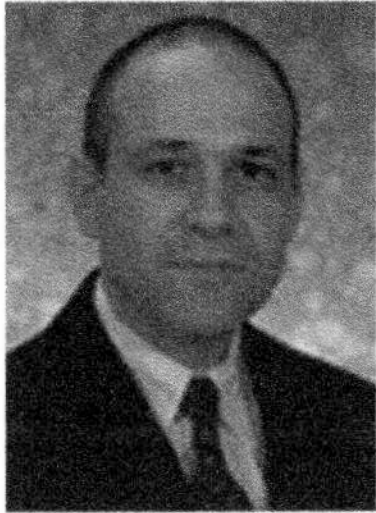

Santos F. Martinez MD, MS
Consulting Editor

Orthobiologics has progressively permeated diverse subspecialties in medicine. Just a few years ago, this was considered a fringe topic with a very select following. Now Orthobiologics is considered a mainstream modality for musculoskeletal and sports medicine practitioners. National and international researchers and practitioners congregate to discuss their latest findings and protocols. There are very few top academic facilities, Sports Medicine meccas, or national Orthopedic conferences that do not offer or include some form of regenerative or Orthobiologic leaning modality training. These approaches have further been enhanced by the refinement and availability of musculoskeletal ultrasound. In fact, there are a handful of US Medical Universities that now provide portable ultrasound training to first-year medical students as a point-of-care modality. Caution certainly is advised in following the science when offering what is a truly justifiable innovative treatment option versus exploitation with unproven strategies. Dr Podesta and Dr Khadavi offer the practitioner a very well thought-out practical format for those of us considering using Orthobiologics in our musculoskeletal practice. There is an insightful transition from the basic sciences to specific pathologic considerations. I commend the Guest Editors and authors for this excellent review for our reading audience.

Santos F. Martinez, MD, MS
Physical Medicine and Rehabilitation
Department of Orthopaedic Surgery and
Biomedical Engineering
University of Tennessee College of Medicine
Campbell Clinic Orthopaedics
Memphis, TN 38104, USA

E-mail address:
smartinez@campbellclinic.com

Phys Med Rehabil Clin N Am 34 (2023) xiii
https://doi.org/10.1016/j.pmr.2022.09.002
1047-9651/23/© 2022 Published by Elsevier Inc.

Foreword

Insights with Friends

Orthobiologics

Santos F. Martinez, MD, MS
Consulting Editor

Orthobiologics has become a very popular topic in subspecialties in medicine. Just a few years ago, this was considered a minor topic with a very select following. Now Orthobiologics is considered a mainstream modality for musculoskeletal and Sports medicine practitioners. National and international researchers and practitioners congregate to discuss their latest findings and protocols. There are very few top athletic facilities, Sports Medicine practices, or national Orthopedic conferences that do not offer or include some form of regenerative or Orthobiologic learning modality training. These approaches have further been enhanced by the refinement and availability of musculoskeletal ultrasound. In fact, there are a handful of US Medical Universities that now provide bedside ultrasound training to first-year medical students as a point-of-care modality. Caution certainly is advised in following the science when deciding what is a truly justifiable innovative treatment option versus exploitation with unproven strategies. Dr [illegible] and Dr [illegible] after the procedure, a very well-thought-out practical format for those of us considering using Orthobiologics in our musculoskeletal practice. There is an insightful transition from the basic science to specific pathologic considerations. I commend the Guest Editors and authors for this excellent review for our reading audience.

Santos F. Martinez, MD, MS
Physical Medicine and Rehabilitation
Department of Orthopaedics
[illegible]
University of Tennessee College of Medicine
Campbell Clinic Orthopaedics
Memphis, TN 38119, USA

E-mail address:
smartinez@campbellclinic.com

Phys Med Rehabil Clin N Am 34 (2023) xiii
https://doi.org/10.1016/j.pmr.2022.09.002
1047-9651/23/© 2022 Published by Elsevier Inc.
pmr.theclinics.com

Preface
Expanding our Knowledge of Orthobiologic Therapies

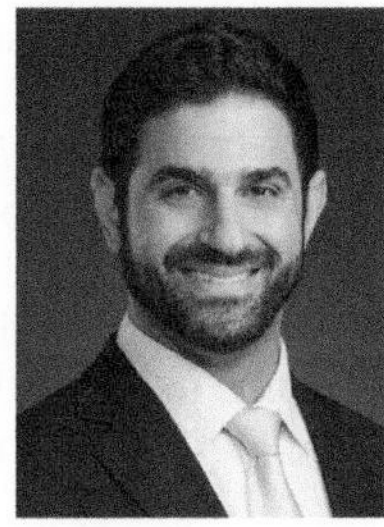

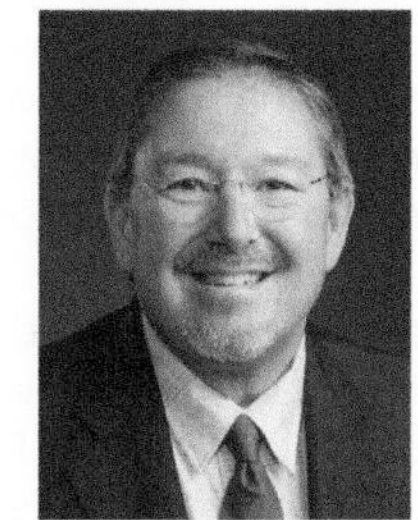

Michael Khadavi, MD, RMSK   Luga Podesta, MD, FAAPMR
Editors

We are extremely excited to present the current issue of *Physical Medicine and Rehabilitation Clinics of North America*, "Regenerative Medicine Update." We have put together an all-star lineup of authors who are some of the world's authorities in the basic science of orthobiologics, cell-based therapies, and the application of these therapies as a first-line treatment, or in combination with surgical procedures to enhance surgical outcomes.

Since the inception of using cell-based therapies to stimulate and enhance the body's innate ability to heal, tremendous effort has been made to understand how the body heals and how we can safely and effectively enhance this healing process. Millions of dollars and countless hours have been spent over the past decade to increase this knowledge base and provide evidence-based, minimally invasive, treatment modalities that are safe and effective. Despite the exponential growth of the field and increasing number of clinicians implementing othobiologic therapies in their practices, we still lack standardization in reporting exactly what we are utilizing, how it was collected, how it was produced, what was the deliverable cellular content, how and where it was administered, and finally, delineating specific rationales pertinent to the initiation and progression of tissue-specific pretreatment and posttreatment rehabilitation.

Therefore, in this publication, we have set out to bring together several of the world's thought-leaders and clinicians in physical medicine and rehabilitation, regenerative medicine, interventional orthopedics, orthopedic surgery, and physical therapy to provide our readers with an update on how these treatment modalities can safely and effectively be applied to our patients for a variety of commonly encountered musculoskeletal conditions within the current restraints recently applied by the FDA.

We are extremely grateful to our contributors, who have invested a great deal of time and effort in researching and writing the most up-to-date evidence-based articles.

Phys Med Rehabil Clin N Am 34 (2023) xv–xvi
https://doi.org/10.1016/j.pmr.2022.09.001
pmr.theclinics.com

Unfortunately, during the preparation of this issue of *Physical Medicine and Rehabilitation Clinics of North America*, we were extremely saddened by the passing of one of our esteemed authors and contributors, Dr Gerald Malanga, on May 14, 2022, at the age of 61. Dr Malangal had an infectious personality. He was also a fierce advocate for what he believed in, research-based, data-driven, evidence-based medicine, minimally invasive orthobiologic treatments, and clinical practices. He was a mentor to many, an accomplished educator, a thought-leader, a brilliant researcher, a collaborator, and a clinician who will be sincerely missed by all that he touched. Our sincere condolences go out to his family, as well as the many colleagues, students, residents, fellows, and patients that were privileged to know him.

We hope that our readers will find this issue of *Physical Medicine and Rehabilitation Clinics of North America* a useful source of information on this ever-changing subject, regenerative medicine.

Personally, we would like to thank our wives, children, and families, for supporting and putting up with us over the past year while we were completing this regenerative medicine update. We would also like to thank Daniel Podesta for his expert assistance with the graphic design and layout of several articles.

Michael Khadavi, MD, RMSK
Kansas City Orthopedic Alliance
10777 Nall Ave, Suite 300
Overland Park, KS 66211, USA

Luga Podesta, MD, FAAPMR
Director Regenerative Sports Medicine
Bluetail Medical Group
Podesta Orthopedic & Sports Medicine Institute
Clinical Assistant Professor
Orlando College of Osteopathic Medicine
1875 Veterans Park Drive, Suite 2201
Naples, FL 34109, USA

E-mail addresses:
mjkhadavi@gmail.com (M. Khadavi)
lugamd13@gmail.com (L. Podesta)

Basic Science of Autologous Orthobiologics

Part 1. Platelet-Rich Plasma

Peter A. Everts, PhD, FRSM[a,*], Payman Sadeghi, MD[b], David R. Smith, MD[c]

KEYWORDS

- Autologous orthobiologics • Platelet-rich plasma • Regenerative medicine
- Platelets • Inflammation • Angiogenesis • Analgesic effects • Immunomodulation

KEY POINTS

- Various autologous orthobiologics methods are used for treating many different musculoskeletal pathologic conditions.
- None of the PRP products is created equal, resulting in potentially different outcome results, with no consensus on standardization and validation.
- PRP preparations have the potential to regulate immunomodulation, lessen pain, repair traumatized and degenerative tissue structures, and improve function.

INTRODUCTION

There is an unmet need for interventional orthobiological procedures, as indicated by an increasing interest and advances in clinical platelet-rich plasma (PRP), bone marrow concentrate (BMC), and adipose tissue concentrate (ATC) applications to various medical fields. To fully exploit the functionalities of autologous orthobiological products that make these clinical applications favorable and finally successful for patients, it is essential to produce high yield cellular products that have the potential to exploit a variety of bioformulations.

The human body has an endogenous system of regeneration through stem cells and progenitor cells, signaling cells, and other cell types because they are found in almost every type of tissue. The term autologous orthobiologics has recently been introduced for the treatment of a variety of musculoskeletal (MSK) disorders with biological preparations such as PRP, BMC, and ATC. Orthobiologics comprise signaling cells and

[a] Gulf Coast Biologics, Research and Scientific Division, Fellow Royal Society of Medicine London, Fort Myers, FL, USA; [b] National Headache Institute and National Stem Cell Clinic, Miami, FL, USA; [c] Kingston Interventional Pain Medicine, Kingston Orthopaedic Pain Institute, Ontario, Canada

* Corresponding author. Veronica S. Shoemaker Boulevard, Suite 1, Fort Myers, FL 33916.
E-mail address: peter@gulfcoastbiologics.com

Phys Med Rehabil Clin N Am 34 (2023) 1–23
https://doi.org/10.1016/j.pmr.2022.08.003

molecules, with the potential to play adjunctive roles in a variety of regenerative medicine treatment plans, by stimulating and enhancing tissue-repair processes. These interventions can be safely executed by well-trained physicians at the point of care (POC). The objectives of regenerative medicine applications are to support the body to form new functional tissues to replace degenerative or defective ones and to provide therapeutic treatment of conditions where conventional therapies are inadequate. To achieve positive treatment outcomes, a solid understanding of the biology of tissue repair, the preparation of orthobiological products, the differences in bioformulations, and their cellular responses to MSK disorders and tissue conditions is mandatory. In particular regarding PRP treatment specimen, where platelets release many platelet growth factors (PGFs), cytokines, proteinases, and chemokines. Additionally, a variety of WBCs can be included in the PRP treatment specimen.[1,2] Many studies and initiatives have tried, unsuccessfully, to standardize and optimize PRP and BMC preparation protocols using an assortment of commercial PRP devices.[3–5]

Importance of Cellular Recovery Rates to Acquire Effective Orthobiological Specimen

It is of the utmost importance that practitioners understand the variables that are involved in the preparation of effective PRP orthobiological products. However, the quality and quantity of PRP products are strongly dependent on the preparation protocols. Nonetheless, the extensive variations in reported PRP preparation conditions, such as the amount of whole blood volume, type of anticoagulant, device physical characteristics, and centrifugal variances make it very difficult to compare PRP outcome results correctly.[6] In particular, the centrifuge performance variations are rarely mentioned, including acceleration and deceleration speed, number of centrifugation steps, and centrifugation duration per cycle. Additionally, the subsequent extraction of the biological products following gravitational cellular density separation is scarcely understood. Piao and colleagues articulated that critical factors for effective PRP cellular yields (similar to BMC preparations) are centrifuge acceleration profiles and time for the maximum recovery rate of platelets and white blood cells (WBCs). Other significant factors affecting maximum cellular yields, and thus platelet concentration, are the total collected volume of whole blood before PRP processing, and the geometrical mathematics and properties of orthobiological device used for cell concentration.[1]

Platelet-rich plasma

Definition. Autologous PRP is a centrifugated and processed liquid fraction of harvested fresh peripheral blood with a platelet concentration above the baseline value.[7] PRP can be characterized as a heterogenous and complex composition of multicellular components in a small volume of plasma, prepared at POC following a phlebotomy procedure (**Box 1**).

Platelet background and properties The underlying scientific rationale for PRP therapy is that an injection of concentrated platelets at tissue sites may initiate repair via the release of many biologically active growth factors, cytokines, lysosomes, and adhesion proteins that are responsible for initiating restorative pathways. In any PRP formulation, platelets are the primary cells.

Platelets are small, anucleate, discoid blood cells (1–3 μm), with an in vivo half-life of 7 days. In adults, the average platelet count ranges from 150 to 350 $\times$ $10^6/\mu$L of circulating blood. Platelets are synthesized in the red bone marrow from megakaryocytes by pinching off from their hematopoietic progenitor cells. Thereafter, platelets are released into the peripheral circulation, in a resting state and on a continuous basis.[8,9]

Box 1
Essentials and considerations of a phlebotomy for whole blood platelet-rich plasma preparation

Proper labeling of relevant syringes with patient information

Sufficient anticoagulant in blood collection syringe.

PPE and aseptic techniques

Harvesting site choice and preparation

Proper blood draw and drawn time

Agitation of blood with anticoagulant during collection

Controlled transfer to PRP device

Follow instructions for use to prepare PRP specimen

On the platelet outside, glycoprotein (GP) receptors and adhesion molecules are present.[10] On the inside, 3 different intraplatelet structures are existing: α-granules, dense granules, and lysosomes.[10]

Platelet α-granule constituents. The α-granules are the most frequently cited intraplatelet structures because they contain, among others, many PGFs (**Table 1**). Less referenced α-granule constituents are the platelet coagulation factors, cytokines and chemokines, and angiogenetic regulators, as displayed in **Table 2**. The overall functions of these specific α granule cytokines and chemokines are to recruit and activate immune cells or induce endothelial cell (EC) inflammation.[11]

Platelet dense-granule constituents. The dense granule constituents encompass serotonin, adenosine diphosphate (ADP) polyphosphates, histamine, and epinephrine. These substances are more implicit as modifiers of platelet activation and thrombus formation.[14] Most importantly, many of these elements have immune cell-modifying effects. Platelet ADP is recognized by dendritic cells (DCs), leading to an increase in antigen endocytosis. DCs are critical for initiating T-cell immune responses and govern the protective immune response,[14] linking the innate and adaptive immune system via inflammatory T helper (Th) 17 cells.[1] Furthermore, platelet serotonin induces T-cell migration and increase monocyte differentiation into DCs.[15] In PRP, these dense granule–derived immune modifiers are highly enriched and have substantial immune regulatory effects.

Platelet-derived angiogenetic factors. The role of platelets in various angiogenetic pathways has been clearly described.[16,17]

In PRP, the overall platelet granules contain an assortment of both proangiogenic growth factors and antiangiogenic proteins and cytokines, targeting the release of specific angiogenetic factors that are involved in new blood vessel formation. In **Table 3**, various platelet contributors in angiogenetic activities are presented.

SUBSTANTIAL INCONSISTENCIES IN PLATELET-RICH PLASMA PRODUCTS

At present, more than 40 commercial PRP devices are available on the market to choose from. Unfortunately, a lack of consensus on standardizing PRP formulations has contributed to a magnitude of different PRP devices, producing dissimilar PRP, or PRP-like products.[18,19] More explicitly, depending on the PRP device used, the platelet concentration may vary significantly, as well as the presence of other

Table 1
Platelet-rich plasma platelet α-granule growth factors and their function[12,14]

Growth factor	Function
Platelet-derived growth factor (PDGF) (3 dimeric isomers AA-BB-AB)	Stimulates chemotaxis and mitogenesis Regulates collagenase secretion and collagen synthesis Mitogenic for mesenchymal cells and osteoblasts in fibroblast—smooth muscle cells Stimulates macrophage and neutrophil chemotaxis Regulator of cell growth and division
Transforming growth factor-β (TGF-β) (5 isomeric forms: β1- β5)	Stimulates undifferentiated mesenchymal cell proliferation Regulates endothelial, fibroblastic, and osteoblastic mitogenesis Regulates collagen synthesis and collagenase secretion Regulator of mitogenic effects of other growth factors Stimulates endothelial chemotaxis and angiogenesis Inhibits macrophage and lymphocyte proliferation
Vascular endothelial growth factor (VEGF) (5 isomeric forms: A–E)	Signaling function to form blood vessels Increases angiogenesis Increase vascular permeability Stimulates mitogenesis specifically for ECs Inducer of lymph-angiogenesis Antiapoptotic effect ECs Promotor of cell migration
Fibroblast growth factor (2 isomers a and b)	Promotes growth and cell proliferation and differentiation of chondrocytes, ECs, and osteoblasts Mitogenic for mesenchymal cells, chondrocytes, and osteoblasts Cell signaling functions in tissue repair
Epidermal growth factor (EGF)	Proliferation of keratinocytes, fibroblasts for collagen production Stimulates mitogenesis for ECs Involved in cell signaling pathways
Connective tissue growth factor (CTGF)	Promotes cartilage regeneration, fibrosis, and platelet adhesion Stimulator of angiogenesis Promotes connective tissue production Involved in extracellular matrix (ECM) remodeling
Hepatocyte growth factor	Regulates cell growth and motility in epithelial/ECs Supportive in epithelial repair and neovascularization Stimulates mitogenesis Stimulator of angiogenesis
Insulin-like growth factor-1	Amplification platelet response Chemotactic for fibroblasts and stimulates protein synthesis Enhances bone formation by proliferation and differentiation of osteoblasts Local supporter of tissue healing
Keratinocyte growth factor	Regulates epithelial migration Regulates epithelial cell proliferation Mitogenic effects on epithelial cells

nonplatelet cellular constituents.[20] Based on literature findings, optimal blood separation is best safeguarded by so-called double-spin PRP protocols capable of creating a layered buffy coat stratum, using dedicated centrifugal protocols and whole blood concentration devices.[21,22] Whereas single-spin devices, also known as plasma-

Table 2
PRP Platelet α-granule chemokines and cytokines and their function[4,13]

Interleukin (IL)-1 (in α and β forms)	Modulator of systemic inflammation Innate immune process regulator Potent regulator cartilage cell function
IL-6	Proinflammation Anti-inflammation Osteoclast formation Activities in innate and adaptive immunity
IL-8	Proinflammatory activity Recruitment of neutrophils Induces chemotaxis Release of lysosomal enzymes Promotes angiogenesis
Platelet factor-4	Regulates leucocytes activation Antiangiogenetic properties
β-Thromboglobulin	Stimulator of mitogenesis Extracellular matrix synthesis Plasminogen activator Synthesis of fibroblasts Regulates platelet production
Macrophage inflammatory protein-1α	Regulate inflammatory functions Immune regulation Bone remodeling Reactive oxygen species (ROS) generation Stimulates leukocyte migration
Neutrophil-activating protein-2	Causes neutrophil degranulation Attractant for neutrophils
Stromal cell–derived factor-α	Calls CD34+ cells, induces their homing Proliferation and differentiation into endothelial progenitor cells stimulating angiogenesis Calls mesenchymal stem cells and leucocytes
Tumor necrosis factor	Regulates monocyte migration, fibroblast Cell proliferation Macrophage activation Angiogenesis
Regulated upon activation, normal T cell expressed and presumably Secreted	Interacts with P-Selectin Mediating in monocyte/macrophage infiltration Active in homing and migration of T cells

PRP devices, prepare a product from the acellular plasma layer, excluding erythrocytes and leukocytes.[1] These single-spin, often referred to as test tube devices, have a low platelet capture rate, because they try to collect as many platelets as possible from the plasma layer, leaving a significant number of platelets behind in the device, when compared with the more advanced double-spin devices.[23] **Fig. 1** shows the differences between a single-spin and a double-spin PRP whole blood separation procedure. A profuse variability in final PRP cellular contents has led to differences in PRP characteristics and cellular compositions and has been recognized in the literature.[24] Marques and colleagues[25] found that inferior treatment outcomes following PRP applications correlated directly with poor quality and inconsistent PRP products. These finding were recently substantiated by the study of Fadadu and colleagues.[5] They reviewed 33 commercially available PRP systems and protocols. They concluded that some of these "PRP" single-spin systems produced

Table 3
Platelet-derived proangiogenetic and antiangiogenetic growth factors and proteins

Proangiogenetic	Antiangiogenetic
TGF-β1	TGF-β1
PDGF	PF4
VEGF	TSP
EGF	Angiostatin
Serotonin	Endostatin
Angiopoietin-1, angiopoietin-2	PAI
MMP-1, MMP-2	CXCL4L
IL-8	TIMPS

Abbreviations: CXCL4L, C-X-C chemokine L4 ligand; MMP, Matrix metalloproteinase; PAI, plasminogen activator inhibitor; PF4, platelet factor 4; TIMPS, Tissue inhibitors of metalloproteinases; TSP, Thrombospondin.

preparations with a platelet count less than that of whole blood. A PRP platelet factor increase compared with baseline of 0.52 was reported using a test tube kit.[24] In contrast, they mentioned that the double-spin PRP devices produce higher platelet concentrations.[5] Magalon and coworkers confirmed the findings of Fadadu and colleagues because they also observed a large heterogeneity among PRP quality and

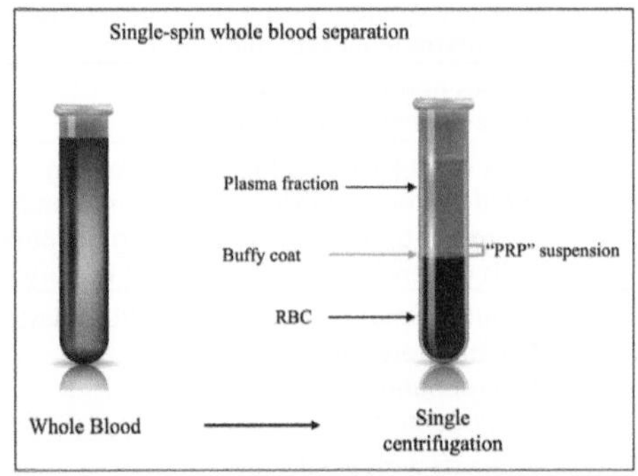

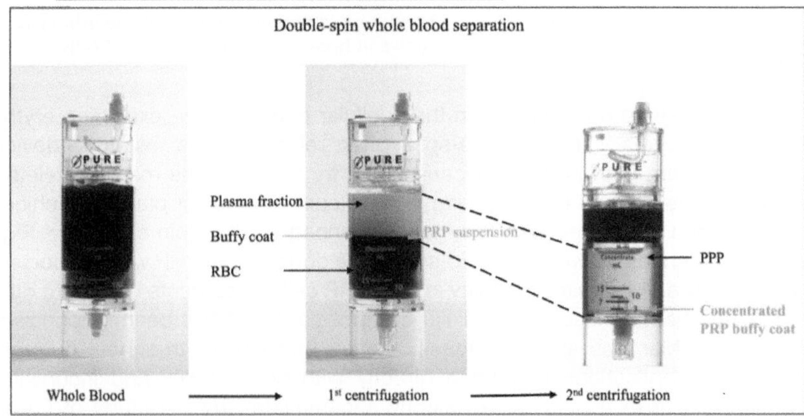

Fig. 1. Single-spin and double-spin whole blood separation. PPP, platelet-poor plasma; PRP, platelet-rich plasma; RBC, red blood cells.

devices. Most notably, it was concluded that the platelet concentration, and therefore the total number of platelets, in PRP treatment specimen is directly correlated with both the predonated whole blood volume before centrifugation and the PRP device centrifugal forces and protocols utilized during the separation steps. Overall, significant differences regarding design concepts, centrifugation parameters, PRP collection volumes, and preparation protocols between single and double-spin PRP devices were noted. It is very likely that these differences lead to distinctive PRP properties and bioformulations, potentially effecting patient outcomes.[26,27] Despite several attempts to characterize and classify PRP and other blood-derived products, a lack of consensus on the standardization of preparation protocols and absence of mentioning bioformulation, continues to contribute to inconsistencies in patient-reported outcomes.[28–33]

CONFUSING PLATELET-RICH PLASMA TERMINOLOGY

Over the years, practitioners, scientists, and companies have suffered from the initial misunderstandings and inadequacies regarding different "PRP" products and terminologies. Consequently, many different PRP bioformulations have been introduced into clinical practice and disappointingly, the literature often lacks detailed description of the PRP formulations,[34] paving the way for a variety of product descriptions and terminologies, as presented in **Box 2**. Of concern is the fact that within a specific group of "PRP-like" products termed platelet-rich fibrin (PRF),[35] many different formulations and preparation protocols are brought to the attention of the practitioner[36] (**Box 3**). It is therefore not surprising that variations in PRP preparations result in

Box 2
Frequently cited platelet-rich plasma terminologies

Advanced PRF (A-PRF)

Autologous conditioned plasma (ACP)

Autologous growth factors (AGF)

Autologous platelet gel (APG)

Clinical PRP (C-PRP)

Fibrin-plasma rich in growth factors (FPRGF)

Leukocyte-poor PRP (LP-PRP)

Leukocyte-rich PRP (LR-PRP)

Platelet-derived factor concentrate (PFC)

Pure PRP (P-PRP)

Platelet fibrin sealant (PFS)

Platelet-leukocyte gel (PLG)

Platelet lysate (PL)

Activated platelet releasate (aPR)

PRF

PRF Matrix

Preparation rich in growth factors

Modified and adapted from Everts et al.[4]

Box 3
Outline of some platelet-rich fibrin formulations

PRF

Injectable leukocyte-PRF (iL-PRF)

Injectable PRF (i-PRF)

A-PRF

Platelets rich in growth factors (PRGF)

Concentrated PRF (c-PRF)

PRF Matrix (PRFM)

Albumen gel PRFM (Al-PRF)

Leukocyte-PRF (L-PRF)

inconsistent patient outcomes.[26,27] Therefore, the true definition of PRP should be termed as small volume of plasma, which is rich in platelets, and not deprived of platelets.

CLINICAL-PLATELET-RICH PLASMA DELINEATED

Many different PRP treatment protocols have evolved during the past decades. Clinical research has stipulated a better understanding of platelet and other cellular physiology. Numerous high-quality systematic reviews, meta-analyses, and randomized controlled trials denote the clinical effectiveness of PRP biotechnology in many medical fields.[4] Currently, C-PRP is portrayed by its absolute platelet concentration, thereby shifting from the initial definition of PRP, a platelet concentration above baseline values,[7] to a minimum platelet concentration of more than $1 \times 10^6/\mu L$, or an approximate 4-fold to 5-fold increase in platelets numbers from baseline.[37] The multifaceted platelet secretome consists of proteins that are released on platelet activation, which can be measured through proteomic-based techniques.[38] This proteomic profiling has increased our current understanding of the functional importance of activities of the platelet granules contents.[39] More specifically, the biological cellular functions of the platelet secretome and other supportive plasma constituents affecting PRP treatment outcomes have become more central to our understanding of PRP treatment mechanisms. Therefore, autologous prepared PRP products should meet specific bioformulative requirements, based on specific pathologic conditions and tissue conditions, capable of contributing to clinically significant outcomes. The authors thought that C-PRP contains a clinically significant supraphysiological number of concentrated platelets to optimize platelet-dosing strategies. Moreover, specific leukocytes should be part of C-PRP bioformulations, based on the indication to treat and tissue specifics. Finally, it is important to note that the treatment specimen should contain minimal, inflammatory, red blood cells (RBCs).[40] These C-PRP qualifications, combined with the activities of an abundance of PGF, platelet proteins, cytokines, and chemokines, hold pivotal roles in (neo) angiogenesis, mitogenesis, chemotaxis, and ultimately ECM formation. Ultimately, these cellular constituents and activities contribute to immunomodulation, pain-killing, regenerative, and tissue repair mechanisms.[10] **Fig. 2** exemplifies some of the effects of PRP platelet activation. In our view, C-PRP preparations should be versatile and compliant to enable the production of different PRP biological formulations, including a significant therapeutic dose of viable platelets. More specifically,

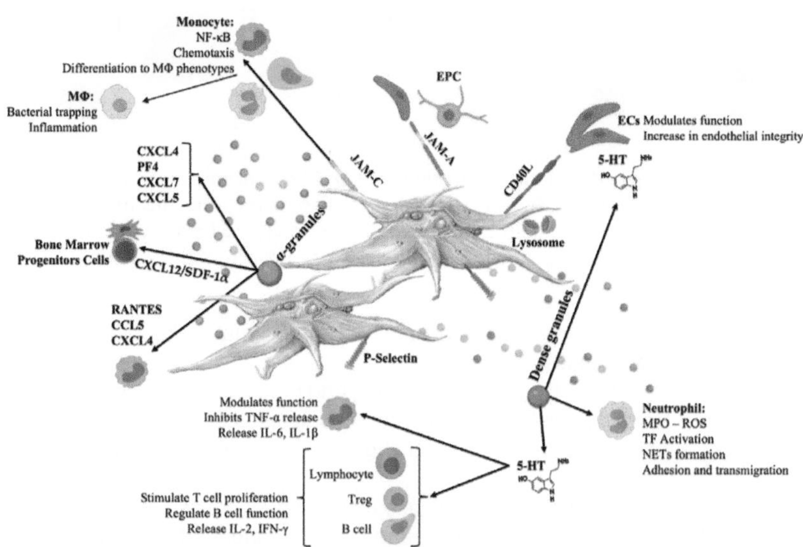

Fig. 2. Molecular and cellular interactions following platelet activation. 5-HT, serotonin; CCL, chemokine ligand; CD40L, cluster of differentiation 40 ligand; C-PRP, clinical platelet-rich plasma; CXCL, chemokine (C-X-C motif) ligand; EC, endothelial cell; EPC, endothelial progenitor cell; IFN-γ, interferon gamma; IL, interleukin; JAM, junctional adhesion molecules type; MPO, myeloperoxidase; NET, neutrophil extracellular traps; NF-κB, nuclear factor kappa B; PF4, platelet factor 4; RANTES, Regulated upon Activation Normal T Cell Expressed and Presumably Secreted; ROS, reactive oxygen species; SDF-1α, stromal cell-derived factor 1 alpha; TF, tissue factor; TNF-α, tumor necrosis factor alpha; Treg, regular T lymphocyte. (*Adapted from* Everts P, Onishi K, Jayaram P, Lana JF, Mautner K. Platelet-Rich Plasma: New Performance Understandings and Therapeutic Considerations in 2020. Int J Mol Sci. 2020 Oct 21;21(20):7794.)

the final cellular PRP treatment vial should be tailored to serve treatment protocols contingent to a variety of MSK pathologic conditions, tissue quality, and duration of the lesion.

A Double-Spin Preparation Method Explained

Because there are many PRP preparation systems on the market and based on the above reasoning to use C-PRP, we emphasize on the preparation essentials to prepare a double-spin PRP treatment specimen. It is critical that physicians meticulously execute PRP preparation protocols and follow each processing step according to the instructions for use. If the treating physician prefers, the platelets can be activated before application. In **Fig. 3**, the various processing steps of a proprietary double-spin device are demonstrated (PurePRP-SP, EmCyte Corporation, Fort Myers FL, USA).

Activated PRP platelets discharge their α and dense granular content, lysosomes, chemokines, and other cytokines, whereby, among others, an abundance of PGFs and 5-hydroxytryptamine (5-HT) is released and combined with the platelet adhesion molecules, a variety of cellular and molecular interactions are mediated. These various platelet-based activities incorporate chemotaxis, cell adhesion, migration, and cell differentiation. C-PRP with a significant load of platelets and thus platelet constituents, play pivotal roles in cell–cell interactions, contributing to angiogenetic,[41] and

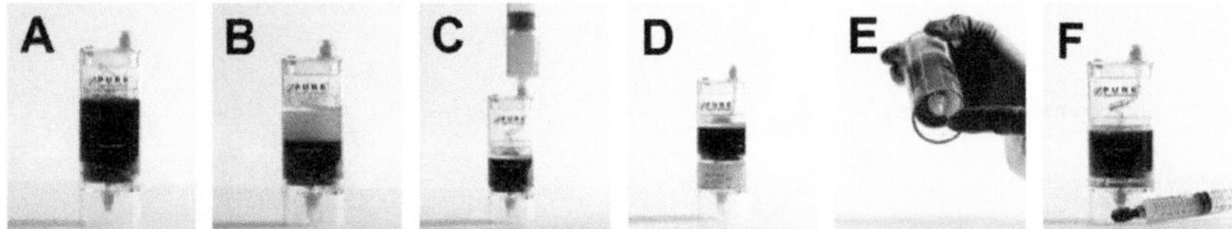

Fig. 3. Processing steps of a double-spin device. (*A*) PRP Concentration device load with blood, (*B*) Situation after first spin, (*C*) Transfer of plasma fraction and intermediate cell layer, (*D*) Situation after second spin, concentrated cells are at the bottom, (*E*) Resuspending the concentrated cells before extraction, (*F*) PRP has bee nevacuated for mthe device.

inflammatory pathways,[42] immunomodulation,[43] and ultimately facilitating in tissue regenerative repair processes.

Platelets interact with neutrophils, monocytes, and macrophages in innate immunity cell interactions. These platelet-leukocyte interactions result in inflammatory contributions through various mechanisms, including neutrophil extracellular traps (NET)-osis.[44]

In inflammatory conditions, C-PRP release a stellar concentration of 5-HT from the dense platelet granules, inciting a wide range of differential effects on a variety of leukocytic and ECs.[45] Furthermore, the liberation of high concentrations of 5-HT have been linked to pain-killing effect following C-PRP applications.[46,47]

Fresh anticoagulated blood is transferred to the PRP device (see **Fig. 3**A). The first centrifugation spin, at a constant speed for a predetermined duration, separates the whole blood in 3 layers (see **Fig. 3**B): a top layer consisting of plasma fraction and platelets, an intermediate thin multicomponent buffy coat layer, including platelets and WBCs, and the bottom layer where most of the RBCs are packed. The upper plasma fraction and intermediate layer are captured after the first spin, leaving RBCs behind (see **Fig. 3**C), and is transferred to the concentration chamber (see **Fig. 3**D) for a second spin, at a constant speed for a particular time to concentrate platelets and particular WBCs, according to their specific densities (see **Fig. 3**E). The concentrated cells are accurately resuspended in a predetermined volume of plasma, based on the intention to treat a specific MSK disorder, and precisely evacuated in an application syringe (see **Fig. 3**F).

It is obvious that the PRP cell yields and composition are strongly associated with both the PRP device design geometry and the associated centrifuge parameters (number of spin cycles, the centrifugation time per spin cycle, centrifuge acceleration, and deceleration profile).[48] Most importantly, these device factors determine the final PRP platelet dose and the potential to produce different bioformulations while safeguarding a viable cellular product.

Cellular Density Separation Principle

Centrifugation procedures are the most frequently used processes in liquid–liquid or solid–liquid separation and is based on the claim that centrifugal forces are much higher than gravitational conditions.[49] During PRP centrifugation processes, the movement of the blood cells is the result of the acting centrifugal forces in the radial direction, gravitational forces in the downward direction, and drag forces in the opposing direction of cellular motion. Therefore, differences in size and density of the whole blood cells are the driving force responsible for the whole blood separation process.[50] Validated double-spin PRP preparation protocols use predetermined centrifugal g-forces and time settings to selectively layer the individual cellular whole blood components, as displayed in **Fig. 4**. The magnification shows the result of

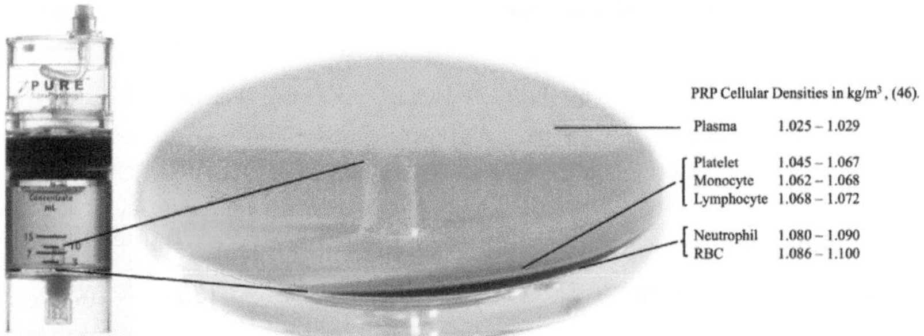
PURE
PRP Cellular Densities in kg/m^3, (46).
Plasma 1.025 – 1.029
Platelet 1.045 – 1.067
Monocyte 1.062 – 1.068
Lymphocyte 1.068 – 1.072
Neutrophil 1.080 – 1.090
RBC 1.086 – 1.100

Fig. 4. PRP cellular density separation after a double-spin procedure. (*From* EmCyte Corporation, Fort Myers FL USA, PurePRP-SP® device, with permission.)

cellular gravitational density separation, according to the specific densities of the individual cells layered down at the bottom of the concentration device. An organized multicomponent, gray, buffy coat layer (indicated between the 2 black lines) with minimal RBCs is exposed. In this example, after a neutrophil poor double-spin PRP procedure, using a 60 mL PRP device, the bioformulation of the extracted PRP revealed a high platelet concentration, increased number of monocytes, and reduces neutrophils, and RBCs; data are shown in **Fig. 5**. The total deliverable platelets (TDP) is calculated by multiplying the PRP volume × platelet concentration while correcting µL to mL: $5.7 \times [(1708 \times 10^3/\mu L) \times (10^3)] = 9739 \times 10^9$. Following this PRP preparation sample, 9739 billion platelets can be delivered to the patient. In this particular PRP preparation, the platelet capture rate was calculated to be 88.65%, whereas more than 97% of neutrophils were removed.

The preparation protocol was in accordance with the findings from Piao.[1]

PLATELET-RICH PLASMA FUNDAMENTALS FOR TISSUE REPAIR AND REGENERATION

The final solution to interventional orthobiological tissue repair is likely to be the administration of autologous multicellular preparations with the potential to intricate the full complexity of biological cell signaling, including all the microenvironmental cues that are needed to regulate the biological mechanisms, as described above. With many different PRP preparations, it has not been possible to provide a pool of cellular and molecular signals and a temporary cell scaffold necessary to initiate tissue repair and regeneration within the same PRP therapeutic product. Substantial progress in the understanding of platelet biology has revealed much about the complexity of PRP therapies. At baseline levels, platelets act as a natural reservoir for PGFs, proteins, cells, and molecules (see **Tables 1** and **2**).

Basic science research has revealed that PRP exerts its effects through many downstream reparative activities, secondary to the release of PGFs, and discharge of a myriad of bioactive factors originating from activated platelets who release their granular contents and interact with other cell types in their new microenvironment.[51] Interventional orthobiological outcomes may vary, depending on the biocellular composition of the applied PRP, the platelet dose (ie, the concentration of PGFs involved in tissue healing responses), the interactions between a variety of platelet factors, and their influence on neighboring cells at the tissue repair site (see **Fig. 3**). Importantly, PRP-mediated effects and proposed mechanisms of repair may vary between the different MSK tissue structures such as tendons, ligament, muscles, and joints.

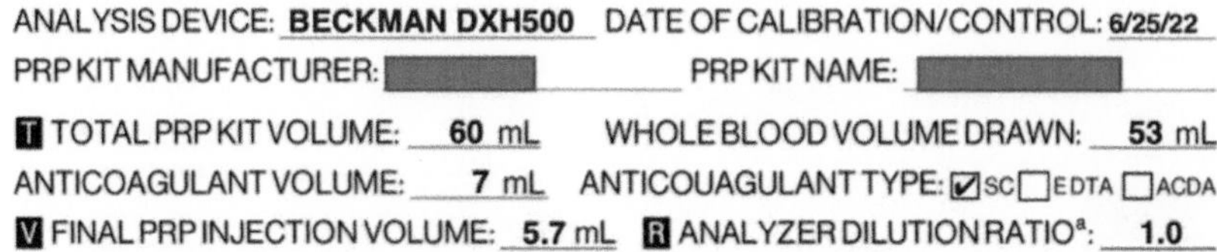
ANALYSIS DEVICE: **BECKMAN DXH500** DATE OF CALIBRATION/CONTROL: **6/25/22**

PRP KIT MANUFACTURER: ▇▇▇ PRP KIT NAME: ▇▇▇

T TOTAL PRP KIT VOLUME: **60 mL** WHOLE BLOOD VOLUME DRAWN: **53 mL**

ANTICOAGULANT VOLUME: **7 mL** ANTICOUAGULANT TYPE: ☑ SC ☐ EDTA ☐ ACDA

V FINAL PRP INJECTION VOLUME: **5.7 mL** **R** ANALYZER DILUTION RATIO[a]: **1.0**

	WHOLE BLOOD ANALYSIS			PRP ANALYSIS	
A	WBC:	**6.18** x10³/µL	A²	WBC:	**13.21** x10³/µL
B	Lymph#:	**2.20** x10³/µL	B²	Lymph#:	**10.64** x10³/µL
C	Mid #:	**0.43** x10³/µL	C²	Mid #:	**1.63** x10³/µL
D	Gran #:	**3.46** x10³/µL	D²	Gran #:	**0.87** x10³/µL
E	Lymph%:	**35.54** %	E²	Lymph%:	**80.52** %
F	Mid %:	**6.93** %	F²	Mid %:	**12.35** %
G	Gran %:	**56.02** %	G²	Gran %:	**6.61** %
H	RBC:	**4.74** x10⁶/µL	H²	RBC:	**0.11** x10⁶/µL
I	HCT:	**42.2** %	I²	HCT:	**1.0** %
J	MPV:	**8.2** fL	J²	MPV:	**9.03** fL
K	PLT:	**183.1** x10³/µL	K²	PLT:	**1708.6** x10³/µL

PCB = (1708.6 x10³/µL x 1.0) ÷ 183.1 x10³/µL = 9.33 **x over baseline**

TDP = (1708.6 x 1.0) X 5.7 = 9,739 **x 10⁶ total deliverable platelets**

RBCr = 100 - [(((0.11 x 1.0) 5.7) ÷ (4.74 x 60)) x100] = 99.78 **% RBCs removed**

TNVr = 100 - [(((0.87 x 1.0) 5.7) ÷ (3.46 x 60)) x100] = 97.61 **% NEUT removed**

PPC = [(1708.6 x 1.0 x 5.7) ÷ (183.1 x 60)] x100 = 88.65 **% platelets captured**

Fig. 5. Hematology analysis report following a double-spin whole blood neutrophil-poor PRP preparation procedure. BL, baseline; Gran, granular neutrophils; HCT, hematocrit; Lymph, lymphocytes; Mid, monocytes; MPV, mean platelet volume; PCB, Platelet Concentration over Baseline; PLT, platelets; PPC, Percentage Platelets Captured; PRP, platelet-rich plasma; RBC, red blood cells; RBCr, Red Blood Cell reduction; TDP, Total Deliverable Platelets; TNVr, Total Neutrophil Volume reduction; WB, whole blood; WBC, white blood cells. (The laboratory data were produced by calibrated laboratory analyzers (Beckham DxH500, Beckham Coulter Inc., Brea CA). [a]If no dilution was utilized value of 1 represents the total Dilution Ratio.

Platelet-Rich Plasma Mimics the Inception of Tissue Repair

PRP formulations should be capable of stimulating cell proliferation, contribute to chemotactic cell migration, stimulate immunomodulatory activities, and support in the activities of mesenchymal and neurotrophic factors.[11,52] C-PRP technologies were designed to mimic the initiation of the healing cascade in a broad application profile,[53] although it is as complex as blood itself and probably more complex than pharmaceutical drugs because it is a living biomaterial. The foremost advantages of PRP include its autologous nature and ingenious preparation techniques. Most importantly, PRP applications are safe, with no known systemic adverse effects, compared with other nonautologous biologics.[54,55] Swelling and pain are often described as adverse effects from a PRP injection. Although rare, there have been reports of posttreatment infection after PRP injection. Nonetheless, the enthusiasm to use PRP in general, is often overshadowed because there are no accepted standardization and classification parameters, or clear regulations. Despite the fact that there is no consensus on optimal and effective PRP bioformulations to treat a diversity of medical maladies, current literature supports the use of PRP in early osteoarthritis (OA) and other MSK disorders.[56,57] The roles of the various leukocytes in PRP preparations have extensively been described by Everts and colleagues.[4] An increase in reports indicate that effective C-PRP treatment outcomes dependent on intrinsic, versatile, and adaptive characteristics of the patient's blood. More precisely, it depends on the bioformulation, dose, and cellular viability of the C-PRP injectate, the interaction with the recipient local microenvironment, and the chronicity of the impaired tissue.

THE BIOLOGY OF TISSUE REPAIR USING AUTOLOGOUS BIOLOGICS

Tissue repair, wound healing, is a complex biological process, which ultimately should lead to the restoration of tissue integrity. Physiologically, the healing cascade follows distinct phases, based on variety of consecutive cellular activities, with guiding extracellular signaling processes. This complex process incorporates the implementation of, a les known, angiogenesis cascade, with a decisive role for platelets. Both cascades are jointly represented in **Fig. 6**.

The Classical Healing Cascade

The classical healing cascade is divided into the 4 distinct and overlapping, phases: hemostasis, inflammation, reparative (proliferation), and remodeling (maturation)[58] (see **Fig. 6**). The duration of tissue repair relies on the severity of tissue lesion, individual cellular characteristics, and specific healing capabilities of the injured tissue. Furthermore, certain pathophysiological and metabolic factors can affect the tissue repair process (tissue ischemia, hypoxia, infection).[59] It has been demonstrated during the past decade that the application of autologous orthobiological products are capable of directly manipulating tissue repair and inflammatory processes.[20]

The Angiogenesis Cascade in Tissue Repair and the Roles of Platelet Growth Factors

Essential in tissue repair and regenerative processes is the forming of new blood vessels. Angiogenesis plays key roles in tissue repair, recovery from ischemic disease, and tissue regeneration. Adequate physiological combinations and ratios of various angiogenic factors are critical for long-term functional blood vessel formation. Angiogenesis is a vibrant, multistep process with multiple biological mechanisms, including EC migration, proliferation, differentiation, and cell division. It involves the sprouting and organization of microvessels from preexisting blood vessels.

Essential in tissue repair are an adequate angiogenesis cascade of events and platelets. Apart from the classical wound healing cascade, the angiogenesis model of tissue repair has been recognized and described as a 5-phase orderly cascade of molecular and cellular events, as shown in **Fig. 5**. These complex platelet growth factor-receptor, cell–cell, and cell–matrix interactions characterize the angiogenetic events. The administration of C-PRP induces angiogenesis, vasculogenesis, and arteriogenesis through stromal cell-derived factor-1a binding to endothelial progenitor cell receptors. The platelet-mediated angiogenic activities are modulated by a balance between proangiogenetic and antiangiogenetic factors.[60] Based on the biological characteristics of C-PRP, it is fair to assume that the delivery of C-PRP, with a distinct bioformulation and platelet dose, will stimulate the angiogenesis cascade to create

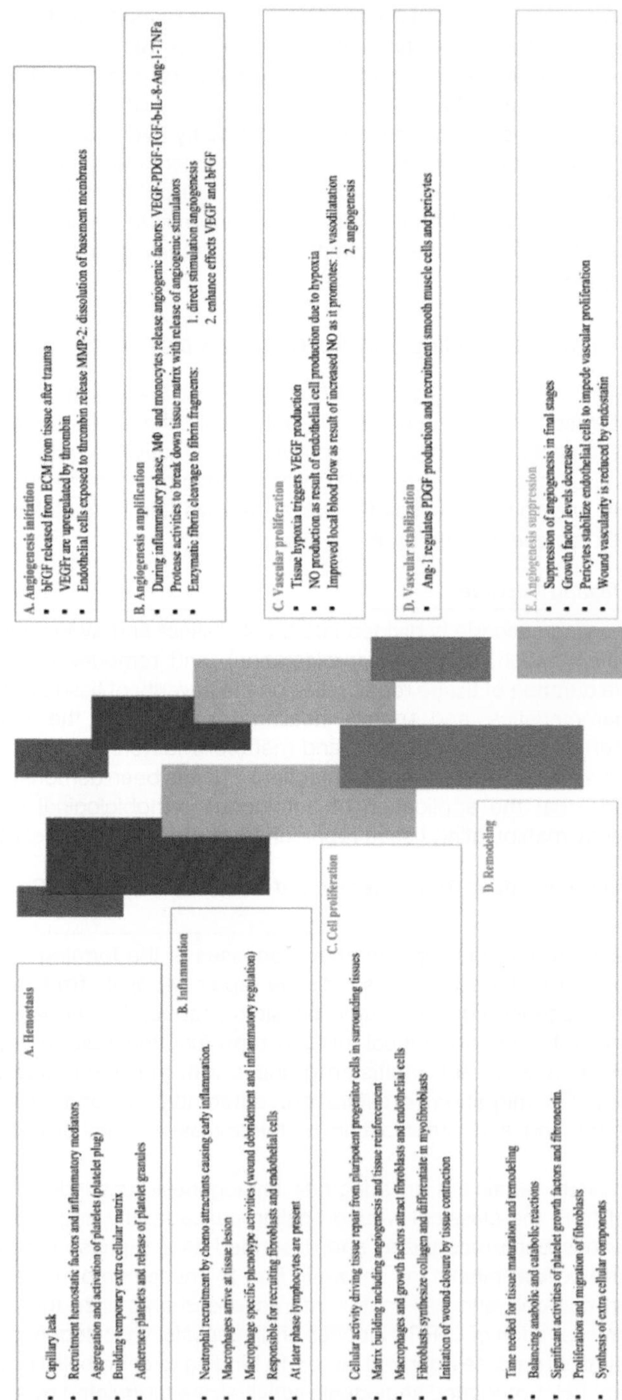

Fig. 6. Parallel between the classical and angiogenesis cascades.

vascular architecture. As a result, blood flow is restored safeguarding the high metabolic activity of tissue repair and tissue regeneration because these new blood vessels allow for the delivery of oxygen and nutrients and the removal of byproducts from the treated tissues.[61] This is of substantial clinical importance because an increase in C-PRP-mediated angiogenesis contributes to the healing of MSK disorders in areas of poor vascularization, such as meniscal tears, tendon injuries, and other areas with poor vascularity.

The role of clinical platelet-rich plasma in immunomodulatory and analgesic effects
In C-PRP formulations, platelets and monocytes are abundantly present, while neutrophils can be present based on the applied PRP preparation protocol. PRP-platelet activation is aggravated by damaged endothelium, exposing collagen and other subendothelial matrix proteins. Under these circumstances, platelet granules undergo regulated exocytosis and release their contents into the microenvironment.[62,63] In damaged and degenerated tissues, the expression of local platelet cell surface integrins, GPs, and selectins stimulate platelet aggregation and adhesion. This is important since these platelet surface molecules have been implicated in the formation of platelet–leukocyte complexes where they hold significant roles in inflammatory processes.[42] Activated PRP-platelets will express P-selectin, which in turn will bind to its specific ligands on monocytes and eventually neutrophils, initiating intracellular signaling, resulting in the stabilization of the neutrophil–platelet cell–cell interaction.[64]

Platelet–Neutrophil Interactions in Immune System

The role of the innate immune system is to nonspecifically identify intruding microbes or tissue fragments and stimulate their clearance. In homeostatic conditions, platelets are among the first cells to detect endothelial injury and microbial pathogens because they gain access or invade the bloodstream or tissues. At injury sites, and PRP injection sites, platelets aggregate and release platelet agonists, leading to further platelet activation and the expression of platelet chemokine receptors, which results in a rapid accumulation of platelets at the site of injury or infection.[65] Neutrophils, monocytes, and DCs, the most common innate immune cells in peripheral blood, are recruited for an adequate early-phase immune response. In PRP used orthobiological therapies, these platelet–leukocyte interactions regulate inflammation, wound healing, and tissue repair. More precisely, specific platelet receptors stimulate platelet–neutrophil interactions,[66] regulating the so-called leukocyte oxidative burst by modulating the release of ROS and myeloperoxidase from neutrophils.[67] Furthermore, the platelet–neutrophil interaction, with subsequent neutrophil degranulation, results in the formation of NETs, an essential pathogen killing mechanism for neutrophils, trap bacteria and kill them by NETosis.[44]

Platelet–Monocyte Interactions in Immune System

Following PRP activation at tissue sites, the monocyte fraction migrates to diseased and degenerative tissues where they perform adhesion activities while secreting inflammatory molecules that might alter chemotaxis and modify proteolytic properties.[68] Additionally, platelets can modulate the effector functions of monocytes, a critical mediator of the inflammatory response with the activation and differentiation of immune cells, and they facilitate the endogenous oxidative burst in monocytes, ultimately promoting their differentiation into macrophages.[69] Moreover, platelets promote monocyte and macrophage responses in the maturation of dendritic and natural killer cells, ensuing in explicit T and B lymphocytes responses, with a specific role for the various Th cells.[70] Only a C-PRP formulation with a significant increased concentration of both platelets and monocytes delivered to tissue treatment sites will mimic the natural activity of Th-2 cells to produce IL-4 at the treatment site. Here, IL-4 will encourage macrophage polarization, directing macrophage to the regenerative macrophage 2 phenotype, whereas interferon-γ shifts macrophages toward the inflammatory macrophage 1 phenotype, depending on the dose and timing. Following IL-4 activation, macrophage 2 induces the differentiation of Treg cells to Th2 cells, subsequently producing additional IL-4.[71] Th cells guide macrophage phenotypes to proregenerative phenotypes in response to tissue-derived biologics in an IL-4-dependent manner.[72] Therefore, the use of C-PRP to stimulate immunomodulatory mechanisms with complex cell–cell interactions and functions in inflammation, embraces a unique biological treatment potential.

From platelet concentration to platelet dose as a quality indicator

Giusti and colleagues[73] undoubtedly indicated the need to deliver a high concentration of platelets, 1.5×10^6 platelets/μL to induce a significant angiogenic response. To translate this in vitro research conclusion to clinical practice, clinicians should consider adopting a new quality parameter of delivered PRP. Using platelet concentration as an indicator for dispensed PRP is insufficient because this measure per unit of volume only relates to the effectivity of the procedure of the whole blood concentration device. PRP injectates should be based on a dosing principle, how many platelets are delivered to a tissue site. Platelet dosing should be based on the PRP volume that is dispensed in one treatment site multiplied by the platelet concentration of this PRP volume, where this PRP dose reflects the TDP. A 7 mL C-PRP treatment vial, to induce angiogenesis, as advocated by Giusti and colleagues,[73] should contain 10.5×10^9 TDP. Bansal and associates measured clinical validated outcome effects in patients treated with a single PRP injection.[74] After a dose of 10 billion TDP, a sustained clinical effect was seen during a 1-year period regarding function, pain, and inflammatory markers. Further studies are warranted to understand whether there is a TDP dose-dependency for specific tissue types and condition (acute, chronic), individual MSK pathologic conditions, and duration of disorder.

PLATELETS AND ANALGESIC EFFECTS

Chronic pain is a major public problem and effective pain management is often absent because there is still a lack of understanding in the fundamentals of the mechanisms of pain and how pain can be reliably and safely reduced or eliminated. In C-PRP preparations, activated platelets release many proinflammatory and anti-inflammatory mediators that are proficient in inducing pain but can also reduce inflammation and pain. Once applied, the typical platelet dynamics of PRP have the potential to alter the local microenvironment before tissue repair and regeneration via multiple complex pathways, related to cell proliferation, differentiation, stem cell regulation, and anabolic–catabolic processes.[75] However, based on the bioformulation of the PRP product, several animal and clinical studies concluded a variety of outcomes. PRP dosing and clinical analgesic effects are correlated. Various clinical studies, in a variety of MSK indications, indicated little to no pain relief following PRP treatment,[76,77] whereas others mention reduced or even eliminated pain.[78,79] Not surprisingly, the PRP bioformulation and platelet dose have been identified as key characteristics that contribute to consistent analgesic effects. Other variables effecting pain modulation include the PRP delivery route, application techniques, the use of platelet activation protocols, the bioactivity levels of the released PGFs and cytokines, the types of tissues to which PRP was applied, and the type of injury. Notably, Kuffler addressed the potential of PRP in pain relief in patients suffering from mild-to-severe chronic neuropathic pain, secondary to damaged nonregenerated nerves. The objective of this study was to investigate whether neuropathic pain would decrease or resolve because of PRP's promotion of axonal regeneration and target reinnervation.[80] Strikingly, in treated patients, the neuropathic pain remained eliminated, or reduced, for a minimum of 6 years after the procedure. Furthermore, in all patient's pain started to decrease within 3 weeks after the PRP application. Similar analgesic PRP effects were observed in postsurgical wound care patients.[61] Mohammadi and colleagues stated that the physiological aspects of wound pain were related to vascular injury and skin tissue hypoxia. They conveyed on the importance of neoangiogenesis to optimize tissue oxygenation and nutrient delivery. Interestingly, their study demonstrated that pain reduction in PRP-treated patients was accompanied by significantly higher incidence of angiogenesis. Johal and coworkers concluded that PRP applications contribute to pain reduction following orthopedic indications, particularly in patients treated for lateral epicondylitis and knee OA.[81] Unfortunately, the analysis did not specify the effects of leukocytes, platelet concentration, or the use of exogenous platelet-activating agents because these variables affect the overall PRP effectiveness. In a study on treating patients with lower back pain, the injection of intradiscal PRP revealed that pain killing was significantly correlated with platelet concentration.[82] PRP with higher platelet counts (>1.0 × 106/μL) provoked a more favorable painkilling response, similar to the findings of Bansal.[74] This profound analgesic effect of high PRP platelet concentrations was recently confirmed by the group of Lutz and associates.[83] They demonstrated that clinical pain scores, following intradiscal PRP injections, can be optimized when PRP preparations were used that contained a high dose of platelets (>10 times baseline platelet level), when compared with historical controls who received PRP at a significant lower dose. Furthermore, in patients with the high dose of platelets, a significant higher patient satisfaction rate was observed. Interestingly, Berger and colleagues[84] concluded more effective tenocyte proliferation and migration in an in vitro study when higher platelet concentrations from platelet lysate preparations were used, in a dose-dependent manner.

The optimal PRP platelet dose, and bioformulation, provoking maximal pain relief is yet unknown. However, it seems from clinical research that PRP should contain at least 1.0 × 106/μL platelets to induce pain-killing effects. This is similar to outcomes following a rat tendinopathy model, where complete pain relief was accomplished with a platelet concentration of 1.0 × 106/μL, whereas PRP with half this platelet concentration induced significantly less pain relief.[85]

A ROLE FOR PLATELET SEROTONIN

In 2008, Everts and colleagues[86] were the first to report a randomized controlled trial on the analgesic effects of a 2-spin PRP formulation activated with autologous prepared thrombin in patients following shoulder decompression surgery. A significant reduction in visual analog scale scores for pain, the use of opioid-based pain medication, and a more successful postsurgical rehabilitation were observed. They reflected on the analgesic effects of activated platelets and postulated on the mechanism of high concentration PRP platelet-released serotonin (5-HT) from the dense granules. In C-PRP, the platelet concentration is 5-fold to 7-fold higher than in peripheral blood, meaning that the release of 5-HT from platelets is astronomical, which was confirmed by Sprott and colleagues.[46]

In the periphery, endogenous 5-HT is released from platelets, mast cells, and ECs in response to tissue injury or surgical trauma.[87] Interestingly, multiple neuronal 5-HT receptors have been detected in the periphery, confirming that the 5-HT system interferes with nociceptive transmission at peripheral tissue sites, potentially decreasing and increasing the magnitude of pain following noxious stimulation.[88]

CLINICS CARE POINTS

- Clinical, effective, PRP is described by its absolute platelet concentration of more than $1 \times 10^6/\mu L$, or an approximate 4 to 5-fold increase in platelets numbers from baseline.
- The underlying rationale for PRP therapy is that the delivery of concentrated PRP platelets mimics the initiation of the healing cascade and tissue repair mechanisms via the release of many biologically active factors growth factors, cytokines, lysosomes, and adhesion proteins.
- Variabilities in PRP preparation protocols, like whole blood volume, type of anticoagulant used, the PRP device physical characteristics, and variances in centrifugation, can lead to inconsistent PRP injectates with non-significant patient outcomes.
- Adequate PRP therapies present a unique biological treatment potential to manage pain and inflammation.
- Pain killing effects have been demonstrated when PRP was used in orthopedic and sport medicine indications, in a dose-dependent manner.
- More favorable painkilling responses happened when the PRP platelet concentration was greater than $> 1.0 \times 10^6/\mu L$.Following C-PRP therapies, complex cell-cell interactions transpire, capable of inducing effective immunomodulatory mechanisms.

DISCLOSURE

P. Everts is also acting Chief Scientific Officer of EmCyte Corporation.

REFERENCES

1. Piao L, Park H, Jo CH. Theoretical prediction and validation of cell recovery rates in preparing platelet-rich plasma through a centrifugation. Wang JHC, editor. PLoS One 2017;12(11):e0187509.
2. Xu L, Li G. Circulating mesenchymal stem cells and their clinical implications. J Orthop Transl 2014;2(1):1–7.
3. Magalon J, Brandin T, Francois P, et al. Technical and biological review of authorized medical devices for platelets-rich plasma preparation in the field of regenerative medicine. Platelets 2021;32(2):200–8.
4. Everts P, Onishi K, Jayaram P, et al. Platelet-rich plasma: new performance understandings and therapeutic considerations in 2020. Int J Mol Sci 2020;21(20): 7794.
5. Fadadu PP, Mazzola AJ, Hunter CW, et al. Review of concentration yields in commercially available platelet-rich plasma (PRP) systems: a call for PRP standardization. Reg Anesth Pain Med 2019;44(6):652–9.
6. Chahla J, Cinque ME, Piuzzi NS, et al. A call for standardization in platelet-rich plasma preparation protocols and composition reporting. The J Bone and Joint Surg 2017;99(20):1769–79.
7. Marx RE. Platelet-Rich Plasma (PRP): What Is PRP and What Is Not PRP? Implant Dent 2001;10(4):225–8.
8. Andia I, Atilano L, Maffulli N. Moving toward targeting the right phenotype with the right platelet-rich plasma (PRP) formulation for knee osteoarthritis. Ther Adv Musculoskelet Dis 2021;13. 1759720X2110043.

9. Collins T, Alexander D, Barkatali B. Platelet-rich plasma: a narrative review. EFORT Open Rev 2021;6(4):225–35.
10. Everts PAM, Knape JTA, Weibrich G, et al. Platelet-rich plasma and platelet gel: a review. J Extra Corpor Technol 2007;14:174–87.
11. Zheng C, Zhu Q, Liu X, et al. Effect of platelet-rich plasma (PRP) concentration on proliferation, neurotrophic function and migration of Schwann cells *in vitro*: Effect of platelet-rich plasma on Schwann cells. J Tissue Eng Regen Med 2016;10(5): 428–36.
12. Blair P. Platelet α–granules: Basic biology and clinical correlates. 2010;29.
13. Chen Y, Zhong H, Zhao Y, et al. Role of platelet biomarkers in inflammatory response. Biomark Res 2020;8(1):28.
14. Iberg CA, Hawiger D. Natural and Induced Tolerogenic Dendritic Cells. J Immunol 2020;204(4):733–44.
15. Ganor Y, Besser M, Ben-Zakay N, et al. Human T cells express a functional ionotropic glutamate receptor GluR3, and glutamate by itself triggers integrin-mediated adhesion to laminin and fibronectin and chemotactic migration. J Immunol Baltim Md 1950 2003;170(8):4362–72.
16. Baka S, Clamp AR, Jayson GC. A review of the latest clinical compounds to inhibit VEGF in pathological angiogenesis. Expert Opin Ther Targets 2006; 10(6):867–76.
17. Walsh TG, Metharom P, Berndt MC. The functional role of platelets in the regulation of angiogenesis. Platelets 2015;26(3):199–211.
18. Mazzucco L, Balbo V, Cattana E, et al. Not every PRP-gel is born equal Evaluation of growth factor availability for tissues through four PRP-gel preparations: Fibrinet®, RegenPRP-Kit®, Plateltex® and one manual procedure. Vox Sang 2009;97(2):110–8.
19. Everts PAM, Hoffmann J, Weibrich G, et al. Differences in platelet growth factor release and leucocyte kinetics during autologous platelet gel formation. Transfus Med 2006;16(5):363–8.
20. dos Santos RG, Santos GS, Alkass N, et al. The regenerative mechanisms of platelet-rich plasma: a review. Cytokine 2021;144:155560.
21. Roh YH, Kim W, Park KU, et al. Cytokine-release kinetics of platelet-rich plasma according to various activation protocols. Bone Jt Res 2016;5(2):37–45.
22. Oh JH, Kim W, Park KU, et al. Comparison of the cellular composition and cytokine-release kinetics of various platelet-rich plasma preparations. Am J Sports Med 2015;43(12):3062–70.
23. Fitzpatrick J, Bulsara MK, McCrory PR, et al. Analysis of platelet-rich plasma extraction: variations in platelet and blood components between 4 common commercial kits. Orthop J Sports Med 2017;5(1). 232596711667527.
24. Magalon J, Chateau AL, Bertrand B, et al. DEPA classification: a proposal for standardising PRP use and a retrospective application of available devices. BMJ Open Sport Exerc Med 2016;2(1):e000060.
25. Marques LF, Stessuk T, Camargo ICC, et al. Platelet-rich plasma (PRP): Methodological aspects and clinical applications. Platelets 2015;26(2):101–13.
26. Bennell KL, Paterson KL, Metcalf BR, et al. Effect of intra-articular platelet-rich plasma vs placebo injection on pain and medial tibial cartilage volume in patients with knee osteoarthritis: the restore randomized clinical trial. JAMA 2021;326(20): 2021.
27. Hurley ET, Lim Fat D, Moran CJ, et al. The efficacy of platelet-rich plasma and platelet-rich fibrin in arthroscopic rotator cuff repair: a meta-analysis of randomized controlled trials. Am J Sports Med 2019;47(3):753–61.

28. Ehrenfest D.M.D., Andia I., Zumstein M.A., et al. Classification of platelet concentrates (Platelet-Rich Plasma-PRP, Platelet-Rich Fibrin-PRF) for topical and infiltrative use in orthopedic and sports medicine: current consensus, clinical implications and perspectives, Muscles, Ligaments and Tendons, 4 (1), 2014, 3-9.
29. DeLong JM, Russell RP, Mazzocca AD. Platelet-rich plasma: the PAW classification system. Arthrosc J Arthrosc Relat Surg 2012;28(7):998–1009.
30. Mishra A, Harmon K, Woodall J, et al. Sports medicine applications of platelet rich plasma. Curr Pharm Biotechnol 2012;13(7):1185–95.
31. Mautner K, Malanga GA, Smith J, et al. A call for a standard classification system for future biologic research: the rationale for new PRP nomenclature. PM&R 2015; 7:S53–9.
32. Lana JFSD, Purita J, Paulus C, et al. Contributions for classification of platelet rich plasma – proposal of a new classification: MARSPILL. Regen Med 2017;12(5): 565–74.
33. Harrison P, the Subcommittee on Platelet Physiology. The use of platelets in regenerative medicine and proposal for a new classification system: guidance from the SSC of the ISTH. J Thromb Haemost 2018;16(9):1895–900.
34. Everts PAM, van Zundert A, Schönberger JPAM, et al. What do we use: platelet-rich plasma or platelet-leukocyte gel? J Biomed Mater Res A 2008;85A(4): 1135–6.
35. Pavlovic V, Ciric M, Jovanovic V, et al. Platelet Rich Plasma: a short overview of certain bioactive components. Open Med 2016;11(1):242–7. https://doi.org/10.1515/med-2016-0048.
36. Miron RJ, Chai J, Fujioka-Kobayashi M, et al. Evaluation of 24 protocols for the production of platelet-rich fibrin. BMC Oral Health 2020;20(1):310.
37. Haunschild ED, Huddleston HP, Chahla J, et al. Platelet-rich plasma augmentation in meniscal repair surgery: a systematic review of comparative studies. Arthrosc J Arthrosc Relat Surg 2020;36(6):1765–74.
38. Cengiz IF, Pereira H, Espregueira-Mendes J, et al. The clinical use of biologics in the knee lesions: does the patient benefit? Curr Rev Musculoskelet Med 2019; 12(3):406–14.
39. Tuakli-Wosornu YA, Terry A, Boachie-Adjei K, et al. Lumbar intradiskal platelet-rich plasma (PRP) injections: a prospective, double-blind, randomized controlled study. PM&R 2016;8(1):1–10.
40. Everts PA, Malanga GA, Paul RV, et al. Assessing clinical implications and perspectives of the pathophysiological effects of erythrocytes and plasma free hemoglobin in autologous biologics for use in musculoskeletal regenerative medicine therapies. A Review Regen Ther 2019;11:56–64.
41. Herr N, Bode C, Duerschmied D. The Effects of Serotonin in Immune Cells. Front Cardiovasc Med 2017;4:48.
42. Bennett JS. Structure and function of the platelet integrin IIb 3. J Clin Invest 2005; 115(12):3363–9.
43. Dale DC, Boxer L, Liles WC. The phagocytes: neutrophils and monocytes. Blood 2008;112(4):935–45.
44. Clark SR, Ma AC, Tavener SA, et al. Platelet TLR4 activates neutrophil extracellular traps to ensnare bacteria in septic blood. Nat Med 2007;13(4):463–9.
45. Duerschmied D, Suidan GL, Demers M, et al. Platelet serotonin promotes the recruitment of neutrophils to sites of acute inflammation in mice. Blood 2013; 121(6):1008–15.
46. Sprott H, Franke S, Kluge H, et al. Pain treatment of fibromyalgia by acupuncture. Rheumatol Int 1998;18(1):35–6.

47. Kuffler D. Variables affecting the potential efficacy of PRP in providing chronic pain relief. J Pain Res 2018;12:109–16.
48. Lueptow RM, Hübler W. Sedimentation of a suspension in a centrifugal field. J Biomech Eng 1991;113(4):485–91.
49. Perez AGM, Lana JFSD, Rodrigues AA, et al. Relevant aspects of centrifugation step in the preparation of platelet-rich plasma. ISRN Hematol 2014;2014:1–8.
50. Jo C.H., Roh Y.H., Kim J.E., et al. Optimizing Platelet-Rich Plasma Gel Formation by Varying Time and Gravitational Forces During Centrifugation, J of Oral Implant, 34, 5, 2013, 525-532.
51. Middleton KK, Barro V, Muller B, et al. Evaluation of the Effects of Platelet-Rich Plasma (PRP) Therapy Involved in the Healing of Sports-Related Soft Tissue Injuries. The Iowa Orthopaedic J 2012;32:150–63.
52. Xu J, Gou L, Zhang P, et al. Platelet-rich plasma and regenerative dentistry. Aust Dent J 2020;65(2):131–42.
53. Andia I, Maffulli N. A contemporary view of platelet-rich plasma therapies: moving toward refined clinical protocols and precise indications. Regen Med 2018;13(6): 717–28.
54. Puzzitiello RN, Patel BH, Forlenza EM, et al. Adverse impact of corticosteroids on rotator cuff tendon health and repair: a systematic review of basic science studies. Arthrosc Sports Med Rehabil 2020;2(2):e161–9.
55. Kumar A, Kadamb AG, Kadamb KG. Hope, hype, hurdles and future perspective for prp, prp versus hyaluronic acid injection in osteoarthritis of the knee, Bio Ortho J, 2, (1), 2020, e1-e12.
56. Hohmann E, Tetsworth K, Glatt V. Is platelet-rich plasma effective for the treatment of knee osteoarthritis? A systematic review and meta-analysis of level 1 and 2 randomized controlled trials. Eur J Orthop Surg Traumatol 2020. https://doi.org/10.1007/s00590-020-02623-4.
57. Madhi MI, Yausep OE, Khamdan K, et al. The use of PRP in treatment of achilles tendinopathy: a systematic review of literature. study design: systematic review of literature. Ann Med Surg 2020;55:320–6.
58. Sinno H, Prakash S. Complements and the wound healing cascade: an updated review. Plast Surg Int 2013;2013:1–7.
59. Broughton G, Janis JE, Attinger CE. The basic science of wound healing. Plast Reconstr Surg 2006;117(SUPPLEMENT):12S–34S.
60. Bir SC, Esaki J, Marui A, et al. Therapeutic treatment with sustained-release platelet-rich plasma restores blood perfusion by augmenting ischemia-induced angiogenesis and arteriogenesis in diabetic mice. J Vasc Res 2011;48(3): 195–205.
61. Mohammadi S, Nasiri S, Mohammadi MH, et al. Evaluation of platelet-rich plasma gel potential in acceleration of wound healing duration in patients underwent pilonidal sinus surgery: a randomized controlled parallel clinical trial. Transfus Apher Sci 2017;56(2):226–32.
62. Morrell CN, Aggrey AA, Chapman LM, et al. Emerging roles for platelets as immune and inflammatory cells. Blood 2014;123(18):2759–67.
63. Thon JN, Peters CG, Machlus KR, et al. T granules in human platelets function in TLR9 organization and signaling. J Cell Biol 2012;198(4):561–74.
64. Weber C, Springer TA. Neutrophil Accumulation on Activated, Surface-adherent Platelets in Flow Is Mediated by Interaction of Mac-1 with Fibrinogen Bound to IIb[illegible]3 and Stimulated by Platelet-activating Factor. J. Clin. Invest. 1997;100(8): 2085–93.

65. Clemetson K, Clemetson J, Proudfoot A, et al. Functional expression of CCR1, CCR3, CCR4, and CXCR4 chemokine receptors on human platelets. Blood 2000;96(13):4046–54.
66. Vasina EM, Cauwenberghs S, Feijge MAH, et al. Microparticles from apoptotic platelets promote resident macrophage differentiation. Cell Death Dis 2011; 2(9):e211.
67. Moojen DJF, Schure RM, Overdevest EP, et al. Antimicrobial activity of platelet-leukocyte gel againstStaphylococcus aureus. J Orthop Res 2008;26(3):404–10.
68. Kapur R, Zufferey A, Boilard E, et al. Nouvelle cuisine: platelets served with inflammation. J Immunol 2015;194(12):5579–87.
69. Scheuerer B, Ernst M, Dürrbaum-Landmann I, et al. The CXC-chemokine platelet factor 4 promotes monocyte survival and induces monocyte differentiation into macrophages. Blood 2000;95(4):1158–66.
70. Gaudino SJ, Kumar P. Cross-talk between antigen presenting cells and T cells impacts intestinal homeostasis, bacterial infections, and tumorigenesis. Front Immunol 2019;10:360.
71. Kaiko GE, Horvat JC, Beagley KW, et al. Immunological decision-making: how does the immune system decide to mount a helper T-cell response? Immunology 2008;123(3):326–38.
72. Sadtler K, Estrellas K, Allen BW, et al. Developing a pro-regenerative biomaterial scaffold microenvironment requires T helper 2 cells. Science 2016;352(6283): 366–70.
73. Giusti I, Rughetti A, D'Ascenzo S, et al. Identification of an optimal concentration of platelet gel for promoting angiogenesis in human endothelial cells. Transfusion (Paris) 2009;49(4):771–8.
74. Bansal H, Leon J, Pont JL, et al. Platelet-rich Plasma (PRP) in osteoarthritis (OA) knee: Correct dose critical for long term clinical efficacy. Scientific Reports 2021; 11:3971. https://doi.org/10.1038/s41598-021-83025-2.
75. Alsousou J, Thompson M, Hulley P, et al. The biology of platelet-rich plasma and its application in trauma and orthopaedic surgery: a review of the literature. J Bone Joint Surg Br 2009;91-B(8):987–96.
76. Fu CJ, Sun JB, Bi ZG, et al. Evaluation of platelet-rich plasma and fibrin matrix to assist in healing and repair of rotator cuff injuries: a systematic review and meta-analysis. Clin Rehabil 2017;31(2):158–72.
77. Verhaegen F, Brys P, Debeer P. Rotator cuff healing after needling of a calcific deposit using platelet-rich plasma augmentation: a randomized, prospective clinical trial. J Shoulder Elbow Surg 2016;25(2):169—173.
78. Urits I, Smoots D, Franscioni H, et al. Injection techniques for common chronic pain conditions of the foot: a comprehensive review. Pain Ther 2020;9(1):145–60.
79. Lin MT, Wei KC, Wu CH. Effectiveness of platelet-rich plasma injection in rotator cuff tendinopathy: a systematic review and meta-analysis of randomized controlled trials. Diagnostics 2020;10(4):189.
80. Kuffler DP. Platelet-rich plasma promotes axon regeneration, wound healing, and pain reduction: fact or fiction. Mol Neurobiol 2015;52(2):990–1014.
81. Johal H, Khan M, Yung S hang P, et al. Impact of platelet-rich plasma use on pain in orthopaedic surgery: a systematic review and meta-analysis. Sports Health Multidiscip Approach 2019;11(4):355–66.
82. Jain D, Goyal T, Verma N, et al. Intradiscal platelet-rich plasma injection for discogenic low back pain and correlation with platelet concentration: a prospective clinical trial. Pain Med 2020;21(11):2719–25.

83. Lutz C, Cheng J, Prysak M, et al. Clinical outcomes following intradiscal injections of higher-concentration platelet-rich plasma in patients with chronic lumbar discogenic pain. Int Orthop 2022;http://link.springer.com/10.1007/s00590-020-02623-4.
84. Berger DR, Centeno CJ, Steinmetz NJ. Platelet lysates from aged donors promote human tenocyte proliferation and migration in a concentration-dependent manner. Bone Jt Res 2019;8(1):32–40.
85. Yoshida M, Funasaki H, Marumo K. Efficacy of autologous leukocyte-reduced platelet-rich plasma therapy for patellar tendinopathy in a rat treadmill model. Muscles Ligaments Tendons J 2016;6(2):205–15.
86. Everts PA, Devilee RJJ, Brown Mahoney C, et al. Exogenous application of platelet-leukocyte gel during open subacromial decompression contributes to improved patient outcome. Eur Surg Res 2008;40(2):203–10.
87. Sommer C. Serotonin in pain and analgesia: actions in the periphery. Mol Neurobiol 2004;30(2):117—125.
88. Wu WP, Hao JX, Xu XJ, et al. The very-high-efficacy 5-HT1A receptor agonist, F 13640, preempts the development of allodynia-like behaviors in rats with spinal cord injury. Eur J Pharmacol 2003;478(2–3):131–7.

Basic Science of Autologous Orthobiologics

Part 2. Mesenchymal Stem Cells

Peter A. Everts, PhD, FRSM[a,*], Alberto J. Panero, DO[b]

KEYWORDS

- Autologous orthobiologics • Regenerative medicine
- Bone marrow aspirate concentrate • Adipose tissue concentrate
- Mesenchymal stem cell • Inflammation • Angiogenesis • Immunomodulation

KEY POINTS

- Various autologous orthobiologics methods are used for treating many different musculoskeletal pathologies.
- None of the bone marrow concentrate and adipose tissue concentrate products are created equal, resulting in potentially different outcome results, with no consensus on standardization and validation.
- Mesenchymal stem cell-based preparations have the potential to regulate immunomodulation, lessen pain, repair traumatized and degenerative tissue structures, and improve function.

INTRODUCTION

The objectives of regenerative medicine applications are to support the body to form new functional tissues to replace degenerative or defective ones and to provide therapeutic treatment for conditions where conventional therapies are inadequate. The human body has an endogenous system of regeneration through stem- and progenitor cells, signaling cells, and other cell types, as they are found in almost every type of tissue. Interventional orthobiological treatment options using autologous prepared stem cell products can be safely executed by well-trained physicians at the point of care (POC).

This article is not meant to be exhaustive, but our aims are to shed light on the bone marrow (BM) and adipose progenitor and stem cell mechanisms and highlight some of their distinct features and how they relate to clinical applications.

[a] Gulf Coast Biologics, Research and Scientific Division, Royal Society of Medicine London, Fort Myers, FL, USA; [b] BIOS Orthopedic Institute, 2277 Fair Oaks Blvd, Suite 415, Sacramento, CA 95825, USA

* Corresponding author. Veronica S. Shoemaker Boulevard, Suite 1, Fort Myers, FL 33916.
E-mail address: peter@gulfcoastbiologics.com

Phys Med Rehabil Clin N Am 34 (2023) 25–47
https://doi.org/10.1016/j.pmr.2022.08.004
pmr.theclinics.com

WHAT ARE STEM CELLS?

Becker and colleagues[1] conducted experiments that lead to the discovery of stem cells in 1963. After injecting BM cells into irradiated mice, nodules developed in proportion to the number of BM cells injected, and they concluded that each nodule arose from a single marrow cell. At a later stage, they produced evidence that these cells were capable of endless self-renewal, which is as we know now, a fundamental feature of stem cells. A stem cell is a type of cell that is nonspecific and thus not specialized in its function, compared with mature tissue cells, which are functionally specific. Generally, we recognize embryonic and non-embryonic stem cells (ESCs), with two defining properties. First, they have the capacity for self-renewal, therefore giving rise to more stem cells. Second, they can differentiate into different lineages under appropriate conditions. ESCs are obtained from 5- to 12-day-old embryos, and they are pluripotent and have high plasticity as they can differentiate into ectoderm, mesoderm, and endoderm layers. Non- ESCs are multipotent, and it seems that they can form multiple cell lineages that form an whole tissue, usually specific to one germ layer, for example, adult stem cells.[2] The capability for stem cell potency, in combination with the relative ease to prepare BM stem cell injectates, is an invaluable property for regenerative medicine cell-based therapies in general and more specifically to treat, a variety of musculoskeletal disorders (MSK-D), spinal pathologies, chronic wounds, and critical limb ischemia (CLI).

Non-embryotic Autologous Adult Stem Cells

Non-ESCs are undifferentiated, and their proliferation potential compared with embryogenic stem cells is limited, as they have lost their pluripotent capability, placing them lower in the stem cell hierarchy. Nonetheless, it has been suggested that non-ESCs maintain their multipotent differentiation potential. As they are categorized as allogenic products, they are commercially prepared from several allogenic sources, like amniotic fluid, umbilical cord, and Wharton's jelly.[3]

Allogeneic products must be produced according to the FDA's criteria of minimal manipulation and should not include any combination products nor be dependent on the metabolic activity of living cells, including mesenchymal stem cells (MSCs). However, the FDA does not allow the use of these products in orthobiological applications. In this article, we only deliberate on non-embryotic, autologous adult bone marrow aspirate (BMA) and adipose tissue (AT)-derived progenitor/stem cells and other stromal cells.

PART 2. BONE MARROW CONCENTRATE

Introduction

Clinicians using platelet-rich plasma (PRP) have a growing interest in using autologous BM preparations, as it is well acknowledged that red BM is a plentiful and heterogenous source of cells that are residing in the trabecular part of flat and long bones.[4] Extracted BM is processed to prepare a BMC therapeutic orthobiologic treatment specimen. The rationale to use BMC is its unique composition of concentrated MSCs and their progenitor cells, myeloid and lymphoid cells, which play pivotal roles in tissue regenerative and repair processes. BMC is prepared after minimal manipulative density centrifugation of a freshly extracted, viable, volume of BMA using a dedicated centrifuge, like PRP preparations. BMC preparation can be safely executed by well-trained physicians, at POC. It has been shown extensively that well-prepared BMCs are capable to affect the local microenvironment very effectively in numerous MSK maladies.[5] We will deliberate on the BM cellular content, their interconnectivity, and typical biological characteristics. In addition, we deliberate on BMA harvesting and BMC preparation techniques, and allude on the effects of BMC concerning immunomodulatory effects, angiogenesis, and platelet trophic effects.

Understanding Bone Marrow Tissue

Friedenstein and colleagues[6] were the first to report on the isolation of BM-derived stem cells from BM stroma. They incubated BM in plastic culture dishes and identified MSCs as colony-forming unit fibroblasts. The BM stroma is made up of a network of fibroblast-like cells and includes a subpopulation of multipotent cells that can generate the mesenchyme, known as the mass of tissue that develops mainly from the mesoderm of the embryo subpopulation. The cells are referred to as bone marrow mesenchymal stem cells (BM-MSCs).[7] The *Friedenstein* culture method revealed that MSCs can differentiate into several connective tissue cell types,[8] described first by Pittenger and colleagues.[9] We recognize two categories of BM tissue, the red and yellow BM. Depending on aging, red-BM is altered into yellow-BM. In adults, the red-BM is a rich source of BM-derived cells and is present in most skeletal system bones, in particular in the anterior and posterior iliac crest. Other anatomic areas include the proximal tibia, spine vertebrae, and humerus, calcaneus, ribs, and near the point of attachment of long bones of legs and arms. However, it has been well recognized that the iliac crest is the site of preference, as it contains many BM-MSCs compared with other extraction sites.[10] In the well-shielded environment, an estimate of 500 billion BM cells per day can be produced, in particular erythrocytes, granulocytes, and platelets.[11] Orthobiological and other regenerative medicine applications have a focus on the use of the red BM, as it contains myeloid and lymphoid stem cells, and MSCs. In contrast, the yellow marrow consists primarily of fat cells with poor vascularity and is deprived of the multipotential MSCs.[12]

BM-MSCs grafting can advance tissue repair, manage inflammatory conditions, reduce pain, and patient function after injury, and may offer solutions to musculoskeletal pathologies, spinal disorders, chronic wound care, and CLI, by changing the local microenvironment to facilitate tissue regeneration.

Bone marrow cellular content

The cellular content of BMC is more complex and distinct compared with PRP, as it contains, among other cells, MSCs and hematopoietic stem cells (HSCs) with their specific multipotential progenitor cells. BM-MSCs, and adipose MSCs, meet the criteria for MSCs as defined by the International Society for Cellular Therapy (ISCT).[13] Traditionally, these adult stem cells are recognized for their ability to self-renew and differentiation potential into various other cells and tissues. When used as a BMC injectate, the objective is toward contributing to tissue repair and immunomodulatory functions.

HSCs are composed of adult hematopoietic progenitor stem cells that are accountable for executing a phenomenon termed hematopoiesis, generating all types of blood cells. MSCs are known to express a range of cell-lineage-specific antigens. MSC progenitor cells give rise to cells of mesodermal lineages, including osteoblasts, chondrocytes, tenocytes, endothelial cells, myocytes, fibroblasts, nerves, and adipocytes.[14] This cell differentiation potential is a fundamental characteristic for using BMC in orthobiological treatment indications.[7] Furthermore, BMC includes endothelial cells, cells at different developmental stages (including pre-osteoblasts, osteoblasts, and osteocytes), juvenile platelets (megakaryocyte), platelets, red blood cells (RBCs), and various other nucleated cells, and cytokines[15] (**Fig. 1**). However, it is important to understand that the number of BM-MSCs is low, it is estimated to vary between 0.01 to 0.02% of the total BM cell volume.[9]

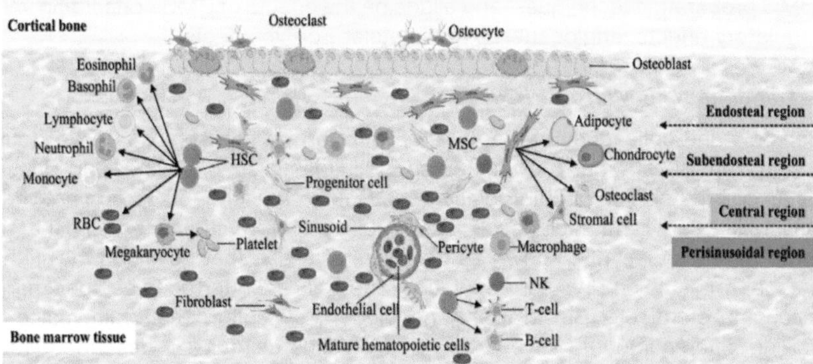

Fig. 1. Impression of the heterogenous cellular content of bone marrow tissue and region segmentation.

Bone marrow structure

Bone is an organ composed of cortical, trabecular bone, cartilage, hematopoietic, and connective tissues. In the BM cavity, the BM tissue is a soft structure, similar to the peripheral blood. In general, BM consists of a hematopoietic component (parenchyma) and a vascular component (stroma). It is composed of a lattice of fine bone plates filled, with hematopoietic marrow, fat cells, a variety of collagen fibrils, calcium, phosphate deposits, and arterial-venous sinusoidal blood vessels. In this well-shielded environment, an estimate of 500 billion cells per day can be produced and released into the peripheral circulation, in particular erythrocytes, granulocytes, and platelets[16]

Bone marrow regions

According to the model of Lambertsen and Weis, the trabecular bone cavity can be segmented into four regions.[17] It has been recognized that most of the MSCs are located in the endosteal–subendosteal region.[18,19]

The BM niche, first described by Schofield,[20] is a dynamic and complex milieu containing a large variety of cells from MSC and HSC lineages. Both stem cells are in a dormant state by producing quiescence and maintenance factors. They are capable of self-renewal, proliferation, and differentiation. MSCs differentiate in various progenitor cells and thereafter they potentially differentiate further in several cell types, like adipocytes, chondrocytes, osteoblasts, and marrow stromal cells. HSCs are multipotent cells that can develop into all types of blood cells. The myeloid progenitor lineages give rise to RBCs, granulocytes, monocytes, and megakaryocytes which mature to platelets. The lymphoid-lineage cells give rise to lymphocytes and include T, B, and natural killer cells. BM cells communicate locally through cell–cell interactions and across greater distances via soluble factors released into the marrow. The four BM cavity regions are indicated.[17] MSCs close to the inner bone surface in the endosteal niche, and in the subendosteal region.[18,19] MSCs diligently interact with bone-lining osteoblasts, HSCs, and other marrow stromal cells. Furthermore, MSCs, presented as pericytes, and HSCs are near the sinusoid vascular network in the perisinusoidal region. MSCs are influenced in both niches by HSCs and non-hematopoietic cells such as fibroblast, macrophages, and endothelial cells.[21] These processes are regulated in the various BM niches by complex biochemical and mechanical signaling via soluble ligands (platelet-derived CXC chemokine ligand 4 [CXCL4], CXC chemokine ligand 12 [CXCL12], and stem cell factor [SCF]), transforming growth factor-β (TGF-β), and direct cell–cell interactions.[22]

Bone marrow niches

Stem cell niches are defined as specific cellular and molecular microenvironments regulating stem cell and progenitor functions and response to stress signals by activating cascades of events[23–26] (**Box 1**). This three-dimensional microenvironment is thought to control genes and properties that define "stemness," including the control and balance between quiescence, cell signaling mechanisms, self-renewal, proliferation, and differentiation of diverse cell types.[27–29] MSCs originating from their specific and original BM niche, are frequently applied as orthobiological product in other cellular, diseased tissue types where they engage in tissue repair and regeneration by differentiating into the cell types present and typical of this specifically treated tissue environment.[30]

Considerations When Extracting Bone Marrow

BM is relatively easy to harvest, largely available, and dispensable. Obviously, it is important that the BMA procedure is performed impeccably to obtain an optimal quality of viable BM tissue.[5,31] In humans, the most common anatomic location to obtain BM is the iliac crest, but other BMA sites have been used.[32] Recently, McDaniel and co-workers, reported that all studied anatomic BM harvesting locations contained MSCs, but the iliac crest was the most abundant source of MSCs,[11] in particular posterior superior iliac spine (PSIS).[15,33,34] Several BM harvesting systems are available, each with their own design features creating different marrow cellular extraction dynamics. Of significant concern is the aspiration of peripheral blood from the deeper marrow regions, diluting the cellular content. In **Fig. 2**, the position of a BM aspiration needle is illustrated. Innovative BM needle harvesting systems are aimed toward less peripheral blood aspiration while yielding higher BMA cell content.[35] During the harvesting procedure, device manipulation should be limited to avoid tissue trauma using the sharp trocar, as this will increase the risk for neurovascular injury, bleeding, tearing of lateral gluteal muscle origins, and post-procedural pain. To conclude, it is fair to assume that the cell viability and cellular yields, prior BMA processing, determines the ultimate quality and cell ratios of the BMC product.

Image-guided bone marrow extraction

It is imperative to precisely locate the donor BMA site, as most of the MSCs are in the endosteal and subendosteal region. During the BMA procedure, precise delivery of local anesthetics and safe trocar placement are mostly ideally accomplished by using image guidance, using ultrasound or fluoroscopy.[5,36]

Box 1 **Bone marrow classical niches**
Mesenchymal stem cell niche
Hematopoietic stem cell niche
Endosteal niche
Perivascular niche
Megakaryocyte niche

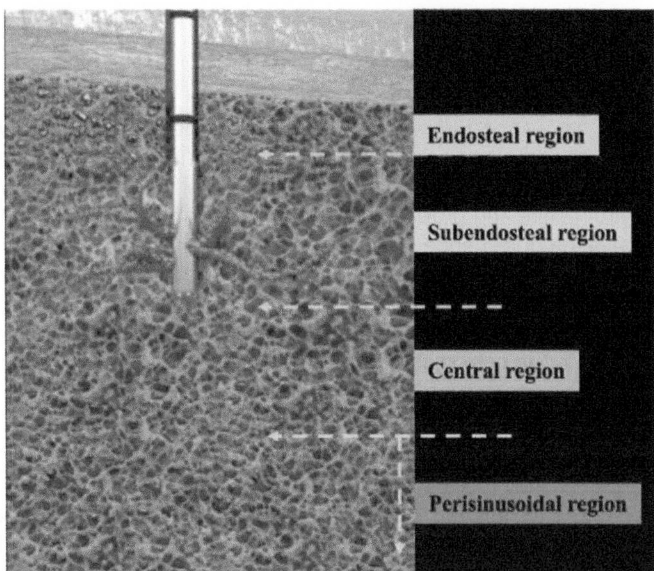

Fig. 2. Illustration of BM aspiration device in subendosteal region.

The choice for bone marrow aspirate collection syringes

Harvesting of MSCs requires a significant negative pressure in the marrow cavity to liberate MSCs from their environment. Theoretically, large-volume BMA collection syringes produce a stronger negative pressure and should therefore harvest more MSCs. However, Hernigou and colleagues[18] found that the aspiration of only 10% to 20% of a full syringe volume resulted in a higher MSC concentration in both 10- and 50-mL syringes and that the number of MSCs decreased as the syringe was further filled. They recommended using smaller syringes and ditto smaller aspiration volumes to acquire higher MSC concentrations when compared with larger aspiration volumes.[37]

In **Fig. 2**, the aspiration needle passed the cortical bone and is positioned in the subendosteal region of the marrow cavity. The illustration indicates the subdivisions in the BM cavity, showing the endosteal, subendosteal, central, and perisinusoidal regions (Adapted and modified from Lambertsen and Weis[17]). The endosteal and subendosteal regions compose the endosteal niche, harboring the proliferative and quiescent HSC-MSC niches.[27] Note: the marrow tissue is extracted only via the side holes of the harvesting cannula, as the distal tip is closed. This reduces peripheral blood contamination and thus BM-MSC dilution.[15]

This is in accordance with the physical equation, "Negative Pressure = Pull Force/ Plunger Surface Area." This translates to the fact that with the same pull force and a smaller diameter syringe plunger, a higher negative pressure is created.[38] Overall, there is a trend toward using 10- or 12-mL collection syringes while using a quick, sharp, and intermittent pull technique to extract small BM volumes from different intra-trabecular sites through the orifices of the harvesting needle.[32] Subsequently, this results in turbulence, as measured by the Reynolds shear stress (RSS) metric.[39] Consequently, high RSS results in RBC damage, presented by RBC deformability followed by the release of its inflammatory hemoglobin components heme and iron, measured as a percentage of hemolysis.[40] Fortunately, more MSCs tend to be

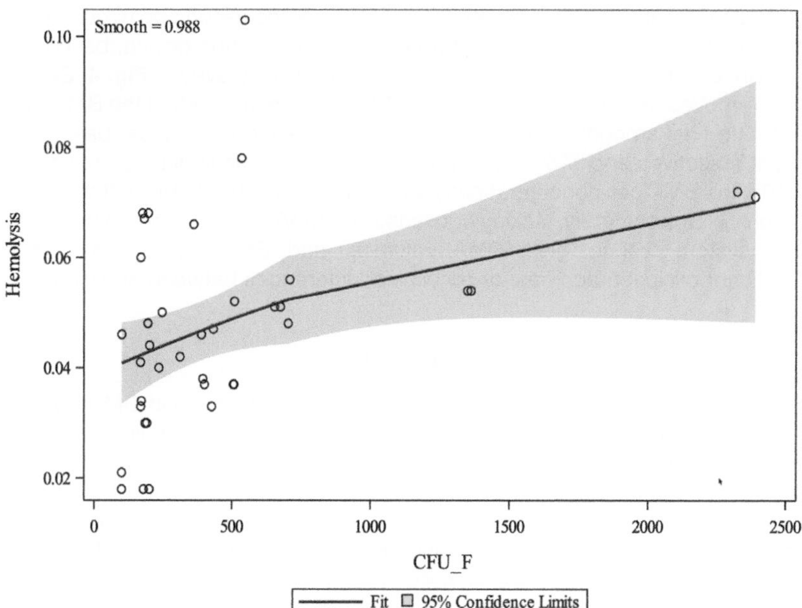

Fig. 3. Regression analysis colony-forming unit fibroblasts and percentage of hemolysis in BMA samples. Statistical analysis is showing a positive regression correlation ($P = .0007$) between the percentage of hemolysis and the number of MSCs in extracted BM vials. Data are generated from 41 patients who participated in a clinical study (manuscript in preparation).

liberated from their bony environment when higher shear forces, with more hemolysis, are used. There seem to be a positive correlation between the percentage of hemolysis and the number of MSCs in a BMA vial, as indicated in **Fig. 3**.

An additional advantage of using smaller syringes is that anticoagulation vigilance can be better managed during aspiration to avoid clotting.

Bone Marrow Aspirate Centrifugation Processing Essentials

Before BM extraction, harvesting needle, syringes, and other processing accessories should be thoroughly rinsed with heparin to prevent BM from clotting. Collected BMA can be filtered to remove microparticles, bone fragments, microaggregates, and fat. The acquired heterogenous cellular BMA volume is pervasively distributed in the concentration device.

It is our belief that the production of BMC, to attain high cell yields, is safeguarded by using two-spin density gradient centrifugation techniques, using dedicated and approved disposable concentration devices. These processing steps are very similar to two-spin PRP preparation methods, with a clear cell layer separation of the BM cellular content.[5] Briefly, after the first centrifugation spin, the BMA is sequestered in a BM plasma fraction (BMPF), containing a buffy coat layer and RBCs. The BMPF is aspirated, immediately followed by a separate collection of 2 mL of RBCs, to collect potentially the MSCs that are attached to the RBC pack. Importantly, avoiding collecting a minimal fraction of the RBC layer will lead to significantly reduced MSCs numbers in the final BMC product, as the MSC and RBC cellular density range is relatively close (PE Internal communications with BioSciences Laboratories). The BMPF and RBC volume are transferred for a second centrifugal spin cycle to the concentration compartment of the same device. After the second spin, concentrated BM cells are typically attached at bottom of the concentration device, based on the specific BM cellular densities after the second spin, as displayed in **Fig. 4**. Excessive BMPF is removed, leaving behind a specific BMPF for resuspending the BMC cellular content. The final amount of the BMC volume is subject to variance, based on the treatment objectives and MSC dosing requirements. By manipulating the volume of the BMPF, the BMC cell concentrations can be more than 10-fold the native BMA concentrations.[15] Unfortunately, lacking consensus on BMA aspiration techniques, centrifugation system technologies, BMA volumes, and BMC dosing can result in nonsignificant clinical outcomes, or no clinical differences between applying PRP or BMC.[41,42]

Bone Marrow Mesenchymal Stem Cell Aptitudes

MSCs are multipotent stem cells that can be obtained from adult BM stroma, AT, synovium, periosteum, and trabecular bone. Their typical features like relative ease of extraction from their environment, self-renewal, multipotentiality, mechanisms to preserve the undifferentiated stem state, and the regulation of lineage-specific differentiation, created a great attractiveness for regenerative medicine autologous therapeutic applications and tissue engineering opportunities.[14,43,44] These MSC proficiencies have led to the use of BMC-MSC-based technologies as a potential strategy for treating various pathologies and diseases, as they encourage the above-mentioned biological processes. Furthermore, when concentrated BM-MSCs are released at tissue sites, they synthesize cytokines and trophic mediators, improve cell recruitment, and increase cell-signaling, instituting a regenerative microenvironment for tissue repair, as they participate in (neo)angiogenesis, immunomodulation, and inflammatory processes.[45]

Immunomodulatory effects

In parallel with their major role as undifferentiated cell reserves, MSCs have immunomodulatory functions which are exerted by direct cell-to-cell contact, secretion of cytokines, and/or by a combination of both mechanisms. MSCs have been shown to exert profound anti-inflammatory and immunomodulatory effects on almost all the

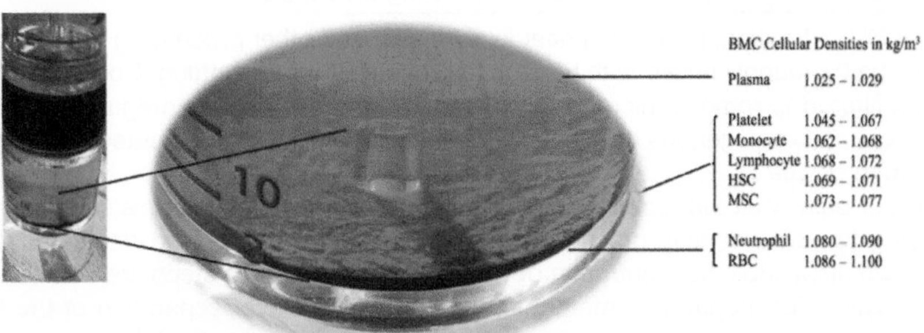
BMC Cellular Densities in kg/m³
Plasma 1.025 – 1.029
Platelet 1.045 – 1.067
Monocyte 1.062 – 1.068
Lymphocyte 1.068 – 1.072
HSC 1.069 – 1.071
MSC 1.073 – 1.077
Neutrophil 1.080 – 1.090
RBC 1.086 – 1.100
10

Fig. 4. BMC cellular density separation after a double-spin procedure. Fig. 4. Illustrates at the bottom of the BMC device the organized multicomponent bone marrow concentrated buffy coat layer (indicated by the *blue lines*), containing high concentrations of platelets, mononuclear cells (including HSCs and MSCs and their progenitors), granulocytes, and RBCs. The second BMC centrifugation step is based on the differences of the densities of the individual cells, following gravitational separation by centrifugation. (*From* EmCyte Corporation, Fort Myers, FL, USA, PureBMC-SP® device, with permission).

cells of the innate and adaptive immune systems via a variety of mechanisms, notably cytokine and chemokine secretion.[80] The immunosuppressive capabilities of MSCs are only exploited when they are exposed to sufficiently high concentrations of pro-inflammatory cytokines, like interferon-gamma (IFN-γ), tissue necrosis factor α (TNF- α), and interleukins α (IL-1α). For MSCs to become "immunosuppressants," they need to be triggered by inflammatory cytokines, and the inflammatory environment is then a crucial factor for MSCs to exert their immunomodulatory effects. These are wielded by blocking apoptosis of native and activated neutrophils, aside from decreasing neutrophils from binding to vascular endothelial cells and the mobilization of neutrophils to the area of damage.[46] However, the mechanisms by which MSCs are mobilized and recruited to damaged sites are not known. In addition, how they survive and differentiate into distinct cell types is still not clear. Once MSCs have been applied to the local environment of injured or degenerated tissues, numerous factors stimulate the release of many growth factors by MSCs. These growth factors stimulate the development of fibroblasts, endothelial cells, and tissue progenitor cells.[25] It is credible to state that the use of MSCs and their potential in immunomodulation in regenerative medicine applications hold great promise.[47,48]

Angiogenetic effect

MSC paracrine trophic factors are potentially important in maintaining endothelial integrity and promoting angiogenesis through their ability to regulate endothelial cell proliferation and ECM production.[48] Furthermore, endothelial cell permeability is reduced, and MSCs inhibit interactions between leukocytes and endothelial cells.[49] Apart from MSC trophic factors, fibroblasts have fundamental functions in maintaining tissue integrity and promote tissue healing through their secretion of cytokines that support ECM building. These endothelial and angiogenetic capabilities have been shown in clinical studies addressing chronic wound healing[50] and recovery from post-myocardial infarction.[51]

Trophic effects

PRP growth factors are crucial proteins that are involved in the BMC reparative processes and their role is to stimulate the various MSC reparative functions, a phenomenon termed PRP trophic effects. The diversity of PGFs and other cytokines involved in BMC trophic processes can initiate tissue repair by decreasing cell apoptosis, and anabolic and anti-inflammatory effects. Furthermore, they stimulate cell proliferation, differentiation, and angiogenesis via paracrine and autocrine pathways.[52,53] Explicitly in OA treatments, PGF plays a specific role in cartilage regeneration and maintaining homeostasis via MSC proliferation and the inhibition of IL-1-induced chondrocyte apoptosis and inflammation.[47] Also, three TGF-β isoforms are active in stimulating chondrogenesis, and inhibiting inflammation, and they express their ability to promote MSC-associated tissue healing via inter-molecular actions.[54] MSC trophic effects are associated with PGF activity and the secretion of reparative cytokines. Ideally, all of these cellular factors should be present in the BMA treatment vials and delivered to tissue injury sites to promote optimal MSC-associated therapeutic tissue healing.[55]

Combining bone marrow concentrate and platelet-rich plasma preparations

There is minimal information available on the presence or concentrations of PGFs in BMCs, or the ideal BMC to PRP ratio needed to support BM-MSC trophic actions. Some clinicians mix separately prepared low volume-high platelet concentration PRP specimen with BMCs, to create a potentially more biologically active graft, projected to optimize regenerative medicine treatment outcomes,[56] as few studies have revealed that they can complement each other.[57,58] However, there are minimal safety and efficacy data available indicating that combining high PRP concentrations with BMC is a more effective treatment option.[59] Therefore, we believe that mixing BM-MSCs with high platelet concentrations may not be indicated at this stage.

PART 3. ADIPOSE TISSUE CONCENTRATE

Introduction

MSCs are found in virtually all organs of the human body and comprise a heterogeneous population of cells with multilineage differentiation potential, secreting numerous cytokines and growth factors, capable of stipulating immunomodulatory, angiogenic, anti-inflammatory, and anti-apoptotic effects. MSCs have been isolated from various other sources with the AT, serving as one of the alternatives to BM tissue.[60] Adipose-derived MSCs (A-MSCs) can be easily isolated following ATC preparations.[61] A-MSCs and BM-MSCs share many biological characteristics[62] However, there are some differences in their immunophenotype, differentiation potential, transcriptome, proteome, and immunomodulatory activity.[63] Some of these differences may represent specific features of BM-MSCs and A-MSCs. Despite minor differences between these MSC populations, A-MSCs seem to be as effective as BM-MSCs in clinical application, and, in some cases, may be better suited than BM-MSCs.[64]

Understanding Adipose Tissue

Aside from PRP and BMC preparations, AT has been used as a cell-based therapy in orthobiological and regenerative medicine procedures to create an ATC, harvested, and prepared at point-of-care in an office setting. Autologous AT is a heterogeneous biological source of various cellular tissue components. Furthermore, concentrated AT provides clinicians with a physiologic 3D multicellular scaffold, including adipose stem cells (ASCs) and stromal cells. Both autologous and allogeneic ATC have been used successfully in clinical trials to treat a variety of conditions, including MSK disorders.[61] Like BM-MSCs, A-MSCs can differentiate into cells of mesodermal (osteoblasts, adipocytes, and chondrocytes), endodermal (hepatocytes, pancreatic cells), and ectodermal (neurons) primary layers.[65] These similar features are of high interest when treating MSK disorders.

Adipose Tissue Structure

AT is a highly vascularized connective tissue, abundantly present throughout the human body. White adipose tissue (WAT) is responsible for energy storage and plays a pivotal physiologic role in maintaining metabolic homeostasis in the body by releasing several adipocytokines, growth factors, and cytokines that may act in an endocrine or paracrine manner.[66] Brown-AT plays a significant role in thermogenesis by dispersing energy by producing heat to ensure body temperature regulation[67]

Adipose tissue as a source of stem cells

Zuk and colleagues performed the first characterization of adult stem cells, isolated from lipoaspirates, showing that ASC derived from WAT lipoaspirate shows MSC and differential capacity.[68–70] A-MSCs have a high proliferation capacity and multilineage cell differentiation potential, capable of differentiating into adipogenic, chondrogenic, myogenic, osteogenic, and neurogenic cells.[71] These AT characteristics, combined with an abundance of MSCs when compared with BM-MSCs, have great potential in clinical orthobiological tissue repair applications.[63,72] Furthermore, Yun and colleagues[73] described the A-MSC mediated effects on the reduction of pro-inflammatory cytokines, chemokines, cellular apoptosis, and collagenases.

Stromal vascular fraction. The use of AT in orthobiological applications is based on the separation of the vascular stroma contained in ATC, allowing for access to A-MSCs.[74,75] SVF is a heterogeneous collection of cells contained within AT which can be isolated using different tissue disruption techniques, like enzymatic digestion, or mechanical emulsification (ME) preparation methods. In **Box 2**, the heterogenous SVF cellular composition is shown, with A-MSCs and SVF cells enclosed in the SVF.

Like the preparation of PRP and BMC, cellular density gradient centrifugation is used to create a viable biological ATC specimen. Centrifugation techniques have proven to be an effective means to produce concentrated AT, whereas adipose infranatant extracellular fluid, residual oil, and debris following effectively separated following a single-spin procedure, as shown in **Fig. 5**. Thereafter, the ATC is collected from the centrifugation tube and subsequently subjected to SVF production (**Fig. 6**).

Enzymatic Digestion Versus Mechanical Emulsification Techniques

Enzymatic digestion techniques use enzymes (collagenase) to isolate A-MSCs and stromal cells from AT by digesting the WAT peptide collagen bonds while destructing extracellular structures. Centrifugation techniques are used to separate the floating adipocytes from the pelleted SVF.[76] Collagenase-based protocols produce an adipose-derived *cellular* SVF (AD-cSVF). Freshly prepared SVF can directly be applicated as an orthobiological product, without the need for further cell separation or in-vitro cell expansion. A-MSCs constitute as much as 1% of SVF cells compared with 0.001% to 0.002% of BM-MSCs.[77] Furthermore, detrimental erythrocytes are usually removed with an enzymatic processing protocol. This is a significant dissimilarity compared with a BMC, which contains a significant number of erythrocytes.[76] In current FDA guidelines, enzymatic cellular prepared SVF products are listed in the "more than manipulated" category, requiring specific human clinical trials to examine efficacy and report on the long-term safety. Another method to produce SVF refers to the definition of adipose-derived *tissue* SVF (AD-tSVF). This method signifies to the cellular population in adipose SVF in a bioactive scaffold or extracellular matrix.[78] For AD-tSVF, the ATC is mechanically sized by a process termed ME. Before

Box 2
SVF cellular distribution

15% to 30% stromal cells:
- AD-MSCs
- Pre-adipocytes
- Fibroblasts

35% to 45% hematopoietic-lineage cells:
- Erythrocytes
- Platelets
- Neutrophils
- Lymphocytes
- Monocytes/macrophages

1% to 15% hematopoietic stem and endothelial progenitor cells

3% to 5% pericytes

10% to 20% endothelial cells

5% to 15% smooth muscle cells

Abbreviation: AD-MSCs, adipose mesenchymal stem cells.

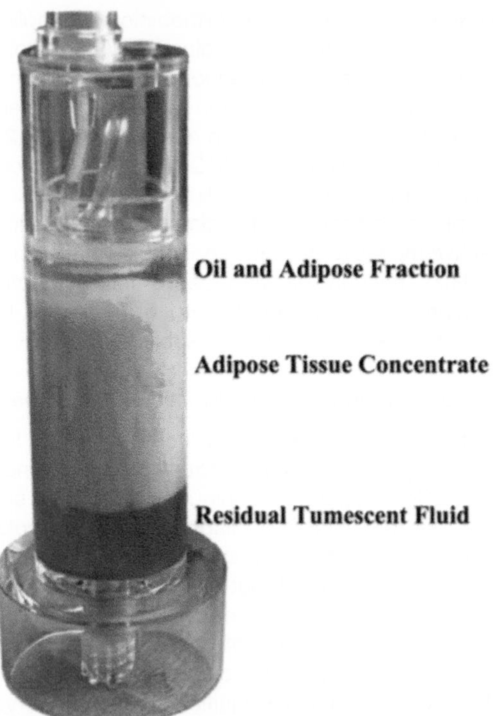

Fig. 5. Centrifugated density separation of adipose tissue. In Fig. 5, the AT is clean and concentrated, following a single centrifugation spin. Typically, with adipose centrifugation, the first, top, layer consists mainly of inflammatory oil and adipose tissue cell residues. The middle layer is comprised ATC, and the third bottom layer contains residual tumescent fluid with some RBCs. (*From* Progenikine® Adipose Concentration System, EmCyte Corporation, Fort Myers FL USA, with permission).

orthobiological application, the AT is sized in different fat dimensions by EM, producing microfat or nanofat, conceivably liberating SVF from the sized fat tissue.

Another method for mechanically isolating A-MSCs, is the use of microfracture adipose tissue graft (MFAT) techniques,[79] without the use of enzymes. With this Lipogems method, the AT is obtained by a significant reduction in size and washing of a lipoaspirate with clusters of about 3 mm. The AT is gently microfractured and washed, leaving pro-inflammatory oil and blood residues behind in the process. The final product contains pericytes retained within an intact stromal vascular niche and is ready to be used.

Adipose harvesting Technique Considerations

AT harvesting is performed using a mini liposuction technique. It involves the removal of subcutaneous fat. The procedure is executed by means of aspiration cannulas, introduced through small skin incisions, and assisted by controlled suction. Its basic principles have been elaborated by Illouz, who was the first to introduce the modern, safe, and widespread method of liposuction with a blunt-tipped cannula as well as subcutaneous infiltration to facilitate adipose breakdown and controlled fat aspiration.[80,81] The procedure preserves neurovascular structures with minimal patient discomfort.[82] In 1985, Klein introduced the tumescent liposuction technique.[83] Later,

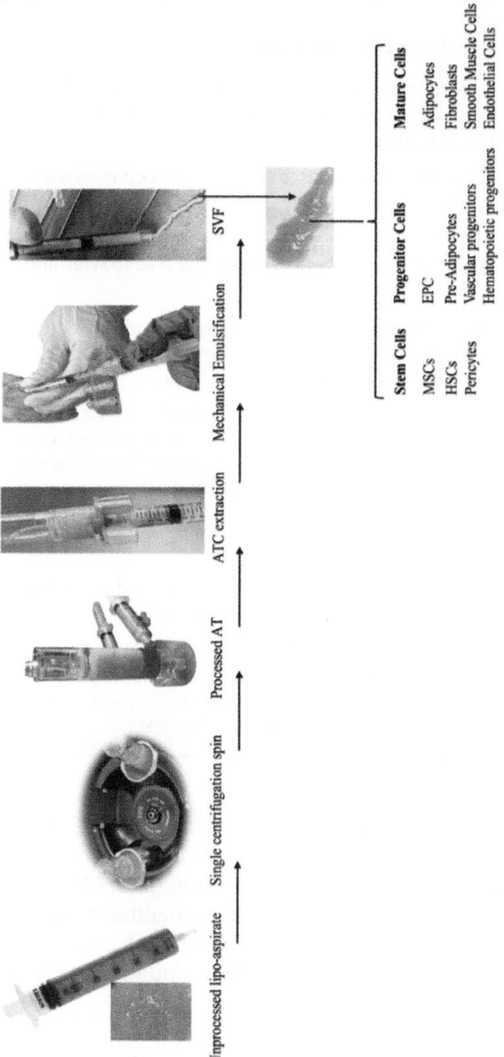

Fig. 6. Schematic picture of SVF production steps.

Coleman introduced a new three-step technique to decrease trauma to AT following liposuction, using manual low negative pressure lipo-aspiration. Harvested WAT is transferred to a dedicated concentration device and centrifugated to concentrate and purify the AT, using minimal processing steps, as illustrated in **Fig. 5**. Finally, the ATC is reinjected as a 3D matrix.[84] Properly executed lipo-aspiration procedures, followed by AT processing and ME will not affect A-MSC cell viability and functionality while yielding significant concentrations of AD-tSVF cells.[85,86] In **Box 3**, detailed ATC preparation steps are presented.

Adipose Tissue Aptitudes

Following ME, the final AT is composed of both cellular and native structural fat fragments.[87,88] Therefore, ME-prepared AD-tSVF is not a 100% concentrated cellular

Box 3
Adipose tissue concentrate preparation steps

A. *Tumescent fluid preparation:* a sterile NaCl solution consisting of anesthetics (lidocaine for pain relieve and epinephrine for blood vessels to constrict to minimize RBC contamination in fat tissue during harvesting).

B. *Tumescent injection:* via small skin cuts, a thin blunt injector needle is injected in the target adipose harvesting area.

C. *W time:* reports indicate to wait at least 20 min before starting the fat harvesting procedure. This time is needed for the fluid to cause the injected area to swell and stiffen, supporting in easy in fat removal.

D. *Adipose harvesting:* with a dedicated harvester cannula, fat tissue is harvested using liposuction, by applying manually negative pressure to a collection syringe fat is removed from the area that was injected with tumescent fluid.

E. *Racking and decanting:* syringes filled with harvested fat is placed in a rack, with plunger in upward direction. After the adipose harvesting, leave all syringes in the in the rack for 10 to 15 min, with the luer connection of the syringe capped. Decant the supernatant (tumescent fluid) by removing the cap, until AT starts to block the luer.

F. *Transfer the decanted fat:* into a disposable processing device and place it in a dedicated centrifuge to concentrate the AT specimen.

G. *Centrifugation protocol*: Density layer separation by centrifugation, producing ATC. Follow the instruction for use of the preparation device to extract ATC.

H. *Mechanical emulsification:* several methods are currently used to emulsify the ATC: a: By moving two syringes back and forward through a restraining device to size the ATC, making it suitable for tissue injection. b: Bead beating of ATC against the hard beads to create cell disruption by physically grinding the fat cells.

product, this is a distinct difference compared with AD-cSVF. The final AD-tSVF treatment specimen is injected into diseased tissue structures enabling, A-MSCs and other SVF cells to initiate the repair process. An advantage of ME-prepared AD-tSVF is its ability to provide both a cellular fraction and a bioactive cellular tissue matrix. Noteworthy, AD-tSVF preparations, and their subsequent applications as a supportive structural tissue, are approved by the FDA following their guidelines[89].

Immunomodulatory effects

AD-tSVF preparations are proficient in secreting anti-inflammatory, or immunosuppressive factors that are capable of exerting immunomodulatory effects.[90] Several studies have compared the immunomodulatory abilities of A-MSCs and BM-MSCs and have shown that they show similar effects when used in chronic inflammatory conditions and autoimmune diseases.[91–93] A-MSCs regulate the immune system via direct cell–cell communication and indirectly through the secretion of soluble mediators, growth factors, and extravascular vesicles.[94,95] They interact with numerous cell types, including immune cells, endothelial cells, pre-adipocytes, hematopoietic cells, nerve cells, endothelial cells, and pericytes surrounding the blood vessels. As a result, the interaction between A-MSCs and immune cells contributes to the activity of T cells, B cells, and macrophages.[96] Indirect cell-cell communication is instigated by A-MSCs when they secrete soluble mediators and extravascular vesicles.[97] The most cited soluble mediators are pro-inflammatory and anti-inflammatory cytokines, adipokines, antioxidative, pro-angiogenic, anti-apoptotic, growth factors (eg, VEGF, FGF, and TGF), and specific interleukins (IL-6, IL-7). Currently, the clinical production of SVF to acquire A-MSCs are subject to investigations addressing their immunomodulatory potential in regenerative medicine. Critical aspects of these studies are the ability to develop standardized preparation protocols to ensure effective and safe use in orthobiological procedures.

Angiogenetic properties of adipose tissue

AT has been intensely studied for the treatment of multiple conditions. In particular, the role of A-MSCs show great potential toward the differentiation of different cell lineages (adipogenic, osteogenic, chondrogenic, and myogenic lineages) while providing immunosuppressive properties and low immunogenicity.[98] In addition, it has been shown that AT produces and secretes various angiogenic factors such as angiopoietin-2 and VEGF, as well as adipokines (leptin and adiponectin), that are capable of modulating angiogenesis and vascular structures.[99] These appearances suggest an auto-regulatory function for angiogenesis in AT. Interestingly, Tran and colleagues[100] concluded that precursor cells in blood vessel walls are capable of differentiating into ECs and/or adipocytes in WAT. They concluded a high adipogenic potential, linking ECs and adipocytes in terms of interchangeability based on cell-cell interactions, enabling them to participate in the

formation of angiogenesis and neo-vascular structures. Therefore, A-MSCs might affect the growth of capillary networks that are required in AT enlargement.[101] Furthermore, by enhancing angiogenesis and vasculogenesis, A-MSCs promote neovascularization, which is fundamental in the treatment of tissue repair and post-ischemic injuries. These findings were confirmed by Miranville and colleagues,[102] revealing the expression of A-MSC surface markers CD34 and CD133 resulting in the EC differentiation, contributing to revascularization.

Not only do A-MSCs stimulate angiogenesis through their differentiation into ECs, but also through paracrine activity, releasing angiogenic factors. More specifically, the cellular components of SVF are rapidly restored to form new vessels in diseased tissue structures following orthobiological injections.[103] Neovascularization is further stimulated by adipose stromal cells, releasing VEGF, TGF-β, and HGF.[104] Moreover, SVF MSCs play a major role in the organization of structural new blood vessels[103] (**Fig. 6**).

Adipose tissue concentrate and tissue repair processes

Tissue repair processes following the release of AD-tSVF to tissues are based on their stromal, multipotent, and hematopoietic cell populations, producing an assortment of angiogenic, hematopoietic, and anti-apoptotic factors, to expedite tissue repair/regeneration, via autocrine and paracrine actions.[61] As the SVF's cellular content holds an AT scaffold, it has the capacity to directly interact with the ECM. Subsequently, this accelerates the repair functions of the nearby cells,[74] and thus contributes to the growth of vascular infrastructures during angiogenesis.[105] It is plausible that various MSK pathologies with tissue voids, like Achilles and rotator cuff tendon ruptures, benefit from a three-dimensional AD-tSVF-centered ECM scaffold, comprising of matrix-secreting fibroblasts and other stromal cells. Synergy between EC populations and adipose stromal cells is a prerequisite in the development of blood vessels.[106] A suitable milieu for tissue repair mechanisms mandates the interaction between angiogenesis and the synthesis of ECM proteins. Additional tissue repair processes are intermediated by leukocytes present in AD-tSVF. Approximately 5% to 15% are MΦ2 anti-inflammatory cells, an important element in controlling the environment for tissue repair, and 10% to 15% of cells are lymphocytes, including regulatory T cells, contributing to tissue immune responses.[107] Hence, the heterogenous composition of AD-tSVF has distinct advantages, as substantiated by the interplay of controlled inflammation with immunomodulatory properties. A-MSCs and other stromal cells are in fact precursors to angiogenetic pathways and ECM formation. Ultimately, these multifaceted cellular processes are capable of tissue repair and function.

Comparing Bone Marrow and Adipose Mesenchymal Stem Cells

Adult MSCs are undifferentiated multipotent cells, characterized by the capacity for self-renewal and the ability to differentiate into various cells of mesenchymal origin, including adipocytes, chondrocytes, myocytes, and osteoblasts, when exposed to specific growth signals.[64] The ISCT proposed clear criteria for the definition of both BM and AT MSCs.[13] When comparing A-MSCs and BM-MSCs, the later have been the most extensively used and investigated MSCs in orthobiological applications. Unfortunately, we do not have a consensus on preparation standards, validation, and quality controls. These deficiencies make it almost impossible to translate basic scientific findings into clinical practice.

Some practitioners mention limitations when extracting BM, like pain and morbidity following BM harvesting. Others cite the scarce amount of BM-MSCs that can be obtained.[9] In this regard, abundant A-MSCs can be isolated from AT by a minimally invasive lipoaspirate procedure.[108] In addition, AT can be harvested from multiple anatomic sites.[109,110] Various studies indicate that BM-MSCs and A-MSCs have comparable cell CD markers and morphology patterns,[86] and both MSC types can undergo multi-lineage differentiation.[111] It has been postulated that due to their similar proliferation and differentiation capacity, A-MSCs are a promising less-invasive alternative to BM-MSCs for orthobiological applications.[112] In a study by Klar and colleagues,[113] cellular data were compared between BMC and SVF. It was concluded that the mononucleated cellular fraction in SVF is richer in stromal cells (15% to 30% of all cells), when compared with BMC. However, most of these studies compared A-MSCs and BM-MSCs obtained from different individuals, and many studies used cellular expansion techniques.[114] In a more recent in vitro donor-matched study, Mohamed-Ahmed and colleagues[64] compared the properties of BM-MSCs and A-MSCs. They reported comparable multi-potencies, morphology, and immunophenotyping for both MSC types. Nevertheless, their tissue-specific differentiation capacity varied. BM-MSCs were superior to A-MSCs in terms of osteogenic and chondrogenic differentiation, whereas A-MSCs had higher proliferation and adipogenic potential. Other studies confirmed that MSCs favorably differentiate into cells of their native microenvironment.[115,116]

CLINICS CARE POINTS

- The bone marrow niche is a dynamic and complex milieu containing a large variety of cells, including MSC's and their progenitors, platelets, leukocytes, and HSC lineages.
- The posterior superior iliac spine (PSISI) is an ideal anatomical site for bone marrow extraction with potentially high MSC counts.
- Two-spin density gradient centrifugation techniques facilitate the production of high cellular yields in bone marrow concentrate (BMC) injectates.
- Bone marrow concentrate and adipose tissue complex are powerful orthobiological products to improve cell recruitment, increase cell-signaling, synthesize cytokines and other tropic mediators to start tissue repair, as they participate in angiogenesis, immunomodulation, and inflammatory processes.

DISCLOSURE

P.A. Everts is also acting Chief Scientific Officer of EmCyte Corporation.

REFERENCES

1. Becker AJ, Mcculloch EA, Till JE. Cytological Demonstration of the Clonal Nature of Spleen Colonies Derived from Transplanted Mouse Marrow Cells. Nature 1963;197(4866):452–4.
2. Lee EH, Hui JHP. The potential of stem cells in orthopaedic surgery. J Bone Joint Surg 2006;88(7):11.
3. Jing B, Yuan H, Yi-Ru W, et al. Comparison of human amniotic fluid-derived and umbilical cord Wharton's Jelly-derived mesenchymal stromal cells: Characterization and myocardial differentiation capacity: Comparison of human amniotic fluid-derived and umbilical cord Wharton's Jelly-derived mesenchymal stromal cells: Characterization and myocardial differentiation capacity. J Geriatr Cardiol 2012;9(2):166–71.
4. Hernigou J, Alves A, Homma Y, et al. Anatomy of the ilium for bone marrow aspiration: map of sectors and implication for safe trocar placement. Int Orthop 2014;38(12):2585–90.
5. Everts P, Flanagan G II, Rothenberg J, et al. The Rationale of Autologously Prepared Bone Marrow Aspirate Concentrate for use in Regenerative Medicine Applications. In: Regenerative Medicine [Working Title] [Internet]. IntechOpen; 2020. https://www.intechopen.com/chapters/71327.
6. Charbord P. Bone Marrow Mesenchymal Stem Cells: Historical Overview and Concepts. Hum Gene Ther 2010;21(9):1045–56.
7. Caplan AI. Mesenchymal stem cells. J Orthop Res 1991;9(5):641–50.
8. Samsonraj RM, Raghunath M, Nurcombe V, et al. Concise Review: Multifaceted Characterization of Human Mesenchymal Stem Cells for Use in Regenerative Medicine: Characterization of Human Mesenchymal Stem Cells. Stem Cells Transl Med 2017;6(12):2173–85.
9. Pittenger MF. Multilineage Potential of Adult Human Mesenchymal Stem Cells. Science 1999;284(5411):143–7.
10. Marx RE, Tursun R. A qualitative and quantitative analysis of autologous human multipotent adult stem cells derived from three anatomic areas by marrow aspiration: tibia, anterior ilium, and posterior ilium. Int J Oral Maxillofac Implants 2013;28(5). e290—4.
11. McDaniel JS, Antebi B, Pilia M, et al. Quantitative Assessment of Optimal Bone Marrow Site for the Isolation of Porcine Mesenchymal Stem Cells. Stem Cells Int 2017;2017:1–10.
12. Gurevitch O, Slavin S, Feldman AG. Conversion of red bone marrow into yellow – Cause and mechanisms. Med Hypotheses 2007;69(3):531–6.
13. Bourin P, Bunnell BA, Casteilla L, et al. Stromal cells from the adipose tissue-derived stromal vascular fraction and culture expanded adipose tissue-derived stromal/stem cells: a joint statement of the International Federation for Adipose Therapeutics and Science (IFATS) and the International Society for Cellular Therapy (ISCT). Cytotherapy 2013;15(6):641–8.
14. Kolf CM, Cho E, Tuan RS. Mesenchymal stromal cells Biology of adult mesenchymal stem cells: regulation of niche, self-renewal and differentiation. Arthritis Res Ther 2007;9(1):204.

15. Mautner K, Jerome MA, Easley K, et al. Laboratory Quantification of Bone Marrow Concentrate Components in Unilateral Versus Bilateral Posterior Superior Iliac Spine Aspiration. J Stem Cell Res Ther 2020;465:10.
16. Hernández-Gil IFT, Gracia MAA, Jerez B. Physiological bases of bone regeneration I. Histology and physiology of bone tissue. Med Oral Patol Oral Cir Bucal 2006;11(1):E47–51.
17. Lambertsen H, Weis L. Studies on the organization and regeneration of bone marrow: Origin, growth, and differentiation of endocloned hematopoietic colonies. Americ J Anatomy 1983;166(4):369–92.
18. Hernigou P, Homma Y, Flouzat Lachaniette CH, et al. Benefits of small volume and small syringe for bone marrow aspirations of mesenchymal stem cells. Int Orthop 2013;37(11):2279–87.
19. Lana JF, da Fonseca LF, Azzini G, et al. Bone Marrow Aspirate Matrix: A Convenient Ally in Regenerative Medicine. Int J Mol Sci 2021;22(5):2762.
20. Schofield R. The relationship between the spleen colony-forming cell and the haemopoietic stem cell. Blood Cells 1978;4(1-2):7–25.
21. Castillo AB, Jacobs CR. Mesenchymal Stem Cell Mechanobiology. Curr Osteoporos Rep 2010;8(2):98–104.
22. Weickert M.T., Hecker J., Buck M., et al., The Role of Bone Marrow Mesenchymal Stem Cells in Myelodysplastic Syndrome and Acute Myeloid Leukemia, Scientific Reports, 11 (1), 2021, 5944.
23. Tamma R, Ribatti D. Bone Niches, Hematopoietic Stem Cells, and Vessel Formation. Int J Mol Sci 2017;18(1):151.
24. Calvi LM, Link DC. The hematopoietic stem cell niche in homeostasis and disease. Blood 2015;126(22):2443–51.
25. Shi Y, Hu G, Su J, et al. Mesenchymal stem cells: a new strategy for immunosuppression and tissue repair. Cell Res 2010;20(5):510–8.
26. Avecilla ST, Hattori K, Heissig B, et al. Chemokine-mediated interaction of hematopoietic progenitors with the bone marrow vascular niche is required for thrombopoiesis. Nat Med 2004;10(1):64–71.
27. Spradling A, Drummond-Barbosa D, Kai T. Stem cells find their niche. Nature 2001;414(6859):98–104.
28. Li L, Xie T. Stem Cell Niche: Structure and Function. Annu Rev Cell Dev Biol 2005;21:605–31.
29. Ehninger A, Trumpp A. The bone marrow stem cell niche grows up: mesenchymal stem cells and macrophages move in. J Exp Med 2011;208(3):421–8.
30. Wu P, Tarasenko YI, Gu Y, et al. Region-specific generation of cholinergic neurons from fetal human neural stem cells grafted in adult rat. Nat Neurosci 2002; 5(12):1271–8.
31. Kunisaki Y, Bruns I, Scheiermann C, et al. Arteriolar niches maintain haematopoietic stem cell quiescence. Nature 2013;502(7473):637–43.
32. Friedlis MF, Centeno CJ. Performing a Better Bone Marrow Aspiration. Phys Med Rehabil Clin N Am 2016;27(4):919–39.
33. Everts PA, Ferrell J, Mahoney CB, et al. A Comparative Quantification in Cellularity of Bone Marrow Aspirated with two New Harvesting Devices, and The Non-equivalent Difference Between A Centrifugated Bone Marrow Concentrate And A Bone Marrow Aspirate As Biological Injectates, Using A Bi-Lateral Patient Model. 10(461):10.
34. Siclari VA, Zhu J, Akiyama K, et al. Mesenchymal progenitors residing close to the bone surface are functionally distinct from those in the central bone marrow. Bone 2013;53(2):575–86.

35. Malanga GA, Buford D, Murrell WD, et al. Bone Marrow Aspirate Concentrate Is Equivalent to PRP for the Treatment of Knee OA at 1 Year: Letter to the Editor. Orthop J Sports Med 2020;8(10). 232596712096070.
36. Hirahara AM, Panero A, Andersen WJ. An MRI Analysis of the Pelvis to Determine the Ideal Method for Ultrasound-Guided Bone Marrow Aspiration from the Iliac Crest. Am J Orthop Belle Mead NJ 2018;47(5). https://doi.org/10.12788/ajo.2018.0038.
37. Batinić D, Marusić M, Pavletić Z, et al. Relationship between differing volumes of bone marrow aspirates and their cellular composition. Bone Marrow Transplant 1990;6(2):103–7.
38. Haseler LJ, Sibbitt RR, Sibbitt WL, et al. Syringe and Needle Size, Syringe Type, Vacuum Generation, and Needle Control in Aspiration Procedures. Cardiovasc Intervent Radiol 2011;34(3):590–600.
39. Jhun CS, Stauffer MA, Reibson JD, et al. Determination of Reynolds Shear Stress Level for Hemolysis. ASAIO J 2018;64(1):63–9.
40. Everts PA, Malanga GA, Paul RV, et al. Assessing clinical implications and perspectives of the pathophysiological effects of erythrocytes and plasma free hemoglobin in autologous biologics for use in musculoskeletal regenerative medicine therapies. A Review. Regen Ther 2019;11:56–64.
41. Piuzzi NS, Hussain ZB, Chahla J, et al. Variability in the Preparation, Reporting, and Use of Bone Marrow Aspirate Concentrate in Musculoskeletal Disorders: A Systematic Review of the Clinical Orthopaedic Literature. J Bone Joint Surg 2018;100(6):517–25.
42. Anz AW, Plummer HA. Bone Marrow Aspirate Concentrate Is Equivalent to Platelet-Rich Plasma for the Treatment of Knee Osteoarthritis at 2 Years: A Prospective Randomized Trial. Am J Sports Med 2022;50(3):12.
43. da Silva Meirelles L, Fontes AM, Covas DT, et al. Mechanisms involved in the therapeutic properties of mesenchymal stem cells. Cytokine Growth Factor Rev 2009;20(5–6):419–27.
44. Cucchiarini M, Venkatesan JK, Ekici M, et al. Human mesenchymal stem cells overexpressing therapeutic genes: From basic science to clinical applications for articular cartilage repair. Biomed Mater Eng 2012;22:197–208.
45. Bashir J, Sherman A, Lee H, et al. Mesenchymal Stem Cell Therapies in the Treatment of Musculoskeletal Diseases. PM&R. 2014;6(1):61–9.
46. Cassatella MA, Mosna F, Micheletti A, et al. Toll-Like Receptor-3-Activated Human Mesenchymal Stromal Cells Significantly Prolong the Survival and Function of Neutrophils. STEM CELLS 2011;29(6):1001–11.
47. Regmi S, Pathak S, Kim JO, et al. Mesenchymal stem cell therapy for the treatment of inflammatory diseases: Challenges, opportunities, and future perspectives. Eur J Cell Biol 2019;98(5–8):151041.
48. Lee JW, Fang X, Krasnodembskaya A, et al. Concise Review: Mesenchymal Stem Cells for Acute Lung Injury: Role of Paracrine Soluble Factors. Stem Cells 2011;29(6):913–9.
49. Giacca M, Zacchigna S. VEGF gene therapy: therapeutic angiogenesis in the clinic and beyond. Gene Ther 2012;19(6):622–9.
50. Chen L, Tredget EE, Wu PYG, et al. Paracrine Factors of Mesenchymal Stem Cells Recruit Macrophages and Endothelial Lineage Cells and Enhance Wound Healing. PLoS ONE 2008;3(4):e1886.
51. Timmers L, Lim SK, Hoefer IE, et al. Human mesenchymal stem cell-conditioned medium improves cardiac function following myocardial infarction. Stem Cell Res 2011;6(3):206–14.

52. Morita Y, Ema H, Nakauchi H. Heterogeneity and hierarchy within the most primitive hematopoietic stem cell compartment. J Exp Med 2010;207(6):1173–82.
53. Caplan AI, Dennis JE. Mesenchymal stem cells as trophic mediators. J Cell Biochem 2006;98(5):1076–84.
54. Hernigou P, Daltro G, Hernigou J. Hip osteonecrosis: stem cells for life or behead and arthroplasty? Int Orthop 2018;42(7):1425–8.
55. Tabatabaee RM, Saberi S, Parvizi J, et al. Combining Concentrated Autologous Bone Marrow Stem Cells Injection With Core Decompression Improves Outcome for Patients with Early-Stage Osteonecrosis of the Femoral Head: A Comparative Study. J Arthroplasty 2015;30(9 Suppl):11—15.
56. Awad ME, Hussein KA, Helwa I, et al. Meta-Analysis and Evidence Base for the Efficacy of Autologous Bone Marrow Mesenchymal Stem Cells in Knee Cartilage Repair: Methodological Guidelines and Quality Assessment. Stem Cells Int 2019;2019:1-15.
57. Zhao T, Yan W, Xu K, et al. Combined treatment with platelet-rich plasma and brain-derived neurotrophic factor-overexpressing bone marrow stromal cells supports axonal remyelination in a rat spinal cord hemi-section model. Cytotherapy 2013;15(7):792–804.
58. Betsch M, Schneppendahl J, Thuns S, et al. Bone Marrow Aspiration Concentrate and Platelet Rich Plasma for Osteochondral Repair in a Porcine Osteochondral Defect Model. PLoS ONE 2013;8(8):e71602.
59. Andia I, Martin JI, Maffulli N. Platelet-rich Plasma and Mesenchymal Stem Cells: Exciting, But ... are we there Yet? Sports Med Arthrosc Rev 2018;26(2):59–63.
60. Ullah I, Subbarao RB, Rho GJ. Human mesenchymal stem cells - current trends and future prospective. Biosci Rep 2015;35(2):e00191.
61. Argentati C, Morena F, Bazzucchi M, et al. Adipose Stem Cell Translational Applications: From Bench-to-Bedside. Int J Mol Sci 2018;19(11):3475.
62. Izadpanah R, Trygg C, Patel B, et al. Biologic properties of mesenchymal stem cells derived from bone marrow and adipose tissue. J Cell Biochem 2006;99(5): 1285–97.
63. Dmitrieva RI, Minullina IR, Bilibina AA, et al. Bone marrow- and subcutaneous adipose tissue-derived mesenchymal stem cells: Differences and similarities. Cell Cycle 2012;11(2):377–83.
64. Mohamed-Ahmed S, Fristad I, Lie SA, et al. Adipose-derived and bone marrow mesenchymal stem cells: a donor-matched comparison. Stem Cell Res Ther 2018;9(1):168.
65. Andrzejewska A, Lukomska B, Janowski M. Concise Review: Mesenchymal Stem Cells: From Roots to Boost: MSCs: From Roots to Boost. STEM CELLS 2019;37(7):855–64.
66. Karastergiou K, Mohamed-Ali V. The autocrine and paracrine roles of adipokines. Mol Cell Endocrinol 2010;318(1–2):69–78.
67. Cinti S. Reversible physiological transdifferentiation in the adipose organ. Proc Nutr Soc 2009;68(4):340–9.
68. Zuk PA, Zhu M, Ashjian P, et al. Human Adipose Tissue Is a Source of Multipotent Stem Cells□D. Mol Biol Cell 2002;13:17.
69. Zuk PA. The Adipose-derived Stem Cell: Looking Back and Looking Ahead. Kellogg D, editor. Mol Biol Cell 2010;21(11):1783–7.
70. Yang HJ, Kim KJ, Kim MK, et al. The Stem Cell Potential and Multipotency of Human Adipose Tissue-Derived Stem Cells Vary by Cell Donor and Are Different from Those of Other Types of Stem Cells. Cells Tissues Organs 2014; 199(5–6):373–83.

71. Wagner SJ, Leiby DA, Roback JD. Existing and Emerging Blood-Borne Pathogens: Impact on the Safety of Blood Transfusion for the Hematology/Oncology Patient. Hematol Clin 2019;33(5):739–48.
72. Baer PC. Adipose-derived mesenchymal stromal/stem cells: An update on their phenotype in vivo and in vitro. World J Stem Cells 2014;6(3):256.
73. Yun S, Ku SK, Kwon YS. Adipose-derived mesenchymal stem cells and platelet-rich plasma synergistically ameliorate the surgical-induced osteoarthritis in Beagle dogs. J Orthop Surg 2016;11(1):9.
74. Brown JC, Shang H, Li Y, et al. Isolation of Adipose-Derived Stromal Vascular Fraction Cells Using a Novel Point-of-Care Device: Cell Characterization and Review of the Literature. Tissue Eng C Methods 2017;23(3):125–35.
75. Gimble JM, Katz AJ, Bunnell BA. Adipose-Derived Stem Cells for Regenerative Medicine. Circ Res 2007;100(9):1249–60.
76. Sugii S, Kida Y, Berggren WT, et al. Feeder-dependent and feeder-independent iPS cell derivation from human and mouse adipose stem cells. Nat Protoc 2011; 6(3):346–58.
77. Varma MJO, Breuls RGM, Schouten TE, et al. Phenotypical and Functional Characterization of Freshly Isolated Adipose Tissue-Derived Stem Cells. Stem Cells Dev 2007;16(1):91–104.
78. Alexander R.W., Understanding Mechanical Emulsification (Nanofat) Versus Enzymatic Isolation of Tissue Stromal Vascular Fraction (tSVF) Cells from Adipose Tissue: Potential Uses in Biocellular Regenerative Medicine, J Prolotherapy, 8, 2016, e947-e960.
79. Tremolada C, Colombo V, Ventura C. Adipose Tissue and Mesenchymal Stem Cells: State of the Art and Lipogems® Technology Development. Curr Stem Cell Rep 2016;2(3):304–12.
80. Simonacci F, Bertozzi N, Grieco MP, et al. From liposuction to adipose-derived stem cells: indications and technique. Acta Bio Med Atenei Parm 2019;90(2): 197–208.
81. Berry M, Davies D. Liposuction: a review of principles and techniques. J Plast Reconstr Amp Aesthet Surg 2011;64(8):985–92.
82. Illouz Y. Body contouring by lipolysis: a 5-year experience with over 3000 cases. Plast Reconstr Surg 1983;72(5):591–7.
83. Klein JA. The Tumescent Technique: Anesthesia and Modified Liposuction Technique. Dermatol Clin 1990;8(3):425–37.
84. Coleman SR. Structural Fat Grafting: More Than a Permanent Filler. Plast Reconstr Surg 2006;118(Suppl):108S–20S.
85. Kurita M, Matsumoto D, Shigeura T, et al. Influences of Centrifugation on Cells and Tissues in Liposuction Aspirates: Optimized Centrifugation for Lipotransfer and Cell Isolation. Plast Reconstr Surg 2008;121(3):1033–41.
86. Gentile P, Calabrese C, De Angelis B, et al. Impact of the Different Preparation Methods to Obtain Human Adipose-Derived Stromal Vascular Fraction Cells (AD-SVFs) and Human Adipose-Derived Mesenchymal Stem Cells (AD-MSCs): Enzymatic Digestion Versus Mechanical Centrifugation. Int J Mol Sci 2019;20(21):5471.
87. Tonnard P, Verpaele A, Peeters G, et al. Nanofat Grafting: Basic Research and Clinical Applications. Plast Reconstr Surg 2013;132(4):1017–26.
88. Bianchi F, Maioli M, Leonardi E, et al. A New Nonenzymatic Method and Device to Obtain a Fat Tissue Derivative Highly Enriched in Pericyte-Like Elements by Mild Mechanical Forces from Human Lipoaspirates. Cell Transpl 2013;22(11): 2063–77.

89. Regulatory Considerations for Human Cells, Tissues, and Cellular and Tissue-Based Products: Minimal Manipulation and Homologous Use; Guidance for. Industry and Food and Drug Administration Staff. Docket 2020. Number: FDA-2017-D-6146.
90. Ong WK, Sugii S. Adipose-derived stem cells: Fatty potentials for therapy. Int J Biochem Cell Biol 2013;45(6):1083–6.
91. Hao T, Chen J, Zhi S, et al. Comparison of bone marrow-vs. adipose tissue-derived mesenchymal stem cells for attenuating liver fibrosis. Exp Ther Med 2017;14(6):5956–64.
92. Pendleton C, Li Q, Chesler DA, et al. Quinones-Hinojosa A. Mesenchymal Stem Cells Derived from Adipose Tissue vs Bone Marrow: In Vitro Comparison of Their Tropism towards Gliomas. PLoS ONE 2013;8(3):e58198.
93. Puissant B, Barreau C, Bourin P, et al. Immunomodulatory effect of human adipose tissue-derived adult stem cells: comparison with bone marrow mesenchymal stem cells. Br J Haematol 2005;129(1):118–29.
94. Fang Y, Zhang Y, Zhou J, et al. Adipose-derived mesenchymal stem cell exosomes: a novel pathway for tissues repair. Cell Tissue Bank 2019;20(2):153–61.
95. Salgado AJ, Reis RL, Sousa NJ, et al. Adipose Tissue Derived Stem Cells Secretome: Soluble Factors and Their Roles in Regenerative Medicine. Curr Stem Cell Res Ther 2010;5(2):103–10.
96. Naik S, Larsen SB, Cowley CJ, et al. Two to Tango: Dialog between Immunity and Stem Cells in Health and Disease. Cell 2018;175(4):908–20.
97. Mitchell R, Mellows B, Sheard J, et al. Secretome of adipose-derived mesenchymal stem cells promotes skeletal muscle regeneration through synergistic action of extracellular vesicle cargo and soluble proteins. Stem Cell Res Ther 2019;10(1):116.
98. Wang K, Yu LY, Jiang LY, et al. The paracrine effects of adipose-derived stem cells on neovascularization and biocompatibility of a macroencapsulation device. Acta Biomater 2015;15:65–76.
99. Sorop O, Olver TD, van de Wouw J, et al. The microcirculation: a key player in obesity-associated cardiovascular disease. Cardiovasc Res 2017;113(9):1035–45.
100. Tran KV, Gealekman O, Frontini A, et al. The Vascular Endothelium of the Adipose Tissue Gives Rise to Both White and Brown Fat Cells. Cell Metab 2012;15(2):222–9.
101. Planat-Benard V, Silvestre JS, Cousin B, et al. Plasticity of Human Adipose Lineage Cells Toward Endothelial Cells: Physiological and Therapeutic Perspectives. Circulation 2004;109(5):656–63.
102. Miranville A, Heeschen C, Sengenès C, et al. Improvement of Postnatal Neovascularization by Human Adipose Tissue-Derived Stem Cells. Circulation 2004;110(3):349–55.
103. Koh YJ, Koh BI, Kim H, et al. Stromal Vascular Fraction From Adipose Tissue Forms Profound Vascular Network Through the Dynamic Reassembly of Blood Endothelial Cells. Arterioscler Thromb Vasc Biol 2011;31(5):1141–50.
104. Rehman J, Traktuev D, Li J, et al. Secretion of Angiogenic and Antiapoptotic Factors by Human Adipose Stromal Cells. Circulation 2004;109(10):1292–8.
105. Bauer AL, Jackson TL, Jiang Y. Topography of Extracellular Matrix Mediates Vascular Morphogenesis and Migration Speeds in Angiogenesis. In: Czirók A, editor. Plos Comput Biol 2009;5(7):e1000445.
106. Docheva D, Müller SA, Majewski M, et al. Biologics for tendon repair. Adv Drug Deliv Rev 2015;84:222–39.

107. Narayanan AS, Page RC, Swanson J. Collagen synthesis by human fibroblasts. Biochem J 1989;260:463–9.
108. Fraser JK, Wulur I, Alfonso Z, et al. Fat tissue: an underappreciated source of stem cells for biotechnology. Trends Biotechnol 2006;24(4):150–4.
109. Oedayrajsingh-Varma MJ, van Ham SM, Knippenberg M, et al. Adipose tissue-derived mesenchymal stem cell yield and growth characteristics are affected by the tissue-harvesting procedure. Cytotherapy 2006;8(2):166–77.
110. Iyyanki T, Hubenak J, Liu J, et al. Harvesting Technique Affects Adipose-Derived Stem Cell Yield. Aesthet Surg J 2015;35(4):467–76.
111. Huang SJ, Fu RH, Shyu WC, et al. Adipose-Derived Stem Cells: Isolation, Characterization, and Differentiation Potential. Cell Transpl 2013;22(4):701–9.
112. De Ugarte DA, Morizono K, Elbarbary A, et al. Comparison of Multi-Lineage Cells from Human Adipose Tissue and Bone Marrow. Cells Tissues Organs 2003;174(3):101–9.
113. Klar AS, Zimoch J, Biedermann T. Skin Tissue Engineering: Application of Adipose-Derived Stem Cells. Biomed Res Int 2017;2017:1–12.
114. Phinney DG, Kopen G, Righter W, et al. Donor variation in the growth properties and osteogenic potential of human marrow stromal cells. J Cell Biochem 1999; 75(3):424–36.
115. Guneta V, Tan NS, Chan SKJ, et al. Comparative study of adipose-derived stem cells and bone marrow-derived stem cells in similar microenvironmental conditions. Exp Cell Res 2016;348(2):155–64.
116. Woo DH, Hwang HS, Shim JH. Comparison of adult stem cells derived from multiple stem cell niches. Biotechnol Lett 2016;38(5):751–9.

Basic Science of Allograft Orthobiologics

Alberto J. Panero, DO[a,*], Peter A. Everts, PhD, FRSM[b], Hirotaka Nakagawa, MD[c], Walter Sussman, DO[d], Xiaofei Qin, PhD[e]

KEYWORDS

• Allografts • Birth tissue-derived products • Amnion • Chorion • Wharton's jelly • Bioactive scaffolds • Demineralized bone matrix

KEY POINTS

- Allograft tissues have the potential to provide orthobiologic treatment due to their cellular, biologic factors, and extracellular matrix proteins.
- Their use can avoid complications from autologous tissue harvests, improve procedural time efficiency, and give patients with comorbidities an alternative to autologous therapies.
- Clinicians must be very familiar with current Federal Drug Administration regulations and stay within the recommendations for allograft tissue use.

INTRODUCTION

Allograft tissues can serve a variety of orthobiologic functions. Each allograft tissue contains a unique set of biochemical and/or structural properties, with some allografts containing a cellular makeup of stem cell or progenitor cells in vivo, along with growth factors and extracellular matrix (ECM) proteins.[1–4] These properties can be used to provide anti-inflammatory effects to reduce pain and improve function resulting from musculoskeletal conditions. In some cases, it is postulated that the progenitor cells may activate the body's innate healing mechanisms through the release of trophic and immunomodulatory factors to promote a healing response.[5–16] Allografts can also be used as bioactive scaffolds to help support the healing process of soft tissues and bone as well as tissue barriers to protect healing tissues after surgical procedures.[17–23]

[a] The BIOS Orthopedic Institute, 2277 Fair Oaks Blvd, Suite 415, Sacramento, CA 95825, USA; [b] Gulf Coast Biologics, Research and Scientific Division, Royal Society of Medicine London, Veronica S. Shoemaker Boulevard, Suite 1, Fort Myers, FL, 33916, USA; [c] Department of Orthopedics and Rehabilitation, Tufts Medical Center, 800 Washington Street, Boston, MA 02111, USA; [d] Boston Sports & Biologics, Department of Orthopedics and Rehabilitation, Tufts Medical Center, 20 Walnut Street Suite 14, Wellesley, MA 02481, USA; [e] Lifenet Health, 1864 Concert Drive, Virginia Beach, 23453, USA

* Corresponding author.
E-mail address: apanero@thebiosinstitute.com

Phys Med Rehabil Clin N Am 34 (2023) 49–61
https://doi.org/10.1016/j.pmr.2022.08.005

Allografts are either derived from birth tissues and live or cadaveric donors. Birth Tissue Derived products include amniotic fluid, sheet products derived from the amniotic sac or umbilical cord, and particulate products derived from the amniotic membrane, the chorion, and the umbilical cord including Wharton's Jelly.[24] Extracellular vesicles (EVs) including exosomes can be isolated from donor blood or bone marrow and have generated great interest in their function in cellular messaging/communication. Cadaveric allografts include demineralized bone matrix, osteochondral grafts, and a variety of tissues including nucleus pulposus and tendon grafts.

These tissues carry tremendous potential in providing patients an option whose own autologous tissues may lack the proper quality to be used for orthobiologic indications, may have contraindications to autologous harvests, or require a scaffold or augmentation to an interventional/surgical procedure. They also carry the potential of providing an off-the-shelf product with specific doses of cellular contents or proteins that can improve procedural time efficiency and allow for consistency in therapeutic responses. Although the potential is present, they lack high-quality studies to support their efficacy and safety. Furthermore, current regulatory guidelines have restricted the use of a variety of products and many of them should only be used in the setting of an Investigational New Drug (IND) research study.

This chapter will highlight the basic anatomy and properties of various allograft tissues that can be deployed to either promote therapeutic responses or provide mechanical support in musculoskeletal conditions.

Birth Tissue-Derived Products

Amniotic Fluid, Amniotic Membrane, Umbilical Cord/Wharton's Jelly, Placental Membrane Sheets.

Anatomy

The placenta, amniotic sac, and umbilical cord have emerged as an area of interest in cell-based therapy and regenerative medicine. The placenta is a discoid organ that provides an interface between the mother and fetus during fetal development (**Fig. 1**). The amniotic membrane covers the placenta, umbilical cord, and amniotic sac, and consists of an outer chorion layer and the thin, innermost amniotic layer (**Fig. 2**). The amnion layer consists of a simple squamous epithelium with an underlying basement membrane and a band of loose connective tissue. The amnion layer is only

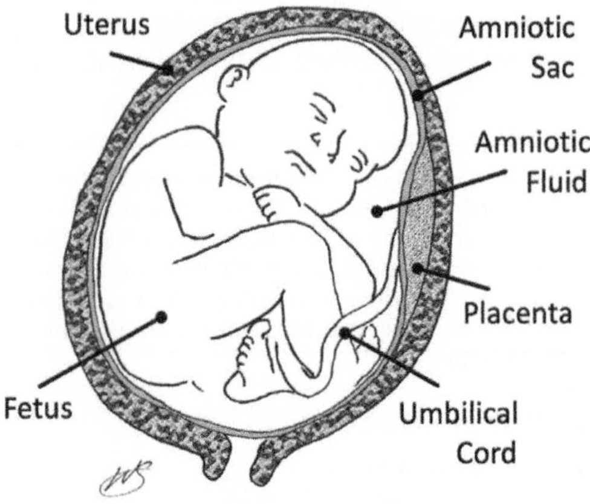

Fig. 1. Umbilical cord, amniotic sac, and placenta.

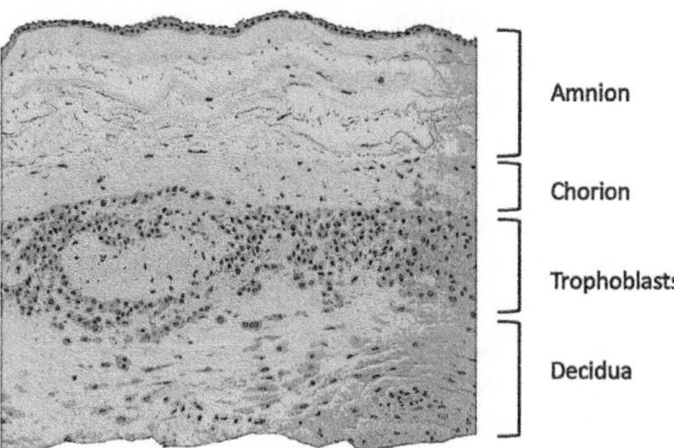

Fig. 2. Histology of the amniotic sac. Image provided by Jeffery Sussman, M.D.

weakly attached to the underlying chorion.[25] Within the amniotic sac, the amniotic fluid envelopes the developing fetus to provide nutritional and immune-modulatory support.[26]

The umbilical cord allows an exchange of blood between mother and fetus to provide oxygenated blood to the fetus and to remove byproducts via maternal circulation. The umbilical cord is made of two umbilical arteries and one umbilical vein surrounded by mucous connective tissue called Wharton's jelly.[27] Its key role is to provide cushion and protection for umbilical vessels.[28] The umbilical cord also contains high amounts of ECM components including collagen, hyaluronic acid, and sulfated proteoglycans.[29]

Harvesting and processing of perinatal tissue

Several preparations of birth tissue-derived products have been described. Harvesting, processing, preservation, and formulation methods of birth tissues have dramatically improved in the past decade to minimize the risk of disease transmission. Placental tissues are harvested with the full consent of the mother.[26,30–32] Typically the placenta, amniotic sac, and umbilical cord are harvested from Cesarian delivery to minimize the risk of potential contamination from normal flora that could occur during vaginal delivery.[32] The collected tissue undergoes meticulous screening protocols for hepatitis B, hepatitis C, syphilis, cytomegalovirus, human immunodeficiency virus, and tuberculosis through regulation by the Federal Drug Administration (FDA) and the American Association of Tissue banks.[33,34]

The placenta, amniotic sac, and umbilical cord are then aseptically processed, cleaned, and optionally separated into individual membrane components before being preserved.[26,32,35] Preservation methods include dehydration, cryopreservation and lyophilization.[30,36,37] Dehydration process removes moisture.[30] Cryopreservation allows for long-term storage of grafts at −80° with a cryoprotectant.[37] This enables membrane grafts to retain a structure more similar to their *in vivo* state.[30] Lyophilization, also known as freeze drying, is a method of dehydration consisting of the removal of water from the tissue by sublimation while minimizing any heat impact on biological factors during dehydration.[36] Lyophilized membrane can be stored at room temperature.[36] The allografts can be micronized to particulate matter to be used as an injectable formulation or can be processed to form sheets of tissue that can be used as tendon, ligament, or nerve wraps.[32,38] The umbilical cord is aseptically processed and typically formulated into an injectable form. Birth tissue products can also be terminally sterilized through E-beam or irradiation to further reduce any potential microbial contamination when cellular viability in the products is not a concern. Birth tissue needs to be prepared according to the FDA's criteria of minimal manipulation and should not include any combination products nor be dependent on the metabolic activity of living cells, including mesenchymal stem cells.

Underlying mechanism

Although the mechanism of action of birth tissue-derived products likely varies depending on the underlying pathology, it is believed to aid in tissue repair by providing key biologic factors including cytokines such as Interleukin-1 Receptor Antagonist (IL-1Ra), growth factors, and protease inhibitors such as Tissue Inhibitors of Metalloproteinases (TIMPs), hyaluronic acid and exosomes, as well as by acting as a scaffold to allow cell adhesion. Perinatal allografts release various growth factors including vascular endothelial growth factors (VEGFs) that promote angiogenesis, basic fibroblast growth factors (bFGF) that promote early tendon healing, and transforming growth factor β (TGF- β) that stimulates the production of ECM.[39,40] *In vitro*, amniotic membrane has been shown to downregulate inflammation by releasing anti-inflammatory cytokines such as interleukin-10 (IL10). The downregulation of inflammation attenuates scar formation around the nerve to prevent adhesion to surrounding tissue.[35,41] Another key mechanism is achieved by anti-catabolic factors, such as protease inhibitors. The large quantity of endogenous protease inhibitors (alpha 2-macroglobulin, TIMP1, TIMP2, TIMP3, and TIMP4) in birth tissue plays a pivotal role in slowing cartilage degeneration progress in cases of osteoarthritis.[35,41] Hyaluronic acid in Wharton's jelly has been shown to have chondroprotective, anti-inflammatory, and analgesic properties when used for knee osteoarthritis.[42]

The capacity for commercial birth-tissue products available in the United States to deliver mesenchymal stem cells has been questioned as it is unclear whether commercial processing, preservation, and formulation techniques affect the viability of the cells in these products. Although amniotic mesenchymal stromal cells have shown to be present in amniotic fluid *in vivo*, the majority of commercial products have shown no living mesenchymal stem cells after commercial processing.[43,44] Despite the lack of viable cells in most commercial products, the clinical benefit of placental-derived products is maintained, suggesting that the effects of these allografts are mediated by matrix proteins, growth factors, and exosomes contained in these tissues. Thus these allografts are more accurately classified as a biologically active biologic scaffolds rather than a mesenchymal "stem cell" product.[39,45]

Although regulatory guidelines can vary from country to country, there are countries outside of the United States, that allow for the culture expansion and manipulation of cells of autologous and allograft tissues. The mesenchymal progenitor or stem cells can be isolated from birth-derived tissues and culture expanded, allowing clinicians to deliver a standardized, homogenous product with low immunogenic properties.[24]

Seemingly promising, there is still great debate as to which birth tissue provides the most efficient source of MSCs and how each tissue will respond to the culture expansion with minimal deterioration in division and growth power, or senescence after multiple cell expansion passages.[20–24,46–49] Furthermore, high-quality clinical trials are lacking to show superiority to the non-expanded allograft counterpart.

To summarize. Therapeutic potential of perinatal tissue in orthopedics

The clinical literatures of the use of birth tissue-derived allografts are overall limited. To date, human studies using amniotic membrane allografts have been published for the treatment of plantar fasciitis, Achilles tendonitis, and knee osteoarthritis. Several randomized controlled studies on the use of amniotic membrane for the treatment of plantar fasciitis seem to suggest that its efficacy is at least equivocal to corticosteroid injections in the short term.[50–52] However, most of these studies were underpowered and lacked long-term follow-up data. Most of the studies for the application of amniotic membrane-derived products in Achilles tendinitis, knee osteoarthritis, and nerve entrapment injuries are limited to case series. Although many studies seem to suggest that amniotic membrane may reduce pain and improve function, additional high-quality supportive data is needed to support the efficacy and safety of placental-derived products. Most studies on Wharton's jelly-derived products are limited to basic science or animal model studies aimed at treating degenerative disk disease, osteoporotic vertebral compression fracture, peripheral nerve injury, and osteoarthritis.[53]

Extracellular Vesicles

What are extracellular vesicles?

Intercellular communication is an important mechanism within multicellular organisms. This is mediated through direct cell–cell contact, transfer of secreted molecules, and the intracellular transfer of EVs.[54]

The latter communication mechanism was not only discovered to occur in apoptotic cells, but also in healthy cells.[55,56]

These membrane vesicles are referred to as microvesicles (ectosomes), microparticles, oncosomes, or exosomes, and collectively they are termed EV. Cells secrete EV in varying in sizes through endosomal pathways and by budding from plasma membranes into the extracellular space.[57] More specifically, the term exosome was initially used for EV ranging in size from 40 to 1000 nm.

Interest in EV, more explicitly exosomes, as a treatment modality for musculoskeletal disorders was recently fueled by the finding that exosomes contain RNA suggesting that their protein and ribonucleic acid (RNA) content might be transferred between cells, establishing intercellular communication.[58] The exosome structures allow for the direct transfer of informative molecules between cells.[59] Initial studies confirmed that both microRNAs (miRNAs) and noncoding RNAs (ncRNAs) are enclosed within exosomes. These molecules, together with other EV complex cargo compositions, consisting among others of hundreds to thousands of different proteins, specific lipids, some DNA, many ncRNAs, and mitochondrial RNA, have the potential to be transferred to recipient cells.

The roles of exosomes in therapeutic treatments

Exosomes are of general interest for their potential roles in cell biology, and for their potential in diagnostics and therapeutic application in tissue repair processes. Initially, exosomes were linked to cellular waste products, however, their possible function is now known to extend beyond waste removal, as they represent a novel mode of cell communication and contribute to a spectrum of biological repair processes in various disease states. Exosomes bear surface molecules that allow them to be targeted to recipient cells, where they deliver their complex cargo loads. Furthermore, exosomes can be therapeutically targeted or engineered as drug delivery systems.[60]

The exact mechanism and regulation of exosome formation can be stimulated by growth factors and cells adjust their exosome production according to their needs, although the mechanisms of action are still not fully understood.[61]

Exosomes in orthobiological preparations

Exosomes are enclosed within single outer cell membranes and are secreted by all cell types. They have been retrieved in blood plasma, urine, semen, saliva, bronchial fluid, cerebral spinal fluid, breast milk, amniotic fluid, synovial fluid, tears, lymph, bile, and gastric acid.[62,63]

Platelet-rich plasma
More interesting regarding clinical orthobiological preparations, exosomes are also secreted by platelet alpha granules, as shown by Heijnen and colleagues.[64] They found exosomes in the platelet releases of prepared platelet-rich plasma (PRP) from fresh whole blood, anticoagulated with sodium citrate, and subsequently activated with thrombin activating peptide. These findings were recently confirmed, with platelet-derived exosomes (PLT-Exos) secreted by platelets.[65] PLT-Exos levels increased following platelet activation by Von Willebrand Factor, tissue factor, and thrombin delivering their cargo to recipient cells, inhibiting inflammation of endothelial cells, among other activities.[66] PRP activation has the potential to lead to the secretion of a high yield of PLT-Exos from small PRP volumes, as determined by nanoflow analysis in a study from Rui and colleagues.[67] However, different platelet activators (like thrombin and calcium) influence the quality and quantity of PRP-Exos, with calcium-activated PRP releasing higher concentrations of exosomes then thrombin. Albeit that the combined mixture of calcium-thrombin released the highest concentrations of microparticles. It is fair to assume that different release profiles influence the PLT-Exos roles in intercellular communication and tissue repair.[67,68]

Bone marrow
Bone marrow tissue with mesenchymal stem cells, and bone marrow stromal cells, contain naturally bone marrow-derived exosomes (BM-Exos) and other EV which are secreted by these various cells.[69] Research made it clear that these BM-Exos are involved in the regulation of skeletal metabolism and extraosseous diseases through modulating intercellular communication and the transfer of vesicle materials. In addition, bone marrow stem cells have been considered a better therapeutic option than adipose mesenchymal stem cells with a higher disease-modifying potential, as shown in an experimental osteoarthritis study.[70]

Exosomes isolation methods
The potential benefits and uses of exosomes and other EVs have been noted in recent experimental models. However, a major hindrance in bringing exosomes into the clinical setting is the lack of standardization in isolation methods. The gold standard for exosome isolation is based on complicated ultracentrifugation-based methods.[57,71]

As with all centrifugation methods, the separation of exosomes and other EVs from the ECM depends on density, size, and shape, with larger and more dense particles sedimenting out first.[72]

The centrifugation parameters for exosome preparations are completely different from what we routinely use for the preparation of orthobiological products, and they cannot mimic ultracentrifuge settings, as they require at some stage 100,000 $\times$ g spins to pellet out exosomes for several hours.[73]

Alternative methods have been introduced and are based on isolation by size, immunoaffinity capture, and precipitation of exosomes. Unfortunately, these techniques also fail in the complete and consistent isolation of exosomes.

To summarize
By way of caveats, the field of exosome technology and clinical application is young and has several "black holes" in data that confound interpretation. For example, EVs of varying size, mode of biogenesis, and cargo can be released from a single cell, and these can change with the physiologic state of the cell. Different cell types may also produce distinct repertoires of vesicles. At current, the focus of this new molecular field is directed toward the development of improved methods of isolation of different EV subtypes.

Exosome research and clinical employment are still in their infancy, an in-depth understanding of subcellular components and mechanisms involved in exosome formation and specific cell-targeting must elucidate on their physiologic and tissue repair activities.

For these reasons the FDA does not approve any exosome products to be used to treat diseases or conditions in humans, other than that they can be used for diagnostics.

Allografts as biologic scaffolds

The progression of musculoskeletal disease or degeneration is a complex process that varies within tissue types and their independent pathologies. However, there is typically an inciting event such as trauma, or repetitive use, where the load exceeds the capacity of the soft tissue or bone. This event leads to a progressive imbalance of anabolic and catabolic processes that results in the improper restoration of the diseased tissue.[74] The tissue is unable to heal and thus starts to lose its mechanical properties, further altering its function and ability to take on a load, releasing more catabolic/inflammatory cytokines that cause pain and further advance degeneration. Creating a negative feedback loop that impedes the tissue to re-establish homeostasis, leading to its own destruction.

Structural allografts derived from a homologous source can be used within the scope of orthobiologic procedures to aid in the restoration of the loss of the tissue's mechanical properties from a structural/mechanical standpoint. Furthermore, these structural allografts may contain biologically active properties that may help interrupt the negative loop created by the degenerative process and restore homeostasis to the tissue environment, promoting or shifting the balance toward healing.

In bone, these imbalances are seen in the form of trabecular fractures or a variety of subchondral reactive changes including edema and cysts, as well as avascular necrosis. The use of bone grafts has provided an efficient tool to treat some of these pathologies.[18–23,46] The graft not only provides mechanical support/scaffolding but also has both osteoconductive and osteoinductive properties.[18–23,46] As autologous bone harvest can create donor site morbidity and is costly, demineralized bone matrix (DBM) is an allograft that can be used in its place. DBM is produced via acid digestion of bone, and retains collagen (predominantly type I), non-collagenous proteins that are osteoinductive, residual calcium phosphate, and residual cellular debris.[18–23,46] In the setting of orthobiologic procedures, DBM can be combined with autologous tissues such as PRP or bone marrow concentrate and delivered percutaneously to treat subchondral pathologies.[18–23,46]

Similarly, in cases of degenerative disk disease in the spine, with time and load, the disk loses its concentration of proteoglycans. This leads to a decrease in intradiscal pressure, and the inability for the disk to hold structured water, leading to altered mechanics and progressive disk degeneration, leading to pain and functional decline.[74] As a reparative strategy, replacing lost disk tissue via the percutaneous delivery of nucleus pulposus allograft tissue intradiscally is being studied, with early positive findings.[74]

Consequently, we hypothesize that future orthobiologic therapies will be centered around the delivery of a bioactive scaffold that can host the deployment of progenitor cells and proper growth factors to either differentiate or signal the host tissue to differentiate into homologous tissue.

Regulatory considerations

The FDA has created the Center for Biologics Evaluation and Research (CBER) to provide guidance on biological products. The Human Cells, Tissues, and Cellular and

Tissue-Based Products (HCT/P) guidance documents were issued in November of 2017 and updated in July of 2020. Allografts must meet the following criteria to be considered an HCT/P and be regulated solely under section 361 of the Public Health Service Act.[48]

1. The HCT/P is minimally manipulated.
2. The HCT/P is intended for homologous use only.
3. The manufacture of the HCT/P does not involve the combination of the cell or tissue component with a drug or device, except for a sterilizing, preserving, or storage agent, if the addition of the agent does not raise new clinical safety concerns with respect to the HCT/P[27]; and
4. Either:
   i. The HCT/P does not have a systemic effect and is not dependent upon the metabolic activity of living cells for its primary function; or
   ii. The HCT/P has a systemic effect or is dependent upon the metabolic activity of living cells for its primary function, and:
      a .is for autologous use
      b. is for allogeneic use in a first or second-degree relative; or
      c. is for reproductive use

If the allograft does not meet the above criteria, then it is regulated under section 351 of the public health service act, and considered a “drug, device, or biological product”. This allograft must then go through the IND pathway or Biologics License Applications (BLA) pathway, requiring strenuous research to prove its safety and efficacy.

The FDA provided allograft manufacturers until May 31, 2021 to determine if they are required to submit an IND or other application based on their guidance. The FDA has since announced the end of the compliance and enforcement policy for certain HCT/Ps). Amniotic sheets are still considered HCT/Ps as they are not more than minimally manipulated and when used homologously with their ability to serve as a barrier in an off-label manner.[48]

Although this has forced many of these products off the market, several manufacturers of particulated birth tissue-derived products have filed for IND and are currently in clinical trials at various stages, primarily for knee osteoarthritis.[47]

With regard to DBM, the FDA has determined that DBM on its own meets the criteria for regulation under 361. However, if combined with products like sodium hyaluronate, glycerol, or calcium phosphate, then they do not qualify that change the consistency of DBM to a putty or paste, those products no longer meet the criteria for section 361 regulation.

SUMMARY

Allograft tissues can provide a valuable tool for orthobiologic treatments due to their cellular contents and structural properties as bioactive scaffolds. The potential to have these products available off-the-shelf may improve time efficiency of procedures while reducing potential complication rates from autologous harvests. Promising as it may, there is the need for level 1 clinical trials to further assess the safety and efficacy of these tissues. Moreover, close attention must be paid to following regulatory guidelines while using these tissues outside of a formal investigational new drug study.

DISCLOSURE

A. Panero is a consultant for Arthrex Inc, received research support from Lifenet Health, is a speaker for Clarius Mobile Health, and has their stock options. He is also a speaker for Ossur Inc, Tenex Health, and Advanced Regenerative Medicine Institute. He is a co-PI for the GID Group—Adipose Research Study in Knee OA. P. Everts is also acting Chief Scientific Officer of EmCyte Corporation.W. Sussman is an educational consultant for Trice Medical and Lipogems Inc.

CLINICS CARE POINTS

- Allograft tissues carry tremendous potential in providing patients an option whose own autologous tissues may lack the proper quality to be used for orthobiologic indications, may have contraindications to autologous harvests, or require a scaffold or augmentation to an interventional/surgical procedure.
- Randomized controlled clicial trials are needed to identify the proper application of each allograft tissue and its efficacy and safety.
- It is imperative to stay up to date with the Federal Drug Administration's recommendations to ensure proper and allowable use of these allograft tissues.

REFERENCES

1. Bottai, et al. Third Trimester Amniotic Fluid Cells with the Capacity to Develop Nerual Phenotypes and with Heterogenicity among sub-populations. Restor Neurol Neurosci 2012;30(1):55–68.
2. Pierce, et al. Collection and characterization of amniotic fluid from scheduled C-section deliverie. Cell Tissue Bank 2016;17(3):413–25.
3. Zia S, et al. Routine Clonal expansion of mesenchymal stem cells derived from amniotic fluid for perinatal applications. Prenat Diagn 2013;33(10):921–8.
4. Panero AJ, Hirahara AM, Andersen WJ, et al. Are Amniotic Fluid Products Stem Cell Therapies? A Study of Amniotic Fluid Preparations for Mesenchymal Stem Cells With Bone Marrow. Am J Sports Med 2019;47(5):1230–5.
5. Kern S, Eichler H, Stoeve J, et al. Comparative analysis of mesenchymal stem cells from bone marrow, umbilical cord blood, or adipose tissue. Stem Cells 2006;24(5):1294–301.
6. Montesinos JJ, Flores-Figueroa E, Castillo-Medina S, et al. Human mesenchymal stromal cells from adult and neonatal sources: comparative analysis of their morphology, immunophenotype, differentiation patterns and neural protein expression. Cytotherapy 2009;11(2):163–76.
7. Moretti P, Hatlapatka T, Marten D, et al. Mesenchymal stromal cells derived from human umbilical cord tissues: primitive cells with potential for clinical and tissue engineering applications. Adv Biochem Eng Biotechnol 2010;123:29–54.
8. Secunda R, Vennila R, Mohanashankar AM, et al. Isolation, expansion and characterization of mesenchymal stem cells from human bone marrow, adipose tissue, umbilical cord blood and matrix: a comparative study. Cytotechnology 2015;67(5):793–807.
9. Zeddou M, Briquet A, Relic B, et al. The umbilical cord matrix is a better source of mesenchymal stem cells (MSC) than the umbilical cord blood. Cell Biol Int 2010; 34(7):693–701.
10. Rebelatto CK, Aguiar AM, Moretao MP, et al. Dissimilar differentiation of mesenchymal stem cells from bone marrow, umbilical cord blood, and adipose tissue. Exp Biol Med (Maywood) 2008;233(7):901–13.

11. Lu LL, Liu YJ, Yang SG, et al. Isolation and characterization of human umbilical cord mesenchymal stem cells with hematopoiesis-supportive function and other potentials. Haematologica 2006;91(8):1017–26.
12. La Rocca G, Anzalone R, Corrao S, et al. Isolation and characterization of Oct-4+/HLA-G+ mesenchymal stem cells from human umbilical cord matrix: differentiation potential and detection of new markers. Histochem Cell Biol 2009;131(2):267–82.
13. Weiss ML, Medicetty S, Bledsoe AR, et al. Human umbilical cord matrix stem cells: preliminary characterization and effect of transplantation in a rodent model of Parkinson's disease. Stem Cells 2006;24(3):781–92.
14. Baksh D, Song L, Tuan RS. Adult mesenchymal stem cells: characterization, differentiation, and application in cell and gene therapy. J Cell Mol Med 2004;8(3):301–16.
15. Baksh D, Yao R, Tuan RS. Comparison of proliferative and multilineage differentiation potential of human mesenchymal stem cells derived from umbilical cord and bone marrow. Stem Cells 2007;25(6):1384–92.
16. Chen MY, Lie PC, Li ZL, et al. Endothelial differentiation of Wharton's jelly-derived mesenchymal stem cells in comparison with bone marrow-derived mesenchymal stem cells. Exp Hematol 2009;37(5):629–40.
17. Kim MJ, Shin KS, Jeon JH, et al. Human chorionic-plate-derived mesenchymal stem cells and Wharton's jelly-derived mesenchymal stem cells: a comparative analysis of their potential as placenta-derived stem cells. Cell Tissue Res 2011;346(1):53–64.
18. Finkemeier CG. Bone-grafting and bone-graft substitutes. J Bone Joint Surg Am 2002;84(3):454–64.
19. Zhang H, Yang L, Yang XG, et al. Demineralized Bone Matrix Carriers and their Clinical Applications: An Overview. Orthop Surg 2019;11(5):725–37.
20. Campana V, Milano G, Pagano E, et al. Bone substitutes in orthopaedic surgery: from basic science to clinical practice. J Mater Sci Mater Med 2014;25(10):2445–61.
21. Gruskin E, Doll BA, Futrell FW, et al. Demineralized bone matrix in bone repair: history and use. Adv Drug Deliv Rev 2012;64(12):1063–77.
22. Urist MR, Dowell TA. Inductive substratum for osteogenesis in pellets of particulate bone matrix. Clin Orthop Relat Res 1968;61:61–78.
23. Senn on the Healing of Aseptic Bone Cavities by Implantation of Antiseptic Decalcified Bone. Ann Surg 1889;10(5):352–68.
24. Martin Fernandez L. Characteristics, Properties, and Functionality of Fetal Membranes: An Overlooked Area in the Field of Parturition. Encyclopedia of Reproduction. 2nd Edition. Elsevier; 2018.
25. Strauss JF 3rd. Extracellular matrix dynamics and fetal membrane rupture. Reprod Sci 2013;20(2):140–53.
26. Hanselman AE, Lalli TA, Santrock RD. Topical Review: Use of Fetal Tissue in Foot and Ankle Surgery. Foot Ankle Spec 2015;8(4):297–304.
27. Ferguson VL, Dodson RB. Bioengineering aspects of the umbilical cord. Eur J Obstet Gynecol Reprod Biol 2009;144(Suppl 1):S108–13.
28. Taghizadeh RR, Cetrulo KJ, Cetrulo CL. Wharton's Jelly stem cells: future clinical applications. Placenta 2011;32(Suppl 4):S311–5.
29. Sobolewski K, Małkowski A, Bańkowski E, et al. Wharton's jelly as a reservoir of peptide growth factors. Placenta 2005;26(10):747–52.
30. Ang J, Liou CD, Schneider HP. The Role of Placental Membrane Allografts in the Surgical Treatment of Tendinopathies. Clin Podiatr Med Surg 2018;35(3):311–21.

31. Riboh JC, Saltzman BM, Yanke AB, et al. Human Amniotic Membrane-Derived Products in Sports Medicine: Basic Science, Early Results, and Potential Clinical Applications. *Am J Sports Med* Sep 2016;44(9):2425–34.
32. Leal-Marin S, Kern T, Hofmann N, et al. Human Amniotic Membrane: A review on tissue engineering, application, and storage. J Biomed Mater Res B Appl Biomater 2021;109(8):1198–215.
33. Kesting MR, Wolff KD, Hohlweg-Majert B, et al. The role of allogenic amniotic membrane in burn treatment. J Burn Care Res 2008;29(6):907–16.
34. Food, Drug Administration HHS. Current good tissue practice for human cell, tissue, and cellular and tissue-based product establishments; inspection and enforcement. Final rule. Fed Regist 2004;69(226):68611–88.
35. Huddleston HP, Cohn MR, Haunschild ED, et al. Amniotic Product Treatments: Clinical and Basic Science Evidence. Curr Rev Musculoskelet Med 2020;13(2): 148–54.
36. Rodriguez-Ares MT, Lopez-Valladares MJ, Tourino R, et al. Effects of lyophilization on human amniotic membrane. Acta Ophthalmol 2009;87(4):396–403.
37. Nakamura T, Yoshitani M, Rigby H, et al. Sterilized, freeze-dried amniotic membrane: a useful substrate for ocular surface reconstruction. Invest Ophthalmol Vis Sci 2004;45(1):93–9.
38. Liu C, Bai J, Yu K, et al. Biological Amnion Prevents Flexor Tendon Adhesion in Zone II: A Controlled, Multicentre Clinical Trial. Biomed Res Int 2019;2019: 2354325.
39. Koob TJ, Rennert R, Zabek N, et al. Biological properties of dehydrated human amnion/chorion composite graft: implications for chronic wound healing. Int Wound J 2013;10(5):493–500.
40. Koob TJ, Lim JJ, Massee M, et al. Angiogenic properties of dehydrated human amnion/chorion allografts: therapeutic potential for soft tissue repair and regeneration. Vasc Cell 2014;6:10.
41. Gaspar MP, Abdelfattah HM, Welch IW, et al. Recurrent cubital tunnel syndrome treated with revision neurolysis and amniotic membrane nerve wrapping. J Shoulder Elbow Surg 2016;25(12):2057–65.
42. Altman RD, Manjoo A, Fierlinger A, et al. The mechanism of action for hyaluronic acid treatment in the osteoarthritic knee: a systematic review. BMC Musculoskelet Disord 2015;16:321.
43. Panero AJ, Hirahara AM, Andersen WJ, et al. Are Amniotic Fluid Products Stem Cell Therapies? A Study of Amniotic Fluid Preparations for Mesenchymal Stem Cells With Bone Marrow Comparison. Am J Sports Med 2019;47(5):1230–5.
44. Becktell L, Matuska AM, Hon S, et al. Proteomic Analysis and Cell Viability of Nine Amnion, Chorion, Umbilical Cord, and Amniotic Fluid-Derived Products. Cartilage 2021;13(2_suppl):495S–507S.
45. Niknejad H, Deihim T, Solati-Hashjin M, et al. The effects of preservation procedures on amniotic membrane's ability to serve as a substrate for cultivation of endothelial cells. Cryobiology 2011;63(3):145–51.
46. Connolly JF. Injectable bone marrow preparations to stimulate osteogenic repair. Clin Orthop Relat Res 1995;313:8–18.
47. U.S. National Library of Medicine. 2022. https://clinicaltrials.gov/ct2/results?cond=Knee+Arthritis&term=amniotic+&cntry=&state=&city=&dist=. [Accessed 12 July 2022].
48. US Department of Health and Human Services, Food and Drug Administration. Regulatory Considerations for Human Cells, Tissues, and Cellular and Tissue-Based Products: Minimal Manipulation and Homologous Use. 2020. Available

at: https://www.fda.gov/regulatory-information/search-fda-guidance-documents/regulatory-considerations-human-cells-tissues-and-cellular-and-tissue-based-products-minimal.
49. Panero AJ, et al. Allograft Tissues (pp 89-101). In: Williams C, Sussman W, Pitts J, editors. Atlas of interventional orthopedics procedures. United States: Elsevier; 2022.
50. Zelen CM, Poka A, Andrews J. Prospective, randomized, blinded, comparative study of injectable micronized dehydrated amniotic/chorionic membrane allograft for plantar fasciitis-a feasibility study. Foot Ankle Int 2013;34(10):1332–9.
51. Cazzell S, Stewart J, Agnew PS, et al. Randomized Controlled Trial of Micronized Dehydrated Human Amnion/Chorion Membrane (dHACM) Injection Compared to Placebo for the Treatment of Plantar Fasciitis. Foot Ankle Int 2018;39(10):1151–61.
52. Hanselman AE, Tidwell JE, Santrock RD. Cryopreserved human amniotic membrane injection for plantar fasciitis: a randomized, controlled, double-blind pilot study. Foot Ankle Int 2015;36(2):151–8.
53. Main BJ, Maffulli N, Valk JA, et al. Umbilical Cord-Derived Wharton's Jelly for Regenerative Medicine Applications: A Systematic Review. Pharmaceuticals (Basel) 2021;14(11).
54. Raposo G, Stoorvogel W. Extracellular Vesicles: Exososomes, microvesicles, and friends. J Cell Biol 2013;200(4):373–83.
55. Hristove M, Erl W, Linder S, et al. Apoptotic bodies from endothelial cells enhance the number and initiate the differentiation of human endothelial progenitor cells in vitro. Blood 2004;104:2761–6.
56. György B, Szabó TG, Pásztói M, et al. Membrane vesicles, current state-of-the-art: emerging role of extracellular vesicles. Cell. Mol. Life Sci. 2011;68:2667–88.
57. Doyle L. Wang M Overview of Extracellular Vesicles, Their Origin, Composition, Purpose, and Methods for Exosome Isolation and Analysis. Cells 2019;8:727.
58. Valadi H. Exosome-mediated transfer of mRNAs and microRNA is a novel mechanism of genetic exchange between cells. Nat Cell Biol 2007;9:654–9.
59. Maas S, Breakenfield X, Weaver A. Extracellular Vesicles: Unique Intercellular Delivery Vehicles. Trends Cell Biol 2017;27(3):172–88.
60. Batrakova E, Kim MS. Using exosomes, naturally-equipped nanocarriers, for drug delivery. J Controlled Release 2015;219:396–405.
61. Borges FT, Melo SA, Özdemir BC, et al. TGF-beta1-containing exosomes from injured epithelial cells activate fibroblasts to initiate tissue regenerative responses and fibrosis. J Am Soc Nephrol 2013;24:385–92.
62. Rabinowits G, Gercel-Taylor C, Day JM, et al. Exosomal MicroRNA: A Diagnostic Marker for Lung Cancer. Clin Lung Cancer 2009;10:42–6.
63. Akers JC, Ramakrishnan V, Kim R, et al. miR-21 in the extracellular vesicles (EVs) of Cerebrospinal Fluid (CSF): A Platform for Glioblastoma Biomarker Development. PLoS ONE 2013;8:e78115.
64. Heijnen H, et al. Activated Platelets Release Two Types of Membrane Vesicles: Microvesicles by Surface Shedding and Exosomes Derived From Exocytosis of Multivesicular Bodies and alpha Granules. Blood 1999;94(11):3791–9.
65. Wei K, et al. Platelet-Derived Exosomes and Atherothrombosis. Front Cardiovasc Med 2022;9:886132.
66. Koupenova M, Clancy L, Corkrey HA, et al. Circulating Platelets as Mediators of Immunity, Inflammation, and Thrombosis. Circ Res 2018;122:337–51.
67. Rui S, et al. Comparison and Investigation of Exosomes Derived from Platelet Rich Plasma Activated by Different Agonist. Cell Transplantation 2021;30:1–13.

68. Milioli M, Ib'añez-Vea M, Sidoli S, et al. Quantitative proteomics analysis of platelet-derived microparticles reveals distinct protein signatures when stimulated by different physiological agonists. J Proteomics 2015;121:56–66.
69. Lyu H, Guo Q, Huang Y, et al. The Role of Bone-Derived Exosomes in Regulating Skeletal Metabolism and Extraosseous Diseases. Front Cell Developmental Biol 2020;8:89.
70. Fazaeli H, et al. A Comparative Study on the Effect of Exosomes Secreted by Mesenchymal Stem Cells Derived from Adipose and Bone Marrow Tissues in the Treatment of Osteoarthritis-Induced Mouse Model. Biomed Res Int Voume 2021;2021:9688138.
71. Muller L, Hong C-S, Stolz DB, et al. Isolation of Biologically-Active Exosomes from Human Plasma. J Immunol Methods 2014;411:55–65.
72. Livshits MA, Khomyakova E, Evtushenko EG, et al. Isolation of exosomes by differential centrifugation: Theoretical analysis of a commonly used protocol. Sci Rep 2015;5:17319.
73. Vlassov AV, Zeringer E, Barta T, et al. Strategies for Isolation of Exosomes. Cold Spring Harb Protoc 2015;2015:319–23.
74. Beall D, et al. VAST Clinical Trial : Safely Supplementing Tissue Lost to Degenerative Disc Disease. Int J Spine Surg 2020;14(2):239–53.

Medical Concerns in Orthobiologics Procedures

Peter C. Yeh, MD[a,b], Prathap Jayaram, MD[c,d,*]

KEYWORDS

• Orthobiologics • Medical concerns • PRP • BMAC • Adipose tissue derivatives

KEY POINTS

- Proper and sterile technique recommended with orthobiologic use to minimize procedural risks.
- No major risks associated with orthobiologic use and transmissible diseases or immune-modulated reactions.
- No major risks associated with orthobiologic use and oncologic process or tumor growth.
- No major drug-to-drug interactions with orthobiologic use but noted nonsteroid anti-inflammatory drugs or antiplatelet medications could affect the therapeutic effects of biological strategies.

INTRODUCTION

Orthobiologics have shown immense treatment potential in many medical fields including sports medicine, musculoskeletal disorders, and pain management, as well as in plastic surgery, cardiac surgery, and dermatology.[1] As with the case of any medical procedures and treatments, there are potential side effects or caveats that physicians and patients should be cognizant of. In this article, we will highlight common medical concerns associated with orthobiologics use.

Although there has been early adoption of biological strategies, standardizing its use has become challenging for several reasons. This has been demonstrated in clinical trials with varying degrees of protocols, such as cell isolation, preparation techniques, and heterogeneity of the patients, and complex mechanisms involved human clinical trials are often challenging to compare.[1,2] Naturally, with continued robust preclinical research and clinical trials paired with collaboration between professional organizations and governing bodies, the clinical use and optimization for

[a] Department of Physical Medicine and Rehabilitation, Vanderbilt University, Nashville, TN, USA; [b] Vanderbilt Stallworth Rehabilitation Hospital, 2201 Children's Way, Suite 1318, Nashville, TN 37212, USA; [c] Department of Orthopedics, Emory University, Atlanta, GA, USA; [d] Department of Rehabilitation Medicine, Emory University, Emory Sports Medicine Complex, 1968 Hawks Lane, Brookhaven, GA 30329, USA
* Corresponding author.
E-mail addresses: Prathap.Jayaram@emory.edu; pjayara4@emory.edu

Phys Med Rehabil Clin N Am 34 (2023) 63–70
https://doi.org/10.1016/j.pmr.2022.08.006

orthobiologics will continue to expand. To this end, there are surrounding parameters that the providing clinician can standardize to reduce adverse events.

Procedural-Related Risks

Procedural-related risks with platelet rich plasma

Platelet Rich Plasma (PRP) has demonstrated an excellent safety profile with no reported major adverse events or reactions.[3] Nevertheless, there are inherent minor risks with venipuncture, which includes but is not limited to ecchymosis, hematoma, the act of piercing the skin leading to pain or anxiety, accidental puncture of arteries, or superficial phlebitis. Skin disinfection techniques using either diluted alcohol solution, aqueous or alcoholic chlorhexidine solutions, or aqueous povidone-iodine solution is recommended.[4] Occasionally, one can get a local inflammatory response to PRP injections itself, such as pain and swelling, which is generally self-limited and does not require treatment in most cases. Meanwhile, postprocedural pain can be a consequence of traumatic venipuncture due to accidental puncture of the brachial artery, superficial phlebitis, or a large hematoma. However, if the venipuncture is performed correctly with appropriate procedure techniques, anatomical knowledge, and proper tools, much of these risks can be minimized.[4,5] In some cases, it may be difficult to obtain blood from a blinded venipuncture. In this scenario, we recommend using ultrasound guidance to properly access the vein of choice.[6]

It is well known that the final PRP product varies given its autologous nature resulting in heterogeneity among the various protocols. This has resulted in a lack of consensus on standardization of PRP preparation protocols, inconsistencies in nomenclature, and other variables such as individual patient age, comorbidities, and circulation.[1,7,8] The injection of PRP itself generally carries minimal risks such as microtrauma or local irritation, often with the local anatomy determining the amount of injection volume and spatial distribution.[9] Theoretically, PRP injections close to large blood vessels can induce thrombi formation through platelet adhesion, aggregation, and fibrin formation.[9] Although no consistent pattern has occurred, there has been a case report where irreversible blindness occurred following periocular PRP injections for skin rejuvenation, thought to be due to ischemia after artery occlusion.[9,10] However with respect to musculoskeletal applications such as knee osteoarthritis, the reported adverse events have been limited to transient joint swelling initially with improvement in overall knee pain.[11]

Procedural-related risks with bone marrow aspiration

With cell-based therapies, the process of bone marrow aspiration (BMA) or lipoaspirate harvesting are more invasive than the venipuncture process associated with preparing PRP. Some risks include infection, bleeding, or breakage of needle. Although the events are rare, the estimated adverse event rate can be upward to 0.07%.[5,12,13] Postoperative bleeding may be attributed to the high vascularity of the sampled tissue but manual pressure or a pressure dressing can be applied to the site until bleeding subsides. Infection risks can be minimized with proper sterile technique and avoiding sampling sites that maybe infected, such as with cellulitis or even osteomyelitis.

Although BMA can be performed with anatomic landmarks alone, many practitioners use image guidance, such as fluoroscopy or ultrasound guidance. The addition of image guidance can increase the accuracy and minimize the need for multiple attempts and procedure duration. It is not uncommon to encounter donor site pain but any increase in chills, fevers, erythema, or discharge should prompt further inquiry.[6] Potential complications vary depending on BMA-harvesting sites. For instance, the posterior iliac spine is the most common location for harvesting BMA, and risks can include sciatic nerve palsy, lateral femoral cutaneous nerve injury, soft tissue injury, and sacroiliac joint injury.[14] If the trocar suddenly loses contact with bone during BMA, visceral injury can occur.[15] Hemorrhage, cardiac tamponade, and death can occur if a needle is misplaced during sternal aspiration, and extreme caution should be exercised if this site is chosen for sampling, underscoring the importance of using image-guided procedure to limit complications. A study by Hernigou and colleagues[15] noted that in 410 cadaveric trocar entries (parallel in various sectors), there were 114 medial or lateral table breaches (28%), with greater risks with inexperienced physicians or patients with a body mass index greater than 30.

Anxiety is another common issue that could occur during BMA or lipoaspiration. Several techniques to reduce anxiety include a thorough explanation before the procedure, reassurance throughout the procedure, distracting music or conversations, or a single oral dose of an anxiolytic.[14] Although most practitioners do not use general anesthesia, those that do should consider the risk and cost of general anesthesia, potential adverse effects from the medications themselves, and if the procedures could be completed without it.[14]

Procedural-related risks with adipose tissue derivatives

Adipose tissue derivatives (ATDs) include microfragmented adipose tissue (MFAT), cultured adipose stem cells, mechanical stromal vascular fracture (SVF), and enzymatic stromal vascular fraction.[16] Lipoaspirate is most commonly obtained from the gluteal and abdominal regions, with other sites including lateral thigh, lateral abdomen, and the greater trochanteric region.[6] Lipoaspiration can often be completed without image guidance but in certain cases, ultrasound can help determine the optimal harvesting site by assessing the thickness of adipose tissue, especially in thinner patients.

Fewer complications occurred since the advent of the microcannula, cell-friendly equipment, and low-volume techniques. Because lipoaspiration harvests a relatively low volume of aspirate, skin dimpling is uncommon. Maione and colleagues[17] reviewed 1000 cosmetic surgery cases using autologous fat graft with a mean aspiration volume of 68 mL, with a follow-up of at least 1 month. Intraoperatively, there were no reported cases of abdominal viscera perforation, major bleeding complications, death, cardiac arrest, or stroke.[17] Postoperatively, there were no cases of pulmonary embolism, sepsis, or deep vein thrombosis.[17] There were 85 donor site complications that consisted of 2 hematomas and 83 local deformities due to fibrosis less than 2 cm in diameter.[17] A 2020 literature review analyzed 20 studies that used the use of nonculture-expanded ATDs, such as MFAT or SVF, to treat nonaxial musculoskeletal conditions.[16] Schroeder and colleagues[16] found that although there was a heterogenous nature of the use of guidance, method of injectate, clinical indications, and outcome measures, there were no reported significant adverse effects.

Transmittable Disease and Immune-Modulated Reactions

PRP and mesenchymal stem cells (MSCs) procedures use autologous products and consist of collecting and concentrating naturally occurring cells from a patient's own body. Consequently, there are minimal risks for transfusion reactions or other immune-modulated reactions.[6] Additionally, the autologous nature alleviates any concerns regarding transmission of diseases such as HIV, hepatitis, or Creutzfeld-Jakob disease, or immunogenic reactions that exist with preparations of allograft or xenograft.[6,18] Although PRP itself may be safe from immunogenic reactions, the use of activating agent theoretically can cause risks, although none has been reported with PRP.

Some PRP-activation methods use calcium chloride and bovine thrombin preparations, which contain bovine factor V.[18] The systemic use of using bovine thrombin to promote clotting in cardiothoracic surgery have reported several cases of coagulopathies resulting from cross-reactivity of antibovine factor V antibodies with human factor V.[18,19] Nevertheless, it is noted the bovine thrombin preparations in those cases were of much higher doses (>10,000 units) than that used to active PRP (<200 units) before application.[18,19] Furthermore, the use, if any, of bovine thrombin before application is generally consumed during clot formation and digested by macrophages, thus the bovine thrombin-activated PRP should not produce antifactor V antibodies.[18,19]

Oncologic Process or Tumor Growth

Contraindications for BMC include bone marrow–derived cancer (lymphoma), non-bone marrow–derived disease, and active systemic infection.[20] Theoretically MSCs can divide into unwanted oncologic cell lineages and could contribute to tumor behavior by influencing the tumor microenvironment and promote angiogenesis; however, this has not been seen with adult-derived MSCs.[21–26]

Hernigou and colleagues[22] followed 1873 patients treated from 1990 to 2006 with bone marrow–derived concentrated cells and found no increased cancer risk in patients after the application of autologous cell-based therapy using bone marrow–derived stromal progenitor cells either at the treatment site or elsewhere in the patients after an average follow-up period of 12.5 years. Although no tumor formation was discovered at the treatment sites on the 7306 magnetic resonance images and 52,430 radiographs, 53 cancers were diagnosed in areas other than the treatment site.[22] In the general population during the same period, the expected number of cancer incidence was between 97 and 108 for the same age and sex distribution.[22] Wakitani and colleagues[23] studied the safety of bone marrow–derived MSCs for the treatment of articular cartilage defects.[23] They monitored 41 patients who received 45 bone marrow MSC injections for 5 to 137 months after procedure and found no occurrences of infection or tumor growth. A longitudinal cohort study by Pak and colleagues[24] assessing the effects of SVF with PRP into various joints in 91 subjects, with an average follow-up of 26.62 months, found no evidence of neoplastic complications in any implantation site.

Centeno and colleagues[25] performed a large prospective study on 339 patients who were treated for various orthopedic conditions with culture-expanded autologous, bone marrow–derived MSCs that were harvested from the posterior superior iliac crest between 2006 and 2010. Follow-up period ranged from 3 to 36 months.[25] Using high-field MRI tracking and complications surveillance, the authors noted that although there were 2 patients who reported the development of cancer, the cancers were not at the reimplant sites and that the percentage of patients developed cancer was not far from the annual rate of cancer in the general population.[25] The most common complaints were pain and swelling (2% of patients), with no reports of infections, and procedure-related complications that were self-limited or remediated with simple therapeutic measures.[25]

Centeno and colleagues[26] subsequently performed a larger prospective multicenter study investigating the safety of autologous stem cell therapy for orthopedic use across 18 sites. A total of 3012 procedures were performed during 9 years with 2372 patients reporting on adverse events (AE). Follow-up ranged from 1 month to 8.8 years with an average of 2.2 years, and 7 reported cases of neoplasm were found, although none occurred at the site of implantation.[26] At the time of the study, according to the National Cancer Institute, the annual incidence of cancer in the US population in 2011 was 0.44% (438 cases per 100,000 individuals), and 0.78% in adults aged 50 to 64 years.[26] In the study, the authors actually observed a lower annual cancer rate (0.14%) among the registry participants than compared with the general population.[26]

Side Effects After Procedure

Potential side effects of the use of orthobiologics after procedure include tenosynovitis and tendonitis, arthralgia, joint stiffness, effusion, swelling, infection, paresthesia, and malaise.[24,27–32] Kuah and colleagues[28] evaluated the safety and tolerability of a single intra-articular injection of in vitro expanded MSCs derived from human donor adipose tissue combined with cell culture supernatant in a double-blind, placebo-controlled, randomized trial in 20 patients with symptomatic Kellgren-Lawrence grade 1-3 knee osteoarthritis with follow-up during 12 months. Although the authors did not find any severe side effects, they noted the presence of mild-to-moderate adverse effects possibly or definitely related to the procedure such as arthralgia, joint effusion, and joint stiffness.[28] Another study followed 91 patients treated with autologous adipose tissue-derived stem cells and PRP for various orthopedic conditions were followed by telephone questionnaires every 6 months for up to 30 months and a postprocedure MRI at 3 months.[24] Postprocedure MRIs performed on one-third of the patients, with the rest of patients declining due to financial costs, did not demonstrate any tumor formation at the implant site.[24] Some complications included pain and swelling in 37% of the treated joints, 0% infection rates, 0% tumor formation, 1% localized skin rash at the site of the injection, 1% hemorrhagic stroke 2 weeks after procedure, and 22% with tendonitis or tenosynovitis.[24] The high rate of joint swelling was thought to be associated with the death of stem cells.[24] Song and colleagues[27] assessed the safety and therapeutic potential of autologous human adipose–derived MSCs in patients with osteoarthritis in 18 patients with a follow-up of 96 weeks. In all, 16 (88%) patients developed adverse events such as swelling, pain, edema, and cramps, although none were classified as severe.[27]

When an instrument or device pierces the skin, it increases risks of infections. Consequently, the authors always recommend a high field of sterility and sterile techniques. A systematic review of the effectiveness of intradiscal biologic treatments for discogenic low back pain found no reports of any major or serious complications although it was noted, there was a dearth of high-quality evidence and limited data to fully comment on the safety given the lower sample sizes.[29] Nevertheless, there have been reports of discitis following intradiscal injection.[30,32] A clinical review of the literature found a small but notable risk for following intradiscal orthobiologic injections of PRP and/or BMC for lumbar disc disease.[32] It is noted that discitis following discography is not uncommon, thus when planning to perform any fluoroscopic-guided procedure that involves injectates into the disc, using a 2-needle technique may help reduce the incidence of infection.[31,32] In the literature, patients have been lost to follow-up, making it difficult to ascertain an accurate risk of complications, an issue that could be addressed with a larger registry and long-term data tracking.

Centeno and colleagues[26] performed a prospective multicenter study investigating the safety of autologous stem cell therapy for orthopedic across 18 sites. A total of 3012 procedures were performed during 9 years with 2372 patients reporting on AEs. Follow-up ranged from 1 month to 8.8 years with an average of 2.2 years. A total of 325 (12.1%) AEs were reported with 38 adjudicated to be definitely related to the procedure (1.6% of the population).[26] The majority of the AEs were postprocedure pain (29% of the AEs) or pain due to degenerative joint disease (28% of the AEs). Other AEs noted in the patients during the follow-up period include neurologic and vascular complications, allergic reactions, cardiac complications, neoplasms, and infections though none of these serious adverse events mentioned below were deemed likely or definitely related to the stem cells or other biologic agents.[26]

Drug-to-Drug Interaction

Generally, there does not seem to be major drug-to-drug interactions with orthobiologics but nonsteroid anti-inflammatory drugs (NSAIDs) or antiplatelet medications could affect the therapeutic effects of biological strategies and even affect healing postprocedure, such as after bone marrow harvesting.[1,14,33] NSAIDs, such as aspirin and naproxen, have also shown to interfere in the growth factor release given their direct inhibition of cyclooxygenase (COX) pathway and can impair platelet function.[34–36] Although there is no literature correlating growth factor release and efficacy of PRP treatment in vivo, studies may provide good reason to recommend holding NSAIDs and aspirin for 7 days before PRP, and use of other analgesics such as acetaminophen for postinjection pain control, if the benefits outweigh the risks.[34] In an open-label fixed sequence study, Jayaram and colleagues[34] noted that a daily intake of 81 mg aspirin reduced the expression of key mediators, such as transforming growht factor B-1 (TGF-β1), platelet derived growth factor (PDGF), and vascular endothelial growth factor (VEGF). These effects were attributed to irreversible inhibition of COX-1 and modifiable inhibition of COX-2, 2 enzymes needed for downstream platelet degranulation. A recent systematic review by Frey and colleagues[33] found that antiplatelet medications may decrease the growth factor release profile in a COX-1-dependent and COX-2-dependent manner, and 8 of the 15 studies found a decrease in growth factors.

SUMMARY

Overall, the use of orthobiologics does not seem to have consistent severe side effects. Nevertheless, generally practitioners can agree that the field can benefit from a more established patient registry that can be used for postmarket quality assessments and follow-up as well as higher quality clinical trials with the benefits of a more standardized classification system.[1,37] The continued evolution of high-quality research with longer follow-up durations will be critical for the future of the field.

DISCLOSURE

The authors have nothing to disclose.

REFERENCES

1. Everts P, Onishi K, Jayaram P, et al. Platelet-rich plasma: new performance understandings and therapeutic considerations in 2020. Int J Mol Sci 2020;21(20):7794.
2. Feisst V, Meidinger S, Locke MB. Stem cells and cloning: advances and applications dovepress from bench to bedside: use of human adipose-derived stem cells. Stem Cells Cloning Adv Appl 2015;8:149–62.
3. Dhillon RS, Schwarz EM, Maloney MD. Platelet-rich plasma therapy - future or trend? Arthritis Res Ther 2010;14(4):219.
4. Ialongo C, Bernardini S. Special issue: responsible writing in science Phlebotomy, a bridge between laboratory and patient. Biochem Med 2016;26(1):17–33.
5. Hjortholm N, Jaddini E, Hałaburda K, et al. Strategies of pain reduction during the bone marrow biopsy. Ann Hematol 2013;92(2):145–9.

6. Malanga G, Abdelshahed D, Jayaram P. Orthobiologic interventions using ultrasound guidance. Phys Med Rehabil Clin N Am 2016;27(3):717–31.
7. Le ADK, Enweze L, DeBaun MR, et al. Current clinical recommendations for use of platelet-rich plasma. Curr Rev Musculoskelet Med 2018;11(4):624–34.
8. dos Santos RG, Santos GS, Alkass N, et al. The regenerative mechanisms of platelet-rich plasma: a review. Cytokine 2021;144:155560.
9. Andia I, Maffulli N. A contemporary view of platelet-rich plasma therapies: moving toward refined clinical protocols and precise indications. Regen Med 2018;13(6): 717–28.
10. Kalyam K, Kavoussi SC, Ehrlich M, et al. Irreversible blindness following periocular autologous platelet-rich plasma skin rejuvenation treatment. Ophthal Plast Reconstr Surg 2017;33(3S):S12–6.
11. Di Martino A, Boffa A, Andriolo L, et al. Leukocyte-rich versus leukocyte-poor platelet-rich plasma for the treatment of knee osteoarthritis: a double-blind randomized trial. Am J Sports Med 2022;(1). 3635465211064303.
12. Bain BJ. Morbidity associated with bone marrow aspiration and trephine biopsy - A review of UK data for 2004. Haematologica 2006;91(9):1293–4.
13. Cole BJ, Gilat R, DiFiori J, et al. The 2020 NBA orthobiologics consensus statement. Orthop J Sport Med 2021;9(5). https://doi.org/10.1177/23259671211002296.
14. Bowen JE. Technical issues in harvesting and concentrating stem cells (bone marrow and adipose). PM R 2015;7(4):S8–18.
15. Hernigou J, Picard L, Alves A, et al. Understanding bone safety zones during bone marrow aspiration from the iliac crest: the sector rule. Int Orthop 2014; 38(11):2377-2284.
16. Schroeder A, Rubin JP, Kokai L, et al. Use of adipose-derived orthobiologics for musculoskeletal injuries: a narrative review. PM R 2020;12(8):805–16.
17. Maione L, Vinci V, Klinger M, et al. Autologous fat graft by needle: analysis of complications after 1000 patients. Ann Plast Surg 2015;74(3):277–80.
18. Alsousou J, Thompson M, Hulley P, et al. The biology of platelet-rich plasma and its application in trauma and orthopaedic surgery: a review of the literature. J Bone Joint Surg Br 2009;91(8):987–96.
19. Cmolik BL, Spero JA, Magovern GJ, et al. Redo cardiac surgery: late bleeding complications from topical thrombin- induced factor V deficiency. J Thorac Cardiovasc Surg 1993;105(2):222–7.
20. Sampson S, Botto-van Bemden A, Aufiero D. Autologous bone marrow concentrate: review and application of a novel intra-articular orthobiologic for cartilage disease. Phys Sportsmed 2013;41(3):7–18.
21. Freese KE, Kokai L, Edwards RP, et al. Adipose-derived stems cells and their role in human cancer development, growth, progression, and metastasis: a systematic review. Cancer Res 2015;75(7):1161–8.
22. Hernigou P, Homma Y, Flouzat-Lachaniette CH, et al. Cancer risk is not increased in patients treated for orthopaedic diseases with autologous bone marrow cell concentrate. J Bone Joint Surg Am 2013;95(24):2215–21.
23. Wakitani S, Okabe T, Horibe S, et al. Safety of autologous bone marrow-derived mesenchymal stem cell transplantation for cartilage repair in 41 patients with 45 joints followed for up to 11 years and 5 months. J Tissue Eng Regen Med 2011; 5(2):146–50.
24. Pak J, Chang JJ, Lee JH, et al. Safety reporting on implantation of autologous adipose tissue-derived stem cells with platelet-rich plasma into human articular joints. BMC Musculoskelet Disord 2013;1(14):337.

25. Centeno C, Schultz J, Cheever M, et al. Safety and complications reporting on the re-implantation of culture-expanded mesenchymal stem cells using autologous platelet lysate technique. Curr Stem Cell Res Ther 2010;5(1):81–93.
26. Centeno CJ, Al-Sayegh H, Freeman MD, et al. A multi-center analysis of adverse events among two thousand, three hundred and seventy two adult patients undergoing adult autologous stem cell therapy for orthopaedic conditions. Int Orthop 2016;40(8):1755–65.
27. Song Y, Du H, Dai C, et al. Human adipose-derived mesenchymal stem cells for osteoarthritis: a pilot study with long-term follow-up and repeated injections. Regen Med 2018;13(3):295–307.
28. Kuah D, Sivell S, Longworth T, et al. Safety, tolerability and efficacy of intra-articular Progenza in knee osteoarthritis: a randomized double-blind placebo-controlled single ascending dose study. J Transl Med 2018;16(1):49.
29. Schneider BJ, Hunt C, Conger A, et al. The effectiveness of intradiscal biologic treatments for discogenic low back pain: a systematic review. Spine J 2022; 22(2):226–37.
30. Beatty NR, Lutz C, Boachie-Adjei K, et al. Spondylodiscitis due to Cutibacterium acnes following lumbosacral intradiscal biologic therapy: a case report. Regen Med 2019;14(9):823–9.
31. Fraser RD, Osti OL, Vernon-Roberts B. Discitis after discography. J Bone Joint Surg Br 1987;69(1):26–35.
32. Jerome MA, Lutz C, Lutz GE. Risks of intradiscal orthobiologic injections: a review of the literature and case series presentation. Int J Spine Surg 2021;15(S1): 26–39.
33. Frey C, Yeh PC, Jayaram P. Effects of antiplatelet and nonsteroidal anti-inflammatory medications on platelet-rich plasma: a systematic review. Orthop J Sport Med 2020;8(4). https://doi.org/10.1177/2325967120912841.
34. Jayaram P, Yeh P, Patel SJ, et al. Effects of aspirin on growth factor release from freshly isolated leukocyte-rich platelet-rich plasma in healthy men: a prospective fixed-sequence controlled laboratory study. Am J Sports Med 2019;47(5):1223–9.
35. Mannava S, Whitney KE, Kennedy MI, et al. The Influence of naproxen on biological factors in leukocyte-rich platelet-rich plasma: a prospective comparative study. Arthrosc - J Arthrosc Relat Surg 2019;35(1):201–10.
36. Schippinger G, Prüller F, Divjak M, et al. Autologous platelet-rich plasma preparations: influence of nonsteroidal anti-inflammatory drugs on platelet function. Orthop J Sport Med 2015;3(6). https://doi.org/10.1177/2325967115588896.
37. Chu CR, Rodeo S, Bhutani N, et al. Optimizing clinical use of biologics in orthopaedic surgery: consensus recommendations from the 2018 AAOS/NIH U-13 conference. J Am Acad Orthop Surg 2019;27(2):e50–63.

Evidence-Based Approach to Orthobiologics for Osteoarthritis and Other Joint Disorders

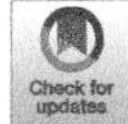

Katarzyna Herman, MD[a,b,c], Alberto Gobbi, MD[a,*]

KEYWORDS

• Osteoarthritis • Orthobiologics • Cartilage

KEY POINTS

- Osteoarthritis and cartilage lesions are a major cause of functional limitations and the goal of biological treatment is to preserve the native joint to delay the onset of OA.
- Biological cell-based cartilage restoration treatment addresses the need for the long-term viability of repaired tissue.
- The treatment of full-thickness cartilage lesions in the knee using a hyaluronic acid-based scaffold with activated bone marrow aspirate concentrate has good to excellent clinical outcomes at long-term follow-up.

INTRODUCTION

Osteoarthritis (OA) is one of the most common joint diseases; characterized mainly by joint pain and functional impairment, owing to articular cartilage degeneration, subchondral bone remodeling, and synovial inflammation.[1] OA affects 7% of the global population and is one the highest cause of years lived with disability worldwide,[2] making it an important problem to solve for the orthopedic surgeon.

Control of the tissue healing is not only limited to the optimization of the biomechanical environment, but also to other coexisting factors such as diabetes, smoking, hypercholesterolemia, or local factors (poor vascularity, tissue degeneration, cell death, and so forth) which can further impair this healing.[3] Over more than 30 years, the orthopedic community has explored ways to use the biologic response of the connective tissues to optimize the healing process. These have resulted in cell-based, cytokine-based, and scaffold-based therapies. This book chapter intends to provide a review of the current status of biological therapies for cartilage injuries and OA in orthopedics.

[a] O.A.S.I. Bioresearch Foundation Gobbi N.P.O, Via G.A. Amadeo, 24, Milan 20133, Italy; [b] Department of Orthopedics and Traumatology, Brothers Hospitallers Hospital, Markiefki 87 Street, 43-600 Katowice, Poland; [c] Department of Medical Rehabilitation, Medical University of Silesia, Ziołowa 45/47 Street, 40-635 Katowice, Poland

* Corresponding author. Via G.A. Amadeo, 24, Milan 20133, Italy.
E-mail address: gobbi@cartilagedoctor.it

Phys Med Rehabil Clin N Am 34 (2023) 71–81
https://doi.org/10.1016/j.pmr.2022.08.019
pmr.theclinics.com

Bone Marrow Stimulation Techniques

Bone marrow stimulation techniques refer to methods using bleeding from subchondral marrow space and further formation of a fibrin clot, which functions as a scaffold for subchondral stem cell migration and consequent formation of fibrocartilage. In general full-thickness cartilage lesion of a surface area < 1 cm^2, without subchondral bone lesions is usually considered an indication for a bone marrow stimulation technique as an isolated procedure.[4] Although, one should be aware that these recommendations should be carefully considered for every patient individually.

Microfracture is probably the most commonly known and used procedure owing to availability, simplicity, and low cost.[5–7] The surgical procedure is fairly uncomplicated; however, there are crucial steps surgeon should be aware of. Firstly, cartilage lesion borders should be thoroughly prepared, loose cartilage should be removed and borders made perpendicular to the subchondral bone. Then using a small diameter chondral awl (1 mm) holes are made and at this point it is vital to maintain the awl perpendicular to the surface not to damage the subchondral plate. Finally, saline pressure is reduced to visualize the release of fat droplets and bleeding that will later form a clot on the defect.[6–9] Studies have shown that this fibrocartilage matrix consists mainly of type I collagen and other noncollagenous proteins, making this tissue more delicate and less elastic, with inferior mechanical properties than normal articular cartilage.[10,11] Newly formed tissue may progressively deteriorate and long-term results of microfracture may not be satisfactory in every patient. In our study, 67 patients treated with microfracture owing to full-thickness cartilage lesions were prospectively followed up for 10 years.[5] All patients reported outcomes increased significantly at 2 years but deteriorated in the long term. Interestingly, patients with smaller lesions ($\leq$400 mm^2) and younger patients ($\leq$30 years) demonstrated significantly improved results in knee injury and osteoarthritis outcome score (KOOS), visual analog scale (VAS), and Marx scores. This suggests that when applied in young patients with smaller lesions, microfracture can offer good clinical outcomes at short-term follow-up. It should be stressed that microfracture may damage the subchondral bone and lead to the formation of microcysts that may accelerate the deterioration of the cartilage and compromise the articular surface for future procedures.[12]

Autologous Matrix-Induced Chondrogenesis (AMIC) is based on the same concept as microfracture but aided with a porcine collagen scaffold.[13] Indications include focal chondral or osteochondral defects with Outerbridge classification grade 3 to 4 with a defect size of approximately 1.0–8.0 cm^2, and patient age of 18 to 55 year old.[3] Scaffold is added after microfractures are conducted to cover the defect and to allow the ingrowth of mesenchymal stem cells (MSCs) from the subchondral bone. AMIC has several advantages, such as no donor site morbidity, the possibility of arthroscopic approach, and low cost compared with autologous chondrocyte implantation (ACI). Good clinical results of AMIC in midterm follow-ups have been described.[14] However, the reliability of these results is limited because of the dwindling number of patients available for the final follow-up evaluation.

Autologous Cartilage Use

In acute lesions use of autologous cartilage is an optimal alternative to repair a cartilage defect. It is described that covering an acute cartilage defect with minced fragments from a large piece of cartilage achieves good clinical results.[15] Authors retrieved a large chondral fragment and minced it into multiple small ones (<1 x 1 $\times$ 1 mm) with a scalpel. First, the cartilage defect is debrided and drilled into the subchondral bone using a 1.4 mm K-wire. Then, minced cartilage fragments are placed into the defect and attached using fibrin glue. This concept has been known since 1980s. The procedure using minced cartilage was modified and combined with various materials to become Cartilage Autograft Implantation System (CAIS).[16] A comparative study looking at different minced cartilage sizes showed that cartilage paste (smaller cartilage size) demonstrated significantly increased extracellular matrix production in contrast with other groups.[17] Consequently, the optimum degree of cartilage fragmentation should always be considered. Stone and colleagues recently reported a 10- to 23-year long-term results in 74 patients treated with Articular Cartilage Paste Graft, the biopsies of the repaired tissue revealed that 14 (48.3%) contained hyaline-like cartilage, 24 (82.8%) fibrocartilage with GAG, 10 (34.5%) fibrocartilage without GAG, and 3 (10.3%)fibrous tissue.[18]

Osteochondral Autograft Transplantation

Osteochondral Autograft Transfer System (OATS) is performed in a single-stage procedure, arthroscopically or through arthrotomy. Cylindrical plugs are harvested from donor sites in nonarticulating regions within the joint. Its main advantage is that it recreates the osteochondral unit in cartilage lesions with damaged subchondral bone, like OCD lesions. This technique is one of the few that has the benefit of restoring the hyaline cartilage. OATS is usually used for lesions smaller than 2 cm^2. One up to 3 osteochondral plugs of varying sizes are harvested and then transferred to the affected area. Authors of a 17-year prospective multicentric study performed in 383 patients found good to excellent results in 91% of femoral mosaicplasty, 86% of tibial, and 74% of patellofemoral mosaicplasty. Interestingly, patellofemoral pain associated with graft harvest was observed in only 5% of cases.[19] Congruent, gliding surfaces of the transplants and satisfactory fibrocartilage coverage of donor sites were seen in second-look arthroscopies. A significant drawback of this procedure is difficult to recreate the anatomic curvature of the articular surface. Wu and colleagues have shown that osteochondral plugs protruding 1 mm resulted in significantly increased contact pressures.[20] Furthermore, treatment using the OAT technique is limited by the availability of autologous tissue, as donor site morbidity is an essential concern if multiple grafts are used.

Autologous Chondrocyte Implantation

ACI consists of 2 steps; first, a piece of healthy cartilage is obtained from a non–weight-bearing area and subsequently expanded in vitro. The second step is grafting of the chondrocyte suspension into the defect.[21] Four generations of ACI have been introduced through the years. First generation, developed by Lars Peterson,[22] consists of infusion of the chondrocyte suspension under periosteal flap. In the second generation, the chondrocyte suspension is injected under a collagen membrane. The third generation also known as matrix-induced autologous chondrocyte implantation (MACI), involves the infusion of the expanded chondrocytes into a scaffold which is further implanted in the cartilage defect. The most recent fourth generation is a one-step procedure with chondrocyte isolation through biopsies and direct implantation. Long-term results with ACI first-generation technique are available with good term results at 20 years follow-up.[23] Some studies report significantly better functional outcomes in patients who underwent second-generation ACI compared with patients with first-generation ACI.[24,25] On the other hand, when comparing MACI against second or first-generation techniques, overall clinical results have not proved superiority with the latest technique.[26]

ACI in comparison with bone marrow stimulating techniques such as microfracture has shown to be superior over time owing to longer-lasting effects. Although the final tissue is still fibrocartilage, it has better quality and is more "hyaline-like" in contrast with the one provided by the microfracture procedure.[27,28] However, when compared with other cell membrane techniques such as the one-step procedure hyaluronic acid combined with bone marrow aspirate, outcomes have not shown statistically significant difference (41).

ACI has proven to offer a durable solution in the treatment of large full-thickness cartilage lesions. However, the need for 2 surgical interventions, the excessive cost for chondrocyte culture, and comparable results compared with one-step biological scaffolds remain the ACI technique's major drawbacks.

Cartilage Allografts

Fresh osteochondral allograft is used mostly in lesions whereby mosaicplasty cannot be performed. The benefits of using allografts include the flexibility of graft sizing and the possibility to treat the entire lesion with a single transplanted plug and no donor site morbidity. Improved patient-reported outcomes can be expected after OCA transplantation, with a survival rate of 78.7% at 10 years, with worse results in cases of patellar lesions and bipolar lesions. Some drawbacks include lower chondrocyte viability owing to storage and processing and potential immunogenic response concerns.[29]

Cell-Based Chondral Scaffolds

Cell-based Chondral Scaffold Allografts consist of hyaline cartilage chondrocytes in a malleable scaffold that can be formed to fill the defect. Because of their "one-time" biological approach, compared with MACI, they are an interesting and accessible alternative to treat cartilage. In general, they have shown good short-term results without significant problems concerning tolerability. Still, there is not enough evidence regarding long-term results. Chondrocytes in human tissue allograft, consisting of juvenile viable hyaline cartilage pieces (DeNovo NT Natural Tissue Graft) have proven to have increased metabolic and proliferative activity when compared with adult chondrocytes,[30] with a proper filling of the defect shown on MRI in addition to good clinical results at over 2-years follow-up.[31] Intriguingly, cells in a cryopreserved viable chondral allograft (Cartiform) shown to stay viable, up to 70%, at 2-years follow-up.[32] An additional option is dehydrated micronized allogeneic cartilage scaffold (BioCartilage) combined with platelet-rich plasma and fibrin glue, although the research on short or long-term outcomes is limited.[33]

Hyaluronic Acid Scaffold with Bone Marrow Aspirate Concentrate Augmentation

HA-BMAC scaffold, developed 30 years ago, allowed the treatment of larger cartilage defects in a one-step surgery. This procedure provided good long-term results and proved its superiority to microfracture owing to continued effect up to 15 years compared with the 2 to 3 years with microfracture. Additionally, it can be used in the case of multiple compartment and extensive lesions or in older patients.[28,34–38] The senior authors' selected technique is a one-stage cartilage repair with a three-dimensional hyaluronic acid-based scaffold (Hyalofast) paired with activated bone marrow aspirate concentrate (HA-BMAC). Compared with 2-step MACI, the clinical outcomes have not shown a significant difference. Additionally, the study showed that there was no relationship between the clinical outcome and the number of Colony Forming Units (CFU) found in bone marrow aspirate, therefore, supporting the rationale of the one-stage treatment.[37]

Every procedure should be preceded with a careful examination under anesthesia to confirm or exclude any limitations in range of motion or ligamentous instability.

The procedure is conducted through a small arthrotomy or arthroscopic depending on the lesion's extent and location. Loose cartilage is removed, stable vertical walls are created around the periphery of the defect with special chondrectomy. Then the calcified cartilage layer must be thoroughly removed without damaging the subchondral plate (**Fig. 1**). The defects are sized with aluminum foil templates and then a matching hyaluronic acid-based scaffold is used to cover the defect. Bone marrow is harvested from the iliac crest and centrifuged to acquire a concentrated bone marrow which is later combined with Batroxobin (Plateltexact-Plateltex S.R.O. Bratislava, SK) to produce a clot. The hyaluronic acid-based scaffold and clot from activated bone marrow aspirate concentrate are blended to create a biologically active construct for cartilage repair (HA-BMAC, **Fig. 2**). The HA-BMAC is positioned on the lesion and secured with fibrin glue. Afterward, the knee is cycled to confirm stability.[39] A technique that is another variation of this procedure was described by Sadlik and colleagues, in which a morselized bone graft is used to fill the lesion and then covered with hyaluronic acid scaffold embedded with BMAC.[40]

BMAC may also be used to treat subchondral bone pathologies. Joint cartilage and subchondral bone function as a unit and over the last few years a debate on the part of subchondral bone purpose has been going on. Bone marrow lesions (BMLs) are focal defects in the subchondral bone and can be diagnosed by magnetic resonance imaging (MRI). The number of pathologies of ischemic, mechanical, and reactive background can be responsible for the formation of these lesions. When evaluating a patient with BML it is vital to assess whether the lesion is reversible and irreversible.[41] Subchondroplasty (SCP) Procedure (Zimmer Biomet) is used to treat bone marrow lesions via the implantation of a bone substitute. A variation of this procedure that uses a biological approach is Osteo-Core-Plasty (Marrow Cellution). This minimally invasive subchondral bone augmentation procedure offers both biological (Bone Marrow) and mechanical (Autologous Bone Core) components to improve the osteochondral unit and boost natural regeneration. This procedure may also be used in the treatment of insufficiency fractures, subchondral cysts, and avascular necrosis[a,.[42]

This method is made of 2 parts, the first being the aspiration of bone marrow and the collection of the bone core grafts. The second involves the application of the material to the defect. Bone marrow is aspirated from the iliac crest, the trocar is advanced into the medullary space and the material is aspirated with a syringe. It is recommended to change the trocar direction throughout aspiration to obtain bone marrow aspirate

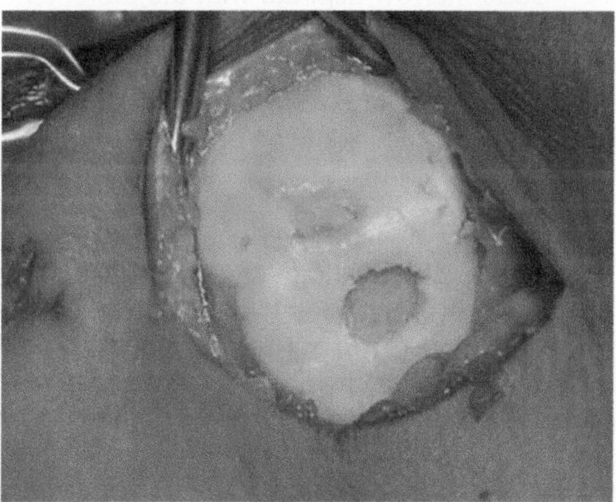

Fig. 1. A hyaluronic acid based scaffold combined with activated BMAC forming a sticky clot ready to be implanted in the prepared lesion site.

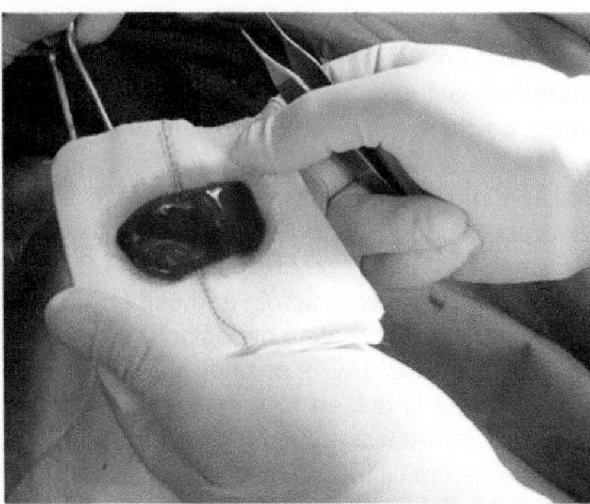

Fig. 2. Two cartilage lesions on the patella. The lesions have been prepared for HA-BMAC implantation, the loose cartilage has been removed and borders of the lesion made perpendicular to the subchondral bone.

(BMA) from various places. After the collection of the BMA, bone cores can be harvested from the same entry point. The application may be conducted arthroscopically or through an open approach, both require fluoroscopic assistance. Necrotic Tissue Zone is identified under fluoroscopy on AP and lateral images. In an open technique, the lesion is debrided, and necrotic bone underneath is removed. In an arthroscopic technique, a K-wire is introduced to the target zone from outside the joint and a cannulated drill bit is inserted over the K-Wire. Then Bone Core Graft is delivered to the necrotic zone with Extraction/Delivery Tool in both open and arthroscopic approaches. The bone core graft is pushed with a probe to the target point. Lastly, aspirated BMA is injected into the necrotic site or in the case of an open procedure the BMA Saturated Matrix Scaffold Membrane is used.[43,44]

Although there are systems available that use centrifugation to obtain a concentrated product, the recent data show that there is no for this step. Brozovich and colleagues used flow cytometry to detect MSCs, colony-forming units (CFUs), and cytokine profiling and found a lower concentration of CFUs in BMAC. They concluded that significantly lower CFUs in BMAC may result in a lower potency of MSCs compared with BMA.[42] Bone marrow aspirate with the aforementioned system was demonstrated to include a sufficiently high CFU-fs/mL and CD34+/mL and therefore not require centrifugation. Additionally, the level of CFU-fs/mL was significantly higher in comparison to BMAC in side-by-side evaluation from the same patient. In Osteo-Core plasty, there is no need for centrifugation and the surgeon can precisely apply the aspirate to the target zone.[45]

Biological Treatment in Osteoarthritis

Even though there is a variety of techniques to treat chondral lesions sometimes the onset of OA is inevitable. OA has such a big influence on patients' quality of life it is, therefore, crucial to understand which therapy offers the most. A variety of conservative therapies are available, both drugs and physical therapy, still they usually fail to provide long-term relief. That is why biological therapies have been earning more and more attention.

The most commonly used injectable is hyaluronic acid (HA), but studies have shown that PRP is more efficient both in short-or long-term pain and functional recovery.[46]

PRP contains a large number of growth factors and proteins stored in the alpha granules of platelets which were found to have regenerative and analgesic effect.[47,48] Additionally, studies have shown that platelet-rich plasma (PRP) has an anti-inflammatory effect and counteracts catabolic processes within the joint.[49–51] Injections of PRP can be conducted separately or in cycles of 3 injections, which is the authors preferred method. PRP is obtained from patients' peripheral blood, which is centrifuged in a special processing kit. The PRP is injected into the joint after careful disinfection of the needle entry point. Peak beneficial effect is observed at 6 months after the cycle of injections, but it may last up to 2 years.[52] A meta-analysis of randomized controlled trials using PRP in the treatment of knee OA has shown that statistically significant beneficial effect over placebo is seen at 6 and 12 months.[53] Interestingly a recent study has shown that there are no significant differences between leukocyte rich and leukocyte poor plasma in the treatment of knee AO.[54]

Treatment of joints other than knee has much fewer data to present. In hip for example, the results are promising, offering a short-term relief of symptoms and better outcome than HA injections[55,56] On the contrary, in carpometacarpal OA, better results were observed with HA injections compared with PRP and in ankle OA no significant improvement of pain and function was found when PRP was compared with placebo.[57,58]

Although satisfactory results can be achieved with PRP research on more efficient treatment has been going on for a few years. An autologous microfragmented adipose tissue (MFAT) in contrast to peripheral blood has 25,000 times more reparative cells.[59] MFAT is obtained from adipose tissue from abdominal or supragluteal region with a special lipoaspirate cannula. Lipoaspirate is transferred to the Lipogems device a low-pressure cylindrical system, to get fluid with a concentration of pericytes and MScs. This product is then applied to the joint through an injection or during arthroscopy. Promising results have been shown in literature.[60–62] Moreover, a study comparing leukocyte poor PRP combined with HA and MFAT has shown statistically significant difference favoring AMAT for Tegner and KOOS symptoms at 6 months and Tegner at 12 months of follow-up.62 However, one should be aware that this is a more invasive procedure than a PRP injection.

SUMMARY

OA is a raising burden and many possibilities to treat cartilage lesions and early OA have been reported. To treat cartilage defects, cell therapies using chondrocytes, MSCs, and other cell sources have been used. To obtain the best cartilage quality, these cartilage preserving/regenerating techniques combined with alignment correction osteotomy will give the best results. The biology of the articular cartilage must be fully explained before cartilage repair technologies can advance further. Collecting evidence of experimental studies on cartilage repair and early OA treatment will enable us to develop a clinical use of novel techniques for biological healing. Therefore, the use of the most appropriate line of treatment and proper patient selection is key to improving results.

CLINICS CARE POINTS

Pearls

- Adequate and thorough exposure to the cartilage lesion is crucial and may be problematic in the patellofemoral compartment. Use traction as needed to get a comfortable working space.

- If dimensions of the cartilage defect are difficult to measure, use an aluminum foil (or similar material) template to assist with accurate scaffold size matching.
- The hyaluronic acid-based scaffold is symmetric; after creating the HA-BMAC graft, implantation may proceed with either side placed against the subchondral bone.

Pitfalls

- Arthroscopic cartilage repair should proceed only in cases whereby the entirety of the defect can be appreciated and treated in a minimally invasive manner; repair should be performed in an open manner otherwise.
- Confirm secure graft seating within the cartilage defect by cycling the knee under arthroscopic visualization; failure to do so may increase the risk of graft delamination in the postoperative period.

DISCLOSURE

The Authors have nothing to disclose.

REFERENCES

1. Hunter DJ, March L, Chew M. Osteoarthritis in 2020 and beyond: a Lancet Commission. Lancet [Internet] 2020;396(10264):1711–2.
2. Global Burden of Disease Collaborative Network. Global Burden of Disease Study 2019 (GBD 2019) results. 2020. http://ghdx.healthdata.org/gbd-results-tool. [Accessed 10 December 2021].
3. Gobbi A, Lane JG. Bio-orthopaedics: A new approach. Cham, Switzerland: Springer Nature Switzerland AG; 2017. p. 1–696.
4. Chahla J, Stone J, Mandelbaum BR. How to Manage Cartilage Injuries? Arthroscopy-j Arthrosc Relat Surg 2019;35(10):2771–3.
5. Gobbi A, Karnatzikos G, Kumar A. Long-term results after microfracture treatment for full-thickness knee chondral lesions in athletes. Knee Surg Sports Traumatol Arthrosc 2014;22(9):1986–96.
6. Steadman JR, Rodkey WG, Briggs KK. Microfracture to treat full-thickness chondral defects: surgical technique, rehabilitation, and outcomes. J Knee Surg 2002; 15(3):170–6.
7. Gobbi A, Lane JG, Dallo I. Editorial Commentary: Cartilage Restoration—What Is Currently Available? Arthrosc - J Arthrosc Relat Surg 2020;36(6):1625–8.
8. Hoemann CD, Gosselin Y, Chen H, et al. Characterization of initial microfracture defects in human condyles. J Knee Surg 2013;26(5):347–55.
9. Gobbi A, Herman K, Grabowski R, et al. Primary Anterior Cruciate Ligament Repair With Hyaluronic Scaffold and Autogenous Bone Marrow Aspirate Augmentation in Adolescents With Open Physes. Arthrosc Tech 2019;8(12): e1561–8.
10. Mithoefer K, Mcadams T, Williams RJ, et al. Clinical efficacy of the microfracture technique for articular cartilage repair in the knee: An evidence-based systematic analysis. Am J Sports Med 2009;37(10):2053–63.
11. Gobbi A, Whyte GP. One-Stage Cartilage Repair Using a Hyaluronic Acid-Based Scaffold with Activated Bone Marrow-Derived Mesenchymal Stem Cells Compared with Microfracture. Am J Sports Med 2016;44(11):2846–54.
12. Frank RM, Cotter EJ, Nassar I, et al. Failure of Bone Marrow Stimulation Techniques. Sports Med Arthrosc Rev 2017;25(1):2–9.
13. Behery O, Siston RA, Harris JD, et al. Treatment of cartilage defects of the knee: Expanding on the existing algorithm. Clin J Sport Med 2014;24:21–30.

14. Gille J, Behrens P, Volpi P, et al. Outcome of Autologous Matrix Induced Chondrogenesis (AMIC) in cartilage knee surgery: Data of the AMIC Registry. Arch Orthop Trauma Surg 2013;133(1):87–93.
15. Salzmann GM, Baumann GA, Preiss S. Spontaneous Minced Cartilage Procedure for Unexpectedly Large Femoral Condyle Surface Defect. Case Rep Orthop 2016;2016:1–3.
16. Bonasia DE, Marmotti A, Rosso F, et al. Use of chondral fragments for one stage cartilage repair: A systematic review. World J Orthop 2015;6(11):1006–11.
17. Marmotti A, Bruzzone M, Bonasia DE, et al. One-step osteochondral repair with cartilage fragments in a composite scaffold. Knee Surg Sports Traumatol Arthrosc 2012;20(12):2590–601.
18. Stone KR, Pelsis JR, Na K, et al. Articular cartilage paste graft for severe osteochondral lesions of the knee: a 10- to 23-year follow-up study. Knee Surg Sports Traumatol Arthrosc 2017;25(12):3824–33.
19. Hangody L, Dobos J, Balo E, et al. Clinical experiences with autologous osteochondral mosaicplasty in an athletic population: a 17-year prospective multicenter study. Am J Sports Med 2010;38(6):1125–33.
20. Wu JZ, Herzog W, Hasler EM. Inadequate placement of osteochondral plugs may induce abnormal stress-strain distributions in articular cartilage –finite element simulations. Med Eng Phys 2002;24(2):85–97.
21. Gobbi A, Lane JG, Dallo I. Editorial Commentary: Cartilage Restoration—What Is Currently Available? Arthrosc. J Arthrosc Relat Surg 2020;36(6):1625–8.
22. Brittberg M, Lindahl A, Nilsson A, et al. Treatment of deep cartilage defects in the knee with autologous chondrocyte transplantation. N Engl J Med 1994;331(14): 889–95.
23. Peterson L, Vasiliadis HS, Brittberg M, et al. Autologous chondrocyte implantation: A long-term follow-up. Am J Sports Med 2010;38(6):1117–24.
24. McCarthy HS, Roberts S. A histological comparison of the repair tissue formed when using either Chondrogide(®) or periosteum during autologous chondrocyte implantation. Osteoarthr Cartil 2013;21(12):2048–57.
25. Niemeyer P, Salzmann G, Feucht M, et al. First-generation versus second-generation autologous chondrocyte implantation for treatment of cartilage defects of the knee: a matched-pair analysis on long-term clinical outcome. Int Orthop 2014;38(10):2065–70.
26. Goyal D, Goyal A, Keyhani S, et al. Evidence-based status of second- and third-generation autologous chondrocyte implantation over first generation: a systematic review of level I and II studies. Arthrosc 2013;29(11):1872–8.
27. Mistry H, Connock M, Pink J, et al. Autologous chondrocyte implantation in the knee: systematic review and economic evaluation. Health Technol Assess 2017;21(6):V-160.
28. Gobbi A, Chaurasia S, Karnatzikos G, et al. Matrix-Induced Autologous Chondrocyte Implantation versus Multipotent Stem Cells for the Treatment of Large Patellofemoral Chondral Lesions: A Nonrandomized Prospective Trial. Cartilage 2015; 6(2):82–97.
29. Chahla J, Sweet MC, Okoroha KR, et al. Osteochondral Allograft Transplantation in the Patellofemoral Joint: A Systematic Review. Am J Sports Med 2019;47(12): 3009–18.
30. Bonasia DE, Martin JA, Marmotti A, et al. Cocultures of adult and juvenile chondrocytes compared with adult and juvenile chondral fragments: in vitro matrix production. Am J Sports Med 2011;39(11):2355–61.

31. Farr J, Tabet SK, Margerrison E, et al. Clinical, Radiographic, and Histological Outcomes After Cartilage Repair With Particulated Juvenile Articular Cartilage: A 2-Year Prospective Study. Am J Sports Med 2014;42(6):1417–25.
32. Queally JM, Harris E, Handoll HHG, et al. Intramedullary nails for extracapsular hip fractures in adults. Cochrane Database Syst Rev 2014;2014(9).
33. Wang KC, Frank RM, Cotter EJ, et al. Arthroscopic Management of Isolated Tibial Plateau Defect With Microfracture and Micronized Allogeneic Cartilage-Platelet-Rich Plasma Adjunct. Arthrosc Tech 2017;6(5):e1613–8.
34. Kon E, Di Matteo B, Verdonk P, et al. Aragonite-Based Scaffold for the Treatment of Joint Surface Lesions in Mild to Moderate Osteoarthritic Knees: Results of a 2-Year Multicenter Prospective Study. Am J Sports Med 2021;49(3):588–98.
35. Gobbi A, Scotti C, Karnatzikos G, et al. One-step surgery with multipotent stem cells and Hyaluronan-based scaffold for the treatment of full-thickness chondral defects of the knee in patients older than 45 years. Knee Surg Sports Traumatol Arthrosc 2017;25(8):2494–501.
36. Kon E, Filardo G, Shani J, et al. Osteochondral regeneration with a novel aragonite-hyaluronate biphasic scaffold: Up to 12-month follow-up study in a goat model. J Orthop Surg Res 2015;10(1).
37. Gobbi A, Karnatzikos G, Scotti C, et al. One-step cartilage repair with bone marrow aspirate concentrated cells and collagen matrix in full-thickness knee cartilage lesions: results at 2-year follow-up. Cartilage 2011;2(3):286–99.
38. Gobbi A, Karnatzikos G, Sankineani SR. One-step surgery with multipotent stem cells for the treatment of large full-thickness chondral defects of the knee. Am J Sports Med 2014;42(3):648–57.
39. Gobbi A, Whyte GP. Long-term Clinical Outcomes of One-Stage Cartilage Repair in the Knee With Hyaluronic Acid–Based Scaffold Embedded With Mesenchymal Stem Cells Sourced From Bone Marrow Aspirate Concentrate. Am J Sports Med 2019;47(7):1621–8.
40. Sadlik B, Gobbi A, Puszkarz M, et al. Biologic Inlay Osteochondral Reconstruction: Arthroscopic One-Step Osteochondral Lesion Repair in the Knee Using Morselized Bone Grafting and Hyaluronic Acid-Based Scaffold Embedded With. Bone Marrow Aspirate Concentrate 2017;6(2):e383–9.
41. Gobbi A, Alvarez R, Irlandini E, et al. Current Concepts in Subchondral Bone Pathology. Jt Funct Preserv 2022;173–80.
42. Scarpone M, Kuebler D, Chambers A, et al. Isolation of clinically relevant concentrations of bone marrow mesenchymal stem cells without centrifugation 11 Medical and Health Sciences 1103 Clinical Sciences. J Transl Med 2019;17(1):1–10.
43. Gobbi A, Dallo I. *Osteo-Core-Plasty technique for the treatment of a proximal tibial subchondral cystic lesion.* https://aspire-medical.eu/wp-content/uploads/2021/06/Osteo-Core-Plasty_CaseReport_Gobbi-Dallo_Jun21.pdf.
44. Brozovich A, Sinicrope BJ, Bauza G, et al. High Variability of Mesenchymal Stem Cells Obtained via Bone Marrow Aspirate Concentrate Compared With Traditional Bone Marrow Aspiration Technique. Orthop J Sports Med 2021;9(12). 23259671211058459.
45. Szwedowski D, Dallo I, Irlandini E, et al. Osteo-core Plasty: A Minimally Invasive Approach for Subchondral Bone Marrow Lesions of the Knee. Arthrosc Tech 2020;9(11).
46. Tang JZ, Nie MJ, Zhao JZ, et al. Platelet-rich plasma versus hyaluronic acid in the treatment of knee osteoarthritis: a meta-analysis. J Orthop Surg Res 2020; 15(1):403.

47. Asfaha S, Cenac N, Houle S, et al. Protease-activated receptor-4: a novel mechanism of inflamma-tory pain modulation. Br J Pharmacol 2007;150:176–85.
48. Ulrich-Vinther M, Maloney MD, Schwarz EM, et al. Articular cartilage biology. J Am Acad Ort-hop Surg 2003;11:421–30 (Review).
49. Sánchez M, Anitua E, Delgado D, et al. A new strategy to tackle severe knee osteoarthritis: Combination of intra-articular and intraosseous injections of Platelet Rich Plasma. Expert Opin Biol Ther 2016;16(5):627–43.
50. Fortier LA, Barker JU, Strauss EJ, et al. The role of growth factors in cartilage repair. Clin Orthop Relat Res 2011;469(10):2706–15.
51. Cole BJ, Karas V, Hussey K, et al. Hyaluronic Acid Versus Platelet-Rich Plasma: A Prospective, Double-Blind Randomized Controlled Trial Comparing Clinical Outcomes and Effects on Intra-articular Biology for the Treatment of Knee Osteoarthritis. Am J Sports Med 2017;45(2):339–46.
52. Gobbi A, Lad D, Karnatzikos G. The effects of repeated intra-articular PRP injections on clinical outcomes of early osteoarthritis of the knee. Knee Surg Sports Traumatol Arthrosc 2014;23:2170–7.
53. Filardo G, Previtali D, Napoli F, et al. PRP Injections for the Treatment of Knee Osteoarthritis: A Meta-Analysis of Randomized Controlled Trials. Cartilage 2021;13(1_suppl):364S–75S.
54. Belk JW, Houck DA, Littlefield CP, et al. Platelet-Rich Plasma Versus Hyaluronic Acid for Hip Osteoarthritis Yields Similarly Beneficial Short-Term Clinical Outcomes: A Systematic Review and Meta-analysis of Level I and II Randomized Controlled Trials. Arthroscopy 2022;38(6):2035–46.
55. Dallari D, Stagni C, Rani N, et al. Ultrasound-Guided Injection of Platelet-Rich Plasma and Hyaluronic Acid, Separately and in Combination, for Hip Osteoarthritis: A Randomized Controlled Study. Am J Sports Med 2016;44(3):664–71.
56. Di Martino A, Boffa A, Andriolo L, et al. Leukocyte-Rich versus Leukocyte-Poor Platelet-Rich Plasma for the Treatment of Knee Osteoarthritis: A Double-Blind Randomized Trial. Am J Sports Med 2022;50(3):609–17.
57. Abdelsabor Sabaah HM, El Fattah RA, Al Zifzaf D, et al. A Comparative Study for Different Types of Thumb Base Osteoarthritis Injections: A Randomized Controlled Interventional Study. Ortop Traumatol Rehabil 2020;22(6):447–54.
58. Paget LDA, Reurink G, de Vos RJ, et al, PRIMA Study Group. Effect of Platelet-Rich Plasma Injections vs Placebo on Ankle Symptoms and Function in Patients With Ankle Osteoarthritis: A Randomized Clinical Trial. JAMA 2021;326(16):1595–605.
59. Russo A, Screpis D, Di Donato SL, et al. Autologous and micro-fragmented adipose tissue for the treatment of diffuse degenerative knee osteoarthritis. J Exp Orthop 2017;4:33.
60. Baria M, Pedroza A, Kaeding C, et al. Platelet-Rich Plasma Versus Microfragmented Adipose Tissue for Knee Osteoarthritis: A Randomized Controlled Trial. Orthop J Sports Med 2022;10(9). https://doi.org/10.1177/23259671221120678.
61. Gobbi A, Dallo I, Rogers C, et al. Two-year clinical outcomes of autologous microfragmented adipose tissue in elderly patients with knee osteoarthritis: a multicentric, international study. Int Orthop 2021;45(5):1179–88.
62. Dallo I, Szwedowski D, Mobasheri A, et al. A Prospective Study Comparing Leukocyte-Poor Platelet-Rich Plasma Combined with Hyaluronic Acid and Autologous Microfragmented Adipose Tissue in Patients with Early Knee Osteoarthritis. Stem Cell Dev 2021;30:651–9.

An Evidence-Based Approach to Orthobiologics for Tendon Disorders

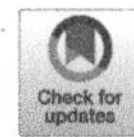

Andre Armando Abadin, DO[a], Jordan Pearl Orr, MD[a], Alexander Raphael Lloyd, MD[a], Phillip Troy Henning, DO[a], Adam Pourcho, DO[b,*]

KEYWORDS

- Tendinopathy • Tendinosis • Orthobiologics • Platelet-rich plasma (PRP
- Mesenchymal signal cells

KEY POINTS

- Orthobiologics are a safe treatment of tendinopathy with minimal reported adverse events.
- Although current studies show promise with treatments involving mesenchymal signal cells, there is a need for high-quality random controlled trials to validate the promising results.
- Platelet-rich plasma is an effective treatment of recalcitrant common extensor tendinopathy and plantar fasciopathy. Leukocyte-rich platelet-rich plasma is the most effective treatment of common extensor tendinopathy.
- Orthobiologics should be considered in refractory cases of tendinopathy or as an adjunct for pain reduction, whereas a patient is undergoing conservative management.

INTRODUCTION

Tendinopathy is a chronic injury to the tendon that affects both athletes and the general population across the spectrum of physical activity.[1] Histology studies have shown that tendinopathy results from a degenerative process rather than an inflammatory process, where type III collagen fibers replace type 1 collagen fibers, resulting in decreased tensile strength.[2,3] Other features of tendinopathy include micro-tearing, disorganized neovascularization, increased matrix metalloproteinases, and lipid deposition.[2,3] Sonographic findings of tendinopathy include thickening of the tendon proper, loss of linear and fibular pattern, hypoechogenicity, and hypervascularization on low-flow color Doppler[4] (**Fig. 1**).

[a] Department of Sports, Spine and Musculoskeletal Medicine, Swedish Medical Center, 1600 E Jefferson Street, Suite 300, Seattle, WA 98122, USA; [b] Elite Sports Performance Medicine, 11545 15th Avenue Northeast, Suite 105, Seattle, WA 98125, USA
* Corresponding author.
E-mail address: espmedicine@yahoo.com

Phys Med Rehabil Clin N Am 34 (2023) 83–103
https://doi.org/10.1016/j.pmr.2022.08.007
pmr.theclinics.com

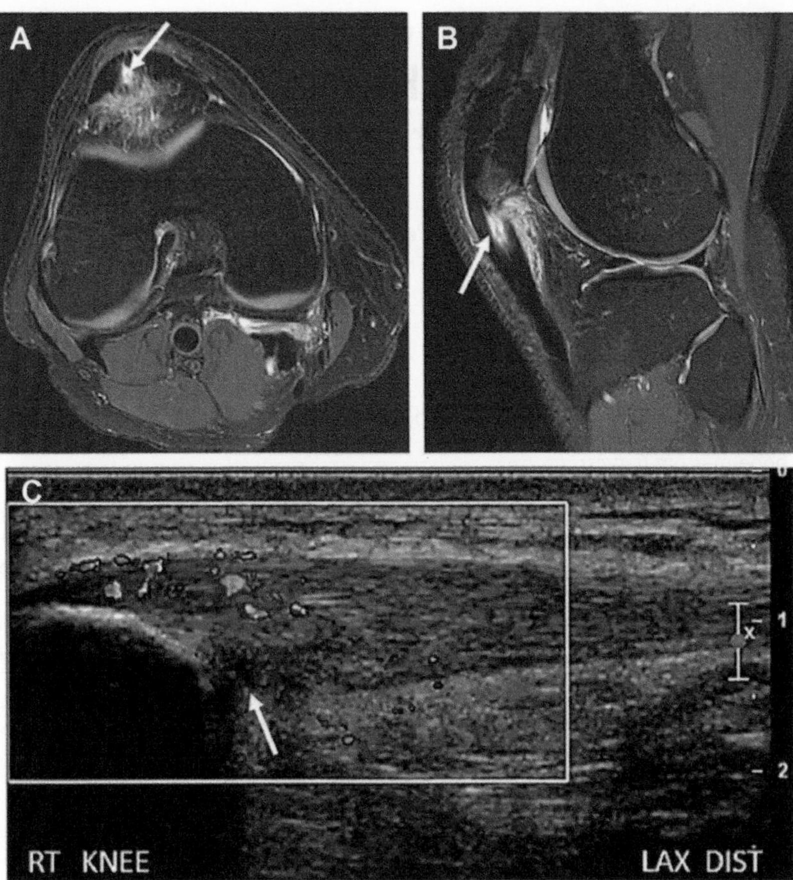

Fig. 1. MRI and ultrasound correlations for patellar tendinosis. (*A*) T2-axial image of the knee demonstrating severe patellar tendinosis with partial tearing (*arrow*). (*B*) T2 sagittal image of the knee in the same patient, again demonstrating severe patellar tendinosis with partial tearing (*arrow*). (*C*) Long axis (*LAX*) ultrasound image of the same knee with distal (DIST) to the right, demonstrating the hypoechoic heterogeneity in area of tendinopathy with partial tearing (*arrow*). Also present is significant neovessel formation throughout affected area of tendon.

Treatments of tendinopathy can be divided into conservative/noninterventional and interventional measures. Conservative treatments include eccentric and/or heavy slow resistance training, topical glyceryl nitrate, oral and topical nonsteroidal anti-inflammatories, night splints, extracorporeal shockwave therapy (ECSWT), and iontophoresis.[5,6] Interventional treatments include dry needling, injections of corticosteroid (CCS), platelet-rich plasma (PRP), and mesenchymal signaling cell (MSC) injections, sclerotherapy, percutaneous ultrasonic tenotomy, and surgical debridement, often with tenotomy and tenodesis[5–7] (**Fig. 2**).The use of orthobiologic injections, specifically PRP and MSCs, for the treatment of tendinopathy has been increasingly studied and used over the past few decades as the understanding of the pathophysiology of tendinopathy continues to expand.[8–10] In vitro studies have demonstrated that PRP increases cell proliferation and differentiation of tenocytes while also inducing type I collagen fiber production.[11,12] This rise in collagen I production increases the type 1

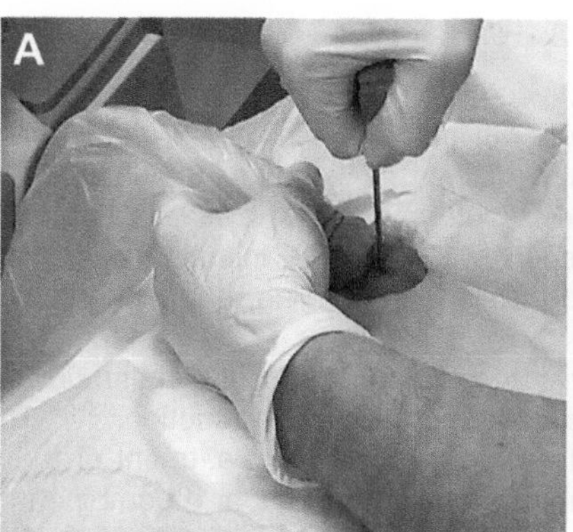

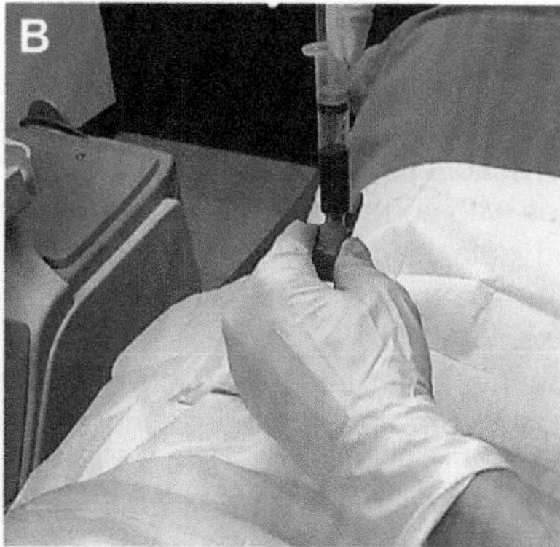

Fig. 2. Bone marrow harvest using ultrasound to guide Jamshidi needle. (*A*) Demonstration of use of curved ultrasound probe to accurately guided Jamshidi needle for posterior iliac crest bone marrow harvest. (*B*) Bone marrow harvest being performed.

to type III ratio, thereby increasing tendon tensile strength, thereby resulting in pain relief and improved function.[11,12] In vitro studies of MSCs on tendons have demonstrated growth factor secretion, resulting in the recruitment of resident MSCs within the tendinopathic tendon, leading to a reduction of apoptosis, and promoted angiogenesis.[13,14] Although injectable MSCs can differentiate into tenocytes, this action does not seem to play a large role in their ability to treat tendinopathy.[13,14] More research in the short- and long-term outcomes of orthobiologics on tendinopathies is ongoing.

This article reviews the current state of research related to the application of orthobiologics in the treatment of tendinopathies. To date, this is an area of emerging research without broad consensus on the clinical application of this treatment intervention, specifically the formulation (eg, leukocyte rich/poor), timing, number of treatments needed, dosing (volume of orthobiologics), and candidate selection criteria. For many tendons, current research on the presence and degree of effectiveness remains limited. These limits highlight both the exciting and growing potential of these autologous treatment options for the treatment of tendinopathy and the need for further research.

Rotator Cuff Tendinopathy

Shoulder pain and dysfunction is a common musculoskeletal complaint commonly seen in both primary care and specialty settings. A recent systematic review found that the prevalence of abnormalities within the rotator cuff tendons was 62% among patients 80 years or older.[15] Physical therapy is effective and remains the primary treatment of rotator cuff tendinopathy (RT).[16] For patients recalcitrant to physical therapy, CCS injections and surgery are offered. Unfortunately, there is a growing body of literature dating back to 1977 when the first meta-analysis on CCS was performed, demonstrating detrimental effects on soft tissues, including tendon rupture.[17] Furthermore, surgery for repair of complete rotator cuff tears does not seem to improve quality of life compared with nonoperative treatments.[18] Recent randomized controlled studies show no difference in long-term outcomes between nonoperative and operative interventions in the management of rotator cuff disease.[19,20] The increase in use of orthobiologics with growing evidence may offer an alternative to CCS injections and possibly surgery.

PLATELET-RICH PLASMA

Much of the preliminary data on the effectiveness of PRP for RT was in conjunction with arthroscopic rotator cuff repair. Postoperatively reports have shown a decrease in pain leading to a decrease in use of pain medicines, as well as better functional outcomes with no reported catastrophic adverse outcomes.[21,22] However, current published data have significant limitations, such as unreported injectate composition and concentration, small sample size, poor follow-up imaging, and lack of control groups.[21,22]

Recent studies into the effects of PRP injected without surgical augmentation have demonstrated varied success in pain reduction and improved function.[23–28] There are two primary injection sites that are typically targeted for treatment of the RT: the subacromial/subdeltoid bursa and the pathologic tendons or a combination of both. In a noncontrolled, prospective cohort study involving 50 shoulders, Rossi and colleagues[23] reported improvement in pain, functional outcomes, and sleep at a 6-month follow-up, following a singular palpation-guided (PG) subacromial leukocyte-rich (LR)-PRP injection. A randomized controlled trial (RCT) from Shams and colleagues[24] involving 40 shoulders compared PG subacromial CCS and PRP injection. Despite not reporting the type of PRP, the PRP group had statistically significant improvements in visual analog scale (VAS) and american shoulder and elbow surgeons standardized shoulder assessment form (ASES) score at 6 months which was maintained through 12 months.[24] Two additional RCTs, by Kwong and colleagues[25] and Thepsoparn and colleagues,[27] comparing ultrasound-guided (USG) injections of PRP to CCS for patients with confirmed tendinopathy or partial tearing, reported greater improvement in pain and functionality starting at 3 months in the PRP cohort.

There is mixed data on the longevity of benefits of the PRP injection, with limited high-quality studies with long-term follow-up. In a randomized, double-blind placebo CT, Kesikburun and colleagues[28] published data from 40 patients comparing USG PRP to saline; concluding that there was no statistically significant difference at 1 year follow-up between the two cohorts. This study was further validated, by Kwong and colleagues,[25] who also published similar findings. This contrasts with a systematic review and meta-analysis, by Hamid and colleagues,[26] which concluded that PRP injections had better pain symptom improvement at 6 and 12 months but limited improvement in shoulder range of motion and functional outcomes when compared with control groups. However, the meta-analysis did note that there were inconsistencies in PRP preparation and type of PRP between the studies reviewed.[26] The most astonishing results for the long-term benefits of PRP was a prospective study by Prodromos and colleagues, in which 71 subjects with MRI-confirmed rotator cuff pathology were followed 2-years post-2 USG unspecified type-PRP (UT-PRP) injection. Quick disabilities of arm, shoulder, and hand (Q-DASH), VAS, and global improvement mean scores improved and were sustained at the 24-month visit with no reported progression to complete rotator cuff tears.[29]

Currently, PRP for the treatment of RT is not a standard treatment. However, in patients who have not adequately responded to traditional conservative treatments, PRP can be considered a treatment option. The available literature indicates that PRP is safe and may be superior to CCS injections with 24 months of follow-up. It seems likely that PRP will become increasingly more available and affordable for patients with RT as higher quality-controlled trials are published. Future studies are needed to help determine how PRP will fit in the RT treatment algorithm.

MESENCHYMAL SIGNALING CELLS

There is a paucity of high-quality RCT for the clinical use of bone marrow-derived MSCs (BM-MSCs) and adipose-derived MSCs (AD-MSCs) in the treatment of musculoskeletal pathology. Much of the early excitement about the potential clinical applications of MSCs was rooted in animal studies.[30,31] Gulotta and colleagues[30] demonstrated improved early supraspinatus tendon to bone healing and greater load to failure with MSC-treated rat models. Oh and colleagues[31] found improved muscle function by electromyography and biomechanical analysis as well as decreased fatty infiltration of the subscapularis following subscapularis repair with intratendinous AD-MSCs injection in rabbit models. There is a paucity of human studies, which are limited to case studies or series, with a few notable exceptions. Hernigou and colleagues[32] published on augmenting surgical outcomes with BM-MSCs. For this study, 45 patients underwent rotator cuff tear repair alone, and 45 patients had a rotator cuff tear augmented with a BM-MSCs injection at the time of the repair.[32] Sonographic assessment of the repair 6 months postoperative revealed 100% of subjects (45/45) with a BM-MSCs augmented repair versus 77% (35/45) that underwent repair alone showed no evidence of recurrent tear.[32] The benefits were sustained at 10-year follow-up where 87% of the BM-MSCs group had no evidence of recurrent tendon tear compared with 44% in the control group.[32]

Similar results were published by Jo and colleagues, who injected AD-MSCs as a conservative treatment for symptomatic partial-thickness rotator cuff tears confirmed by US or MRI. In their uncontrolled study, subjects were divided into three groups: low, mid, and high AD-MSC dosage, as calculated by the number of cells in 3 mL. Outcomes resulted in 77% to 80% significant improvement in pain and function as reported on the shoulder pain and disability index (SPADI) for the high- and mid-dose groups, respectively. In addition, the high-dose group showed significant reductions in pain by 71%, whereas the low- and mid-dose groups' pain reduced by 52%, but this change was not statistically significant.[33] Follow-up MRI and arthroscopies showed evidence of decreased volume of articular- and bursal-sided tearing by as much as 90%.[33] Although all three groups noticed improvements in pain, functionality, and reduction in tears, only the high-dose group showed statistically significant improvements in the SPADI score, VAS, and bursal-side tear size reduction. This dose-dependent response with both BM-MSCs and AD-MSCs has also been seen in other studies, with higher concentrations leading to a reduction in retear rates and improvement in pain and function.[32,33] Neither study reported significant adverse reactions to MSCs injection therapy.

MSCs injections for rotator cuff pathology seem to be safe and well tolerated with few reported side effects and adverse outcomes. However, there is a need for further research with high-quality RCTs with investigational new drug approval to advance our understanding of potential benefits or risks of such treatments.

Common Extensor Tendinopathy

Common extensor tendinopathy (CET) involves the common extensor tendon complex, which attaches at the lateral epicondyle of the humerus. Although commonly called lateral epicondylitis or "tennis elbow," it is more related to chronic attritional breakdown of the CET itself.[34] Typically, patients will complain of pain and functional limitations with activities such as repetitive typing, gripping, carrying, and lifting, which may result in decreased daily function and workplace productivity.[35] Conservative treatment includes rest, activity modification, anti-inflammatory medications, physical or occupational therapy, eccentric strengthening, bracing, extracorporeal, shockwave therapy, and therapeutic injections, among other treatments.[36,37] Traditional surgical treatment consists of tendon debridement by either open or endoscopic approach, sometimes combined with repair and/or decortication.[38] Published surgical series report good to excellent outcomes in 94.6% of patients, depending on the patient population and surgical technique; however, these procedures are complicated by potential for neural injury, wound infection, and loss of joint range of motion.[38–40] Orthobiologics may offer a viable alternative to surgical treatment for recalcitrant cases.

PLATELET-RICH PLASMA

To date, there are more orthobiologic studies on the treatment of CET than any other tendon in the human body. An early double-blind RCT, by Peerbooms and colleagues,[41] compared PRP with CCS injection, demonstrating a superior 25% improvement in the VAS and DASH scores in the PRP group at 1-year follow-up, with sustained improvement at 2 years. A systematic review drew similar conclusions to previous studies, finding PRP injections had improved VAS and DASH scores compared with CCS injections in refractory CET at 2 months.[42] Further evidence was provided by Thanasas and colleagues, in their RCT comparing USG PRP to whole blood (WB). The PRP group had statistically better improvements in pain at 6 weeks, but no differences were seen at 3 and 6 months. There was also no difference in functional score (Liverpool elbow score) between the two groups.[43] This may indicate a role of WB in the treatment of CET.

Moreover, this brings up the question of whether LR-PRP or leukocyte-poor (LP-PRP) results in superior outcomes in CET. In a double-blinded, prospective, multicenter, RCT, Mishra and colleagues[44] reported that LR-PRP provided sustained pain relief and improvement of function when compared with control. Two adverse outcomes related to PRP were reported, which were significant pain for 2 and 4 days after LR-PRP injection.[44] In addition, two recent systematic review meta-analyses concluded that LR-PRP resulted in superior pain relief and functional outcomes compared with LP-PRP, saline, CCSs, and other control groups in the treatment of CET.[45,46] Pain for several days after the injection was the extent of adverse effects related to the injection from the PRP group.[45,46]

Out of all the tendons studied thus far, CET has the most robust data to support good clinical outcomes following PRP injections. It seems prudent to consider the type of PRP being injected for the treatment of CET with LR-PRP being superior to LP-PRP. Ongoing investigations reporting on PRP preparation have improved, making results easier to interpret and compare.[42,45–47] For now, PRP injections have been shown to be safe and more effective than CCS injections for the management of CET.

MESENCHYMAL SIGNALING CELLS

Similar to other tendinopathies mentioned in this article, there is a lack and need of high-quality investigations involving MSCs for the treatment of CET. In a prospective study, Singh and colleagues treated 30 adult patients with recalcitrant CET using PG BM-MSCs. The primary outcome measure was the patient-rated tennis elbow evaluation score at 2, 6, and 12 weeks, in which statistically significant improvements were seen at each time interval.[48] No adverse effects were reported. In another investigation, Lee and colleagues conducted a 12-month prospective pilot study to assess the safety of ADSCs in 12 patients with chronic LE. No adverse effects occurred, and subjects reported less pain and better function. Furthermore, follow-up sonographic imaging had improved echogenicity of structural defects.[49] A systematic review of four studies on the efficacy of MSCs on CET included the aforementioned studies as well as an additional two publications treated with autologous tenocyte injections.[50,51] All studies demonstrated improvement in functional outcomes, minimal adverse events (temporary pain and swelling), with 3/4 studies showing improvement of sonographic or MRI appearance of the CET at follow-up.[52]

MSCs for treatment of CET can be considered safe, with no reported serious adverse outcomes. Although improvements in pain and function haven been reported, there is a paucity of high-quality, double-blinded RCTs. Therefore, no definitive recommendations can be made at this until additional higher quality controlled studies validate the current findings.

Common Flexor/Pronator Tendinopathy

Common flexor/pronator tendinopathy (CFT), also known as "golfer's elbow" or "medial epicondylitis," can be seen with poor swing technique and in other sports or activities, such as rock climbing, where repetitive wrist flexion/pronation, or repetitive gripping/grasping is required.[35,53] Again here, the pathology has nothing to do with the epicondyle itself, but instead is proposed to occur because of excessive loading/strain on a tendon.[54] CFT is less common compared with CET with one epidemiologic study finding it to be three times less common.[53] Conservative treatment is very similar, which includes rest, activity modification, anti-inflammatory medications, physical or occupational therapy, eccentric strengthening, bracing, ECSWT, and therapeutic injections.[55] Surgery is an option if conservative treatments fail to improve symptoms. Surgical results are not as successful as that of CET, possibly due to the relative short course of the tendon complex. Furthermore, the close proximity of the ulnar nerve and ulnar collateral ligament increases the risk of iatrogenic injury.[55] Orthobiologics may represent an alternative to surgical management.

PLATELET-RICH PLASMA

Understandably, given the less frequent pathology of the CFT, there is less research on the use of orthobiologics for treatment of this condition. Suresh and colleagues reported prospective data results on 20 patients with recalcitrant CFT treated with USG injection of 2 mL of autologous blood. At 10-months follow-up, subjects reported a reduction of pain on their VAS score. Objectively, there was improvement of sonographic echotexture with decreased neovessel formation on repeat imaging.[56] No adverse events were reported. In a retrospective case series of 62 patients, Boden and colleagues compared treatment of recalcitrant elbow tendinopathy (medial or lateral) using either Tenex or LP-PRP. Ten out of the 62 subjects had a clinical diagnosis of CFT. Both treatment groups showed significant improvements in the VAS, Q-DASH, and EuroQol-5D regardless of which tendon complex was treated.[57] Similar issues with diagnostic representation were seen in a RCT published by Varshney and colleagues comparing PRP to CCS in the treatment of elbow tendinopathy. Of the 83 subjects in the study, only 20 had CFT. Unfortunately, the investigators did not indicate how many subjects with CFT were in the PRP or CCS groups.[58] Nevertheless, the PRP group had statistically significant improvement in VAS and Mayo performance index at the elbow compared with the CCS group at 6-month follow-up with no adverse outcomes reported for either group.[58]

Given the relative lack of clinical publications on PRP for the treatment of CFT, indications for its use are unclear. What can be stated is that it is safe and seems to be more effective than placebo or CCS injections. Further high-quality studies with long-term follow-up and control for variables are needed to validate these findings.

MESENCHYMAL SIGNALING CELLS

At the time of this publication, there are no peer-reviewed studies on MSCs for the treatment of CFT.

Distal Biceps Tendinopathy

The incidence of distal biceps ruptures is 1.2 per 100,000 patients with most injuries (86%) affecting the dominant arm.[59] This most commonly occurs in males during the fourth decade of life and has a higher incidence in anabolic steroid use.[59] Furthermore, 90% of biceps brachii tendon ruptures occur at the proximal origin of the tissue, whereas only 10% of biceps tendon ruptures with distal biceps tendinosis (DBT) are reported even less frequently.[60] Typically, patients will present with a sudden, sharp pain at the antecubital fossa after forceful eccentric extension of the elbow.[61] Subsequently, the patients can experience weakness and pain with elbow flexion and supination.[61] Owing to its rarity, there is little published on conservative management specifically for DBT, but often similar conservative treatments are used to other upper extremity tendinopathies. For those that failed conservative management, surgery to release, debride, and reattach the distal biceps tendon is a common surgical approach, often with a 3 to 6 month or longer recovery.[61] Again, here orthobiologics may offer an alternative to more invasive surgical procedures.

PLATELET-RICH PLASMA

Given the relatively uncommon occurrence of DBT, the research on the efficacy of PRP on DBT is similarly scarce. Two studies have demonstrated the effectiveness of PRP on DBT.[62,63] Sanli and colleagues published a prospective multicenter cohort study on 12 patients with MRI-confirmed DBT that had failed conservative treatment. All 12 subjects received an USG LR-PRP injection with a mean follow-up of 36 months. The median VAS score improved from 8 to 2.5, and elbow function assessment scores improved from 63 to 90.[62] Similarly, Barker and colleagues[63] reported favorable results on a prospective cohort involving six elbows also demonstrating statistically significant improvement in the Mayo Elbow Performance Score and VAS with a 16-month follow-up. Despite having no adverse outcomes, both studies were limited by a small number of subjects and lacked a placebo control.

PRP for treatment of DBT at most can be considered safe, with no adverse outcomes reported. Although small studies showed statistically significant improvement, the paucity of high-quality RCT makes definitive recommendations difficult. Additional higher quality controlled studies with larger subject sizes would help to validate the current findings.

MESENCHYMAL SIGNALING CELLS

At the time of this publication, there are no peer-reviewed studies on MSCs for the treatment of DBT.

Patellar and Quadriceps Tendinopathy

Jumper's knee is a term labeling anterior knee pain that could be due to patellar or quadriceps tendinopathy.[64] Both of these tendinopathies occur often in athletes that are taller, have increased body weight, and engage in heavier weight training or sports with repetitive explosive movements, such as jumping.[64–66] The prevalence of patellar tendinopathy (PT) is 14.2% in elite athletes[67] and 8.5% in non-elite athletes.[64,68] Quadriceps tendinopathy occurs less frequently at a rate of 0.2% to 2%

in athletes or 25% of those reporting extension activity related pain.[69] Among elite and non-elite athletes, volleyball is the sport with the highest prevalence of PT.[67,68] In 1986, Ferretti concluded that 75% of jumper's knee cases were due to PT and the other quarter of cases was due to QT.[70] Typical conservative treatments consisting of gluteal strengthening, quadriceps strengthening with eccentric loading, stretching, and relative rest have been tried.[65] Arthroscopic surgical debridement has been described with varied success. For patients who have failed conservative management orthobiologics may be a viable treatment option.

PLATELET-RICH PLASMA

In a RCT comparing saline, LP-PRP, and LR-PRP, there was reported statistically significant improvement in the cohort receiving LR-PRP at 12 weeks over other cohorts, with no difference between all cohorts at 1 year.[71] In a double-blind RCT conducted by Dragoo and colleagues,[72] LR-PRP injection was superior to dry needling for PT, with improvements in Victoria Institute of Sports Assessment-Patella scores at 12-week follow-up, but without statistical difference at 26-week follow-up. In a RCT comparing PRP to ECSWT for the treatment of PT, Vetrano and colleagues[66] reported statistically significant higher pain relief in the PRP cohort as reported on VAS and VISA-P with 12-month follow-up. In a nonrandomized study compared PRP with physical therapy with physical therapy alone for the treatment of PT, both groups had statistically significant improvement in pain with no significant difference found between groups.[73] No clinically relevant side effects were noted in any of these studies.[66,71–73]

Unlike PT, there is little research on orthobiologics for the less common QT, with only one case report published. In this publication, a case of QT was treated with a single injection of LR-PRP, with improvement of VAS as well as improvement of imaging appearance on repeat MRI 19 months after the procedure.[74]

Many studies have failed to show that PRP is superior to other conservative management strategies; however, it is safe with few reported side-effects, with some reports of improvement in pain and function. Given the lack of data related to the use of PRP for QT, a formal recommendation cannot be made.

MESENCHYMAL SIGNALING CELLS

MSCs have been less studied for treatment of PT. In a case series of eight patients with PT treated with a single injection of BM-MSCs, Pascual-Garrido and colleagues reported statistically significant improvements in knee injury and osteoarthritis outcome score (KOOS), Tegner, and International Knee Documentation Committee. Seven out of eight patients reported that they were satisfied and would undergo the procedure again when asked at the 5-year follow-up.[75] In another RCT comparing BM-MSCs with LP-PRP for PT, it was reported that both interventions had statistically significant improvements in VAS and VISA-P, but there was no difference between the two groups with 6-month follow-up.[76] There were no adverse effects in either of these studies.[75,76] There are currently no publications on MSCs for QT.

The above studies evaluating MSCs for PT have demonstrated great patient satisfaction and safety but fail to show a statistically significant superiority of MSCs over PRP. Further RCT controlling for aforementioned variables with long-term follow-up are needed to investigate the efficacy of MSCs for PT and QT and validate these findings.

Gluteal Tendinopathy

Gluteal tendinopathy (GT), also known as "greater trochanteric pain syndrome," was previously often referred to as greater trochanteric bursitis. However, the latter has fallen out of favor as inflammation of the lateral hip bursae is rarely the cause for pain.[77] A cross-sectional study performed by Albers and colleagues[78] found that GT was the most prevalent lower limb tendinopathy. GT presents with lateral hip pain that is often provoked with hip abduction or when the patient is side-lying or sitting.[77] The level of disability caused by GT has been equated to that of severe hip osteoarthritis.[79] Patients will often try conservative treatment consisting of offloading, physical therapy, stretching, and gluteal strengthening as well as core strengthening. Patients are often offered CCS injections; however, recent data on CCSs detrimental effects on soft tissues have caused this to go out of favor.[80] Open and endoscopic surgical debridement with or without tenodesis has been described with mixed results.[81] Orthobiologics have been used for treatment and may offer an alternative to more invasive approaches.

PLATELET-RICH PLASMA

Orthobiologics can be considered as a treatment of recalcitrant GT. In a case series of 21 patients with GT, there was statistically significant improvement in pain and function in outcome measures, after patients underwent a single injection with LR-PRP, with no adverse events or outcomes reported.[82] In a level 1 double-blind RCT comparing LR-PRP with CCS for the treatment of GT, Fitzpatrick and colleagues[83] published statistically significant greater improvement in the PRP cohort at 12 weeks, with continued superior improvement in 38 out of 40 patients at 1-year follow-up. Interestingly, Jacobson and colleagues[77] published data on a RCT comparing LR-PRP versus needle tenotomy, demonstrating statistically significant improvement at 1 week, 2 weeks, and 3 months follow-up in both groups, with no significant difference between groups.

Current evidence supports that PRP for GT is a safe treatment option and that it is more effective than CCS, but may not be superior to needle tenotomy alone. Further research with long-term follow-up is needed to delineate these results.

MESENCHYMAL SIGNALING CELLS

At the time of this publication, there are no peer-reviewed studies on MSCs for the treatment of GT.

Proximal Hamstring Tendinopathy

Proximal hamstring tendinopathy (PHT) is becoming increasingly recognized as a causative factor in both sitting and activity-related posterior hip pain. Unlike an acute tear, the pain usually comes on gradually and may be aggravated by repetitive activities, such as running or biking, and worsened by prolonged sitting.[84–86] Approximately 20% of patients with PHT who undergo noninvasive treatment, such as rest and physical therapy, have residual hamstring pain.[87–91] For recalcitrant cases, surgical debridement with or without tenodesis is offered, with varied reported success rates and no uniform approach.[92,93] The increase of orthobiologics may offer a less invasive approach to management.

PLATELET-RICH PLASMA

Multiple case series have shown promising outcomes for PRP as a treatment of PHT. A retrospective case series by Fader and colleagues[94] was conducted on 18 patients that underwent a single USG injection of LR-PRP and found that the average improvement in VAS was 63% postinjection at 6-month follow-up. In a retrospective study of

22 patients, Auriemma and colleagues[95] showed statistically significant improvement in Numeric Pain Rating Scale and Victorian Institute of Sport Assessment-Proximal Hamstring Tendons (VISA-H) 8 months after a single USG LR-PRP injection. In a prospective case series published on 14 patients receiving a single USG injection of PRP, a statistically significant improvement in Lower Extremity Functional Scale (LEFS), and VAS was reported at 12-week follow-up.[96]

Only one double-blinded RCT evaluating PRP as a treatment of PHT has been conducted. In this publication, a single injection of either LR-PRP or WB for the treatment of chronic PHT was performed. At 6-month follow-up, the PRP group reported statistically significant improvement in activities of daily living (ADL) and IHOTT-33 scores from baseline, whereas the WB group failed to show significant change.[97] A pilot prospective cohort study by Levy and colleagues[98] evaluated outcomes of 29 patients with PHT who underwent LR-PRP injection, demonstrating no significant difference in VISA-H at 8 weeks after LR-PRP injection. A significant limitation of this study is that of short follow-up, with many prior studies on other aforementioned tendons indicating a 6 to 12 week range for PRP to demonstrate improvement in tendon pathology. Therefore, a longer term follow-up may have demonstrated improvement in many of these patients.

PRP for PHT has been shown to be safe with no significant reported side effects and improvement in reported outcomes for both pain and function. Future RCT controlling for variables and long-term outcomes are needed to validate these findings.

MESENCHYMAL SIGNALING CELLS

At the time of this publication, there are no peer-reviewed studies on MSCs for the treatment of PHT.

Adductor Tendinopathy

Groin pain can be debilitating in both the athletic and nonathlete populations.[78] In a Dutch general population cross-sectional study, adductor tendinopathy was found to have a prevalence rate of 1.22 (per 1000 person-years).[78] In athletes, adductor tendinopathy is common in those that participate in kicking activities, such as soccer as well as skating sports, such as hockey. The yearly incidence of groin pain in male soccer athletes is estimated to be 10% to 18%.[99] Patients will typically report gradual onset pain in the groin that can radiate into the abdomen. Hernia evaluation should be considered in the differential for this type of pain as often the two can be hard to separate, often occurring in tandem. Conservative treatments can include bracing, rest, stretching, strengthening, and activity restriction. Surgical management with adductor longus release or debridement with or without ilioinguinal nerve ablation/lysis is a consideration for recalcitrant cases with good, reported outcomes.[100] Orthobiologics may offer an alternative or preamble to surgical management.

PLATELET-RICH PLASMA

Currently, there are no RCT and only one case study describing PRP as a treatment of adductor tendinopathy (AddT). In a case report by Singh and colleagues, improvement in pain and function was seen following treatment with two USG UT-PRP injections given 6 weeks apart for a traumatic complete rupture of the adductor longus tendon along its origin in an adult male soccer player. The patient had an improvement in adductor strength from 0/5 to 5/5 posttreatment. The time frame of return to sport after PRP injections was not described.[101]

Given the limited data on PRP injections for AddT, it is difficult at this time to recommend this as a first-line treatment option. RCT with control of variables and long-term follow-up will be needed to justify PRP as a treatment option.

MESENCHYMAL SIGNALING CELLS

At the time of this publication, there are no peer-reviewed studies on MSCs for the treatment of AddT.

There is no data on MSCs and little to no data on PRP for the treatment of adductor tendinopathy. As groin pain is a common and debilitating condition, investigation for the use of orthobiologics in this region is imperative.

Achilles Tendinopathy

Achilles tendinopathy (AT) is a common overuse injury. It is commonly seen in athletes participating in strenuous activities such as long-distance running, sprinting, and jumping.[102] Epidemiologic studies found that AT occurs in 9% of recreational runners and about 6% in nonathletes.[103] AT can be divided into insertional AT and non-insertional or mid-portion AT, of which mid-portion AT is more common.[103] It is important to make this distinction as treatment responsiveness varies between the two, with mid-portion responding better to both conservative and interventional treatments.[104] Patients will typically complain of pain and stiffness at the posterior aspect of their ankle that is worse in the morning, improved with activity, and worse after activity. Common conservative treatments include shoe modifications, heel lifts, oral analgesics, eccentric exercises, deep friction massage, ECSWT, and CCS injections.[103] For those that have failed conservative treatments, surgery can be considered. Surgery usually consists of fractional lengthening of the tendon, debridement, and reattaching with or without grafts.[103] Alternatively, orthobiologics have been offered as a treatment option.

PLATELET-RICH PLASMA

Despite a lack of high-quality studies reporting the use of PRP for mid-portion AT, the efficacy of PRP injections for this diagnosis has recently come into question.[105,106] There is much variability in treatment protocols reported for PRP for AT, which makes interpretation of its effectiveness difficult.[106] Two recent systematic reviews with meta-analysis failed to show a difference in VISA-A scores at 3 and 6 months following PRP injections for AT.[106,107] Both publications also questioned if there was improvement of the tendinous structure following PRP, as there was no statistically significant difference in tendon thickness on MRI or ultrasound.[106,107] Similarly, a recent RCT concluded that there was no statistically significant difference in VISA-A scores between PRP group and sham injection groups at 3-months or 6-months for mid-portion AT.[108] This lack of demonstrated benefit could be explained by the heterogeneity of treatment protocols in each study including variable site of injection, preparation of PRP, volume of injection, use of ultrasound guidance, and adjunct therapies.[106] It is also possible that the mid-portion AT has a different pathogenesis than other tendons treated with PRP and therefore requires a different treatment protocol and approach for effectiveness. For example, one such double-blinded prospective RCT compared 60 male patients with mid-portion AT treated with eccentric loading exercises. The patients were divided into three cohorts, one receiving high-volume peritendinous injection (CCS, local anesthetics, and saline), one receiving four PRP injections spaced 2 weeks apart, and one receiving placebo injection of saline.[109] At 24-week follow-up, the high-volume and PRP injection groups reported superior reduction in the VISA-A, pain, and tendon thickness, when combined with eccentric exercises compared with placebo.[109] No adverse reactions were reported, and no differences were noted between the high-volume and PRP groups at 24-week follow-up.

Regarding insertional AT, only one cohort was available at the time of review. In this retrospective study of 45 patients with insertional AT, the patients were treated with two UT-PRP injections separated 1 week apart or three ECSWT (focused electromagnetic) treatments. Improvement was seen in VAS and VISA-A score at 0-, 2-, 4-, and 6-month follow-up in both treatment arms. There was no difference between the two groups at 6 months, and no adverse reactions were reported.[110]

There are mixed reviews on whether PRP injection is an effective treatment of both insertional and non-insertional AT. For non-insertional AT, PRP injections seem to be safe and may be as effective as high-volume peritendinous injections when used in conjunction with eccentric exercises. No studies highlight which type of PRP or what frequency of injection would be most effective for this region. Further RCT into the effect of controlled post-procedure exercise and volume of injectate with long-term outcomes are needed to better understand these results.

MESENCHYMAL SIGNALING CELLS

MSCs may play a role in the treatment of both mid-portion and insertional AT. One trial conducted in 2017 randomized patients to receive injections of either PRP or stromal vascular fraction (SVF) derived from adipose tissue for treatment of mid-portion AT.[111] A statistically significant greater improvement in VAS and VISA-A scores at 15 and 30 days was seen in the group receiving SVF with improvements seen in both treatment arms.[111] The improvements in VAS and VISA-A in the SVF group continued through 6-month follow-up despite no evidence of improvement in tendon structure or appearance on repeat MRI.[111] In addition, the initial differences in superior outcomes at 1 month reported in the SVF were not seen at 6-month follow up with both groups reporting similar improved outcomes.[111] Similar improvements in VAS were reported in another RCT of 43 subjects (58 tendons) receiving intra-tendinous SVF or PRP for mid-portion AT with 6-month follow-up.[112] A retrospective case review of 15 patients treated with BM-MSCs for either insertional or mid-portion AT reported improvement in numeric pain scale at 48-week follow-up, with the bulk of the improvement occurring at 6-week follow-up.[113] None of the studies mentioned above reported adverse effects with their patients.

MSC injections for AT seem to be safe and well tolerated with no reported adverse outcomes. However, there is a need for more high-quality RCTs, some of which will require an investigational new drug approval if performed in the United States, to advance our understanding of potential benefits or risks of such treatments.

Plantar Fasciopathy

Plantar fasciopathy (PF) is a painful condition that affects millions of people with a prevalence rate of 8%.[114] Although it is commonly seen in runners, it can be seen in other populations such as those with jobs that require excessive standing or walking, people with pes cavus or planus, and people with an elevated body mass index (BMI).[115] Patients usually complain about plantar heel pain that is worse in the morning or after prolonged inactivity. PF is histologically similar to tendinopathy where collagen degeneration, disruption of fibular pattern, and absence of inflammatory cells are found.[116] For this reason, treatments for tendinopathy have been applied as treatment of PF. Conservative treatments include night splints, oral and topical analgesic, stretching, ECSWT, and CCS injections.[115] Complete or partial fascia release is reserved for patients that failed conservative management, but the complications associated with such surgery can include persistent heel pain, nerve damage, and infections.[115,117] The increase of orthobiologics has resulted in a potential alternative treatment to surgical management for patients with recalcitrant cases.

PLATELET-RICH PLASMA

PRP is a common treatment option offered to patients with recalcitrant PF, with many peer-reviewed articles. There are numerous studies that compare the PRP injection with CCS injection for treatment of PF.[118–120] In a prospective RCT, Jain and colleagues[118] treated 60 subjects with a PG CCS or UT-PRP injection while recording Roles–Maudsley Score, VAS, and the American Orthopaedic Foot and Ankle Society (AOFAS) ankle and hind foot score. The groups reported similar improvement at 3 and 6 months, with superior results at 12 months in the PRP group.[118] Similar results were seen in Monto's single-blinded, prospective, randomized, longitudinal case series of 40 patients who received either a USG CCG or UT-PRP injection for treatment of their chronic PF. AOFAS ankle and hind foot scores between the two groups were similar at 3 months, but at 6, 12, and 24 months, the PRP group had statistically significantly higher AOFAS ankle and hind foot scores.[119] Peerbooms and colleagues also performed a single–blind, prospective RCT comparing PG UT-PRP and CCG injections among 115 patients with chronic PF. Foot Function Index Pain scores were statistically improved at the 12-month period in the PRP group compared with the CCG group.[120]

None of the RCTs reported adverse outcomes in the PRP group. Data supporting this trend were also seen in a prospective case series of 40 patients, in which improvement in VAS score at 6 months were seen in both the CCS and PRP group with sustained improvement only in the PRP group at 12-month follow-up.[121] Furthermore, in the same case series, sonographic improvement in thickness, hypoechogenicity, and hyperemia was seen primarily in the PRP group on follow-up imaging.[121] Two recent systematic reviews and meta-analyses in 2021 compared the efficacy of PRP and CCS in the treatment of PF, concluding that there was no difference in treatment outcomes at 1 month and superior outcomes with PRP at 6 months and beyond.[122,123]

There are robust data from multiple RCT and systematic reviews that support the treatment of chronic PF with PRP injections.[118–123] The improvement in pain is apparent at 3 months after the injection, but the benefits remain persistent at least 12 months postinjection. PRP seems a viable treatment option for recalcitrant PF.

MESENCHYMAL SIGNALING CELLS

At the time of this publication, there are no peer-reviewed studies on MSCs for the treatment of PF.

SUMMARY

Many studies have outlined the safety and effectiveness of orthobiologics for the treatment of tendinopathies; however, ample evidence is still lacking to consider these interventions to be standard of care. The most compelling data are for the treatment of CET and PF. PRP and MSCs should be considered in refractory cases of tendinopathy after exhausting conservative measures or could be considered as an adjunct for pain reduction, whereas a patient is undergoing conservative management. Future RCTs, preferably with investigational new drug approval, with long-term follow-up, are imperative to determine the ideal treatment protocol (ie, formulation, number and frequency of injections), type of orthobiologic, and patient characteristics.

DISCLOSURE

The authors have no conflicts of interest to declare that are relevant to the content of this article.

REFERENCES

1. Almekinders LC, Temple JD. Etiology, diagnosis, and treatment of tendonitis: an analysis of the literature. Med Sci Sports Exerc 1998;30:1183–90.
2. Wang JH-C, Guo Q, Li B. Tendon biomechanics and mechanobiology—a mini-review of basic concepts and recent advancements. J Hand Ther 2012;25: 133–41.
3. Jones GC, Corps AN, Pennington CJ, et al. Expression profiling of metalloproteinases and tissue inhibitors of metalloproteinases in normal and degenerate human achilles tendon. Arthritis Rheum 2006;54:832–42.
4. Robinson P. Sonography of common tendon injuries. AJR Am J Roentgenol 2009;193:607–18.
5. Hartley DR, McMahon JJ. The role of strength training for lower extremity tendinopathy. Strength Conditioning J 2018;40:85–95.
6. Irby A, Gutierrez J, Chamberlin C, et al. Clinical management of tendinopathy: a systematic review of systematic reviews evaluating the effectiveness of tendinopathy treatments. Scand. J Med Sci Sports 2020;30:1810–26.
7. Vajapey S, Ghenbot S, Baria MR, et al. Utility of percutaneous ultrasonic tenotomy for tendinopathies: a systematic review. sports health: A Multidisciplinary Approach 2021;13:258–64.
8. Redler LH, Thompson SA, Hsu SH, et al. Platelet-rich plasma therapy: a systematic literature review and evidence for clinical use. Phys Sportsmed 2011;39: 42–51.
9. Engebretsen L, Steffen K, Alsousou J, et al. IOC consensus paper on the use of platelet-rich plasma in sports medicine. Br J Sports Med 2010;44:1072–81.
10. Van Schaik KD, Lee KS. Orthobiologics: diagnosis and treatment of common tendinopathies. Semin Musculoskelet Radiol 2021;25:735–44.
11. Zhou Y, Wang JH-C. PRP Treatment efficacy for tendinopathy: a review of basic science studies. Biomed Res Int 2016;2016:1–8.
12. Alsousou J, Ali A, Willett K, et al. The role of platelet-rich plasma in tissue regeneration. Platelets 2013;24:173–82.
13. Young M. Stem cell applications in tendon disorders: a clinical perspective. Stem Cells Int 2012;2012:1–10.
14. da Silva Meirelles L, Fontes AM, Covas DT, et al. Mechanisms involved in the therapeutic properties of mesenchymal stem cells. Cytokine Growth Factor Rev 2009;20:419–27.
15. Teunis T, Lubberts B, Reilly BT, et al. A systematic review and pooled analysis of the prevalence of rotator cuff disease with increasing age. J Shoulder Elbow Surg 2014;23:1913–21.
16. Kuhn JE. Exercise in the treatment of rotator cuff impingement: a systematic review and a synthesized evidence-based rehabilitation protocol. J Shoulder Elbow Surg 2009;18:138–60.
17. Hoyt CJ, Jay Hoyt C, Halpern AA, et al. Tendon ruptures associated with corticosteroid therapy. Plast Reconstr Surg 1978;62:483.
18. Boorman RS, More KD, Hollinshead RM, et al. What happens to patients when we do not repair their cuff tears? Five-year rotator cuff quality-of-life index

outcomes following nonoperative treatment of patients with full-thickness rotator cuff tears. J Shoulder Elbow Surg 2018;27:444–8.
19. Karjalainen TV, Jain NB, Page CM, et al. Subacromial decompression surgery for rotator cuff disease. Cochrane Database Syst Rev 2019;1:CD005619.
20. Cederqvist S, Flinkkila T, Sormaala M, et al. Non-surgical and surgical treatments for rotator cuff disease: a pragmatic randomised clinical trial with 2-year follow-up after initial rehabilitation. Ann Rheum Dis 2020. https://doi.org/10.1136/annrheumdis-2020–219099.
21. Randelli PS, Arrigoni P, Cabitza P, et al. Autologous platelet rich plasma for arthroscopic rotator cuff repair. A pilot study. Disabil. Rehabil 2008;30:1584–9.
22. Randelli P, Arrigoni P, Ragone V, et al. Platelet rich plasma in arthroscopic rotator cuff repair: a prospective RCT study, 2-year follow-up. J Shoulder Elbow Surg 2011;20:518–28.
23. Rossi LA, Piuzzi N, Giunta D, et al. Subacromial platelet-rich plasma injections decrease pain and improve functional outcomes in patients with refractory rotator cuff tendinopathy. Arthroscopy 2021;37:2745–53.
24. Shams A, El-Sayed M, Gamal O, et al. Subacromial injection of autologous platelet-rich plasma versus corticosteroid for the treatment of symptomatic partial rotator cuff tears. Eur J Orthop Surg Traumatol 2016;26:837–42.
25. Kwong CA, Woodmass JM, Gusnowski EM, et al. Platelet-rich plasma in patients with partial-thickness rotator cuff tears or tendinopathy leads to significantly improved short-term pain relief and function compared with corticosteroid injection: a double-blind randomized controlled trial. Arthroscopy 2021;37:510–7.
26. A. Hamid MS, Sazlina SG. Platelet-rich plasma for rotator cuff tendinopathy: a systematic review and meta-analysis. PLoS One 2021;16:e0251111.
27. Thepsoparn M, Thanphraisan P, Tanpowpong T, et al. Comparison of a platelet-rich plasma injection and a conventional steroid injection for pain relief and functional improvement of partial supraspinatus tears. Orthopaedic J Sports Med 2021;9. 232596712110249.
28. Kesikburun S, Tan AK, Yılmaz B, et al. Platelet-rich plasma injections in the treatment of chronic rotator cuff tendinopathy. Am J Sports Med 2013;41:2609–16.
29. Prodromos CC, Finkle S, Prodromos A, et al. Treatment of Rotator Cuff Tears with platelet rich plasma: a prospective study with 2 year follow-up. BMC Musculoskelet. Disord 2021;22:499.
30. Gulotta LV, Kovacevic D, Packer JD, et al. Bone Marrow–derived mesenchymal stem cells transduced with scleraxis improve rotator cuff healing in a rat model. Am J Sports Med 2011;39:1282–9.
31. Oh JH, Chung SW, Kim SH, et al. 2013 Neer Award: effect of the adipose-derived stem cell for the improvement of fatty degeneration and rotator cuff healing in rabbit model. J Shoulder Elbow Surg 2014;23:445–55.
32. Hernigou P, Lachaniette CHF, Delambre J, et al. Biologic augmentation of rotator cuff repair with mesenchymal stem cells during arthroscopy improves healing and prevents further tears: a case-controlled study. Int Orthop 2014;38:1811–8.
33. Jo CH, Chai JW, Jeong EC, et al. Intratendinous injection of autologous adipose tissue-derived mesenchymal stem cells for the treatment of rotator cuff disease: a first-in-human trial. Stem Cells 2018;36:1441–50.
34. Doran A, Gresham GA, Rushton N, et al. Tennis elbow: a clinicopathologic study of 22 cases followed for 2 years. Acta Orthop. Scand 1990;61:535–8.
35. Shiri R, Viikari-Juntura E. Lateral and medial epicondylitis: role of occupational factors. Best Pract Res Clin Rheumatol 2011;25:43–57.

36. Bhabra G, Wang A, Ebert JR, et al. Lateral elbow tendinopathy: development of a pathophysiology-based treatment algorithm. Orthop J Sports Med 2016;4. 2325967116670635.
37. Radwan YA, ElSobhi G, Badawy WS, et al. Resistant tennis elbow: shock-wave therapy versus percutaneous tenotomy. Int Orthop 2008;32:671–7.
38. Kwon BC, Kim JY, Park K-T. The Nirschl procedure versus arthroscopic extensor carpi radialis brevis débridement for lateral epicondylitis. J Shoulder Elbow Surg 2017;26:118–24.
39. Dunkow PD, Jatti M, Muddu BN. A comparison of open and percutaneous techniques in the surgical treatment of tennis elbow. J Bone Joint Surg Br 2004;86:701–4.
40. Solheim E, Hegna J, Øyen J, et al. arthroscopic treatment of lateral epicondylitis: tenotomy versus debridement. Arthrosc J Arthroscopic Relat Surg 2016;32:578–85.
41. Peerbooms JC, Sluimer J, Bruijn DJ, et al. Positive effect of an autologous platelet concentrate in lateral epicondylitis in a double-blind randomized controlled trial. Am J Sports Med 2010;38:255–62.
42. Kemp JA, Olson MA, Tao MA, et al. Platelet-rich plasma versus corticosteroid injection for the treatment of lateral epicondylitis: a systematic review of systematic reviews. Int J Sports Phys Ther 2021. https://doi.org/10.26603/001c.24148.
43. Thanasas C, Papadimitriou G, Charalambidis C, et al. Platelet-rich plasma versus autologous whole blood for the treatment of chronic lateral elbow epicondylitis. Am J Sports Med 2011;39:2130–4.
44. Mishra AK, Skrepnik NV, Edwards SG, et al. Efficacy of platelet-rich plasma for chronic tennis elbow: a double-blind, prospective, multicenter, randomized controlled trial of 230 patients. Am J Sports Med 2014;42:463–71.
45. Shim JW, Lee J-S, Park Y-B, et al. The effect of leucocyte concentration of platelet-rich plasma on outcomes in patients with lateral epicondylitis: a systematic review and meta-analysis. J Shoulder Elbow Surg 2022;31:634–45.
46. Muthu S, Patel S, Gobbur A, et al. Platelet-rich plasma therapy ensures pain reduction in the management of lateral epicondylitis – a PRISMA-compliant network meta-analysis of randomized controlled trials. Expert Opin Biol Ther 2022;22:1–12.
47. Arirachakaran A, Sukthuayat A, Sisayanarane T, et al. Platelet-rich plasma versus autologous blood versus steroid injection in lateral epicondylitis: systematic review and network meta-analysis. J Orthop Trauma 2016;17:101–12.
48. Singh A, Gangwar D, Singh S. Bone marrow injection: a novel treatment for tennis elbow. J Nat Sci Biol Med 2014;5:389.
49. Lee SY, Kim W, Lim C, et al. Treatment of lateral epicondylosis by using allogeneic adipose-derived mesenchymal stem cells: a pilot study. Stem Cells 2015;33:2995–3005.
50. Wang AW, Bauer S, Goonatillake M, et al. Autologous tenocyte implantation, a novel treatment for partial-thickness rotator cuff tear and tendinopathy in an elite athlete. Case Rep 2013;2013. bcr2012007899.
51. Wang A, Breidahl W, Mackie KE, et al. Autologous tenocyte injection for the treatment of severe, chronic resistant lateral epicondylitis. Am J Sports Med 2013;41:2925–32.
52. Dakkak A, Krill ML, Fogarty A, et al. Stem cell therapy for the management of lateral elbow tendinopathy: a systematic literature review. Sci Sports 2021;36:181–92.

53. Shiri R, Viikari-Juntura E, Varonen H, et al. Prevalence and determinants of lateral and medial epicondylitis: a population study. Am J Epidemiol 2006; 164:1065–74.
54. Pingel J, Lu Y, Fredberg U, et al. 3-D ultrastructure and collagen composition of healthy and overloaded human tendon: evidence of tenocyte and matrix buckling. J Anat 2014;224:548–55.
55. Amin NH, Kumar NS, Schickendantz MS. Medial epicondylitis: evaluation and management. J Am Acad Orthop Surg 2015;23:348–55.
56. Suresh SP, Ali KE, Jones H, et al. Medial epicondylitis: is ultrasound guided autologous blood injection an effective treatment? * Commentary * Commentary. Br J Sports Med 2006;40:935–9.
57. Boden AL, Scott MT, Dalwadi PP, et al. Platelet-rich plasma versus Tenex in the treatment of medial and lateral epicondylitis. J Shoulder Elbow Surg 2019;28: 112–9.
58. Varshney A, Maheshwari R, Juyal A, et al. Autologous platelet-rich plasma versus corticosteroid in the management of elbow epicondylitis: a randomized study. Int J Appl Basic Med Res 2017;7:125–8.
59. Safran MR, Graham SM. Distal biceps tendon ruptures: incidence, demographics, and the effect of smoking. Clin Orthop Relat Res 2002;275–83.
60. Kelly MP, Perkinson SG, Ablove RH, et al. Distal biceps tendon ruptures. Am J Sports Med 2015;43:2012–7.
61. Ramsey ML. Distal biceps tendon injuries: diagnosis and management. J Am Acad Orthop Surg 1999;7:199–207.
62. Sanli I, Morgan B, van Tilborg F, et al. Single injection of platelet-rich plasma (PRP) for the treatment of refractory distal biceps tendonitis: long-term results of a prospective multicenter cohort study. Knee Surg. Sports Traumatol. Arthrosc 2016;24:2308–12.
63. Barker SL, Bell SN, Connell D, et al. Ultrasound-guided platelet-rich plasma injection for distal biceps tendinopathy. Shoulder & Elbow 2015;7:110–4.
64. King D, Yakubek G, Chughtai M, et al. Quadriceps tendinopathy: a review-part 1: epidemiology and diagnosis. Ann Transl Med 2019;7:71.
65. Vander Doelen T, Jelley W. Non-surgical treatment of patellar tendinopathy: a systematic review of randomized controlled trials. J Sci Med Sport 2020;23: 118–24.
66. Vetrano M, Castorina A, Vulpiani MC, et al. Platelet-rich plasma versus focused shock waves in the treatment of Jumper's knee in athletes. Am J Sports Med 2013;41:795–803.
67. Lian ØB, Engebretsen L, et al. Prevalence of jumper's knee among elite athletes from different sports: a cross-sectional study. Am J Sports Med 2005;33:561–7.
68. Zwerver J, Bredeweg SW, Van Den Akker-Scheek I. Prevalence of jumper's knee among nonelite athletes from different sports: a cross-sectional survey. Am J Sports Med 2011;39:1984–8.
69. Sprague A, Epsley S, Silbernagel KG. Distinguishing quadriceps tendinopathy and patellar tendinopathy: semantics or significant? J Orthop Sports Phys Ther 2019;49:627–30.
70. Ferretti A. Epidemiology of jumper's knee. Sports Med 1986;3:289–95.
71. Scott A, LaPrade RF, Harmon KG, et al. Platelet-rich plasma for patellar tendinopathy: a randomized controlled trial of leukocyte-rich PRP or Leukocyte-Poor PRP versus saline. Am J Sports Med 2019;47:1654–61.

72. Dragoo JL, Wasterlain AS, Braun HJ, et al. Platelet-rich plasma as a treatment for patellar tendinopathy: a double-blind, randomized controlled trial. Am J Sports Med 2014;42:610–8.
73. Filardo G, Kon E, Della Villa S, et al. Use of platelet-rich plasma for the treatment of refractory jumper's knee. Int Orthopaedics 2010;34:909–15.
74. Wagner RJ, Zach KN. Platelet-rich plasma injection for quadriceps tendinopathy: a case report. WMJ 2021;120:78–81.
75. Pascual-Garrido C, Rolón A, Makino A. Treatment of chronic patellar tendinopathy with autologous bone marrow stem cells: a 5-year-followup. Stem Cells Int 2012. https://doi.org/10.1155/2012/953510.
76. Rodas G, Soler-Rich R, Rius-Tarruella J, et al. Effect of autologous expanded bone marrow mesenchymal stem cells or leukocyte-poor platelet-rich plasma in chronic patellar tendinopathy (with gap >3 mm): preliminary outcomes after 6 months of a double-blind, randomized, prospective study. Am J Sports Med 2021;49:1492–504.
77. Jacobson JA, Yablon CM, Henning PT, et al. Greater trochanteric pain syndrome: percutaneous tendon fenestration versus platelet-rich plasma injection for treatment of gluteal tendinosis. J Ultrasound Med 2016;35:2413–20.
78. Albers IS, Zwerver J, Diercks RL, et al. Incidence and prevalence of lower extremity tendinopathy in a Dutch general practice population: a cross sectional study. BMC Musculoskelet. Disord 2016;17.
79. Fearon AM, Cook JL, Scarvell JM, et al. Greater trochanteric pain syndrome negatively affects work, physical activity and quality of life: a case control study. J Arthroplasty 2014;29:383–6.
80. Nuelle CW, Cook CR, Stoker AM, et al. In vitro toxicity of local anaesthetics and corticosteroids on supraspinatus tenocyte viability and metabolism. J Orthop Translat 2017;8:20–4.
81. Domb BG, Carreira DS. Endoscopic repair of full-thickness gluteus medius Tears. Arthrosc Tech 2013;2:e77–81.
82. Lee JJ, Harrison JR, Boachie-Adjei K, et al. Platelet-rich plasma injections with needle tenotomy for gluteus medius tendinopathy: a registry study with prospective follow-up. Orthopaedic J Sports Med 2016;4:1–7.
83. Fitzpatrick J, Bulsara MK, O'Donnell J, et al. Leucocyte-rich platelet-rich plasma treatment of gluteus medius and minimus tendinopathy: a double-blind randomized controlled trial with 2-year follow-up. Am J Sports Med 2019;47:1130–7.
84. Engebretsen AH, Myklebust G, Holme I, et al. Intrinsic risk factors for hamstring injuries among male soccer players: a prospective cohort study. Am J Sports Med 2010;38:1147–53.
85. Gabbe BJ, Bennell KL, Finch CF, et al. Predictors of hamstring injury at the elite level of Australian football. Scand J Med Sci Sports 2006;16:7–13.
86. Chumanov ES, Heiderscheit BC, Thelen DG. The effect of speed and influence of individual muscles on hamstring mechanics during the swing phase of sprinting. J Biomech 2007;40:3555–62.
87. Puranen J, Orava S. The hamstring syndrome–a new gluteal sciatica. Ann Chir Gynaecol 1991;80:212–4.
88. Lempainen L, Sarimo J, Mattila K, et al. Proximal hamstring tendinopathy: results of surgical management and histopathologic findings. Am. J Sports Med 2009;37:727–34.
89. Fredericson M, Moore W, Guillet M, et al. High hamstring tendinopathy in runners: meeting the challenges of diagnosis, treatment, and rehabilitation. Phys Sportsmed 2005;33:32–43.

90. Zissen MH, Wallace G, Stevens KJ, et al. High hamstring tendinopathy: MRI and ultrasound imaging and therapeutic efficacy of percutaneous corticosteroid injection. AJR Am J Roentgenol 2010;195:993–8.
91. Sarimo J, Lempainen L, Mattila K, et al. Complete proximal hamstring avulsions: a series of 41 patients with operative treatment. Am J Sports Med 2008;36: 1110–5.
92. Fletcher AN, Lau BC, Mather RC 3rd. Endoscopic proximal hamstring tendon repair for nonretracted tears: an anatomic approach and repair technique. Arthrosc Tech 2020;9:e483–91.
93. Belk JW, Kraeutler MJ, Mei-Dan O, et al. Return to sport after proximal hamstring tendon repair: a systematic review. Orthop J Sports Med 2019;7. 2325967119853218.
94. Fader, R. R. et al. Platelet-rich plasma treatment improves outcomes for chronic proximal hamstring injuries in an athletic population. vol. 4 461–466 (2014).
95. Auriemma MJ, Tenforde AS, Harris A, et al. Platelet-rich plasma for treatment of chronic proximal hamstring tendinopathy. Regen Med 2020;15:1509–18.
96. Krauss J, Nugent R, Bodor M, et al. Clinical medical reviews and case reports therapeutic efficacy of platelet-rich plasma injections in treating chronic high hamstring tendinopathy. Clin Med 2016;1–5.
97. Davenport KL, Campos JS, Nguyen J, et al. Ultrasound-guided intratendinous injections with platelet-rich plasma or autologous whole blood for treatment of proximal hamstring tendinopathy: a double-blind randomized controlled trial. J Ultrasound Med 2015;34:1455–63.
98. Levy GM, Lucas P, Hope N. Efficacy of a platelet-rich plasma injection for the treatment of proximal hamstring tendinopathy: a pilot study. J Sci Med Sport 2019;22:247–52.
99. Hölmich P, Uhrskou P, Ulnits L, et al. Effectiveness of active physical training as treatment for long-standing adductor-related groin pain in athletes: randomised trial. Lancet 1999;353:439–43.
100. Meyers WC, Lanfranco A, Castellanos A. Surgical management of chronic lower abdominal and groin pain in high-performance athletes. Curr Sports Med Rep 2002;1:301–5.
101. Singh JR, Roza R, Bartolozzi AR. Platelet rich plasma therapy in an athlete with adductor longus tendon tear. Univ Penn Orthop J 2010;20:42–3.
102. Järvinen TAH, Kannus P, Maffulli N, et al. Achilles tendon disorders: etiology and epidemiology. Foot Ankle Clin 2005;10:255–66.
103. Li H-Y, Hua Y-H. Achilles tendinopathy: current concepts about the basic science and clinical treatments. Biomed Res Int 2016;2016:1–9.
104. Zhi X, Liu X, Han J, et al. Nonoperative treatment of insertional Achilles tendinopathy: a systematic review. J Orthop Surg Res 2021;16:233.
105. Patricios J, Harmon KG, Drezner J. PRP use in sport and exercise medicine: be wary of science becoming the sham. Br J Sports Med 2022;56:66–7.
106. Nauwelaers A-K, Van Oost L, Peers K. Evidence for the use of PRP in chronic midsubstance Achilles tendinopathy: a systematic review with meta-analysis. Foot Ankle Surg 2021;27:486–95.
107. Chen J, Wan Y, Jiang H. The effect of platelet-rich plasma injection on chronic Achilles tendinopathy and acute Achilles tendon rupture. Platelets 2021; 33:1–11.
108. Kearney RS, Ji C, Warwick J, et al. Effect of platelet-rich plasma injection vs sham injection on tendon dysfunction in patients with chronic midportion achilles tendinopathy. JAMA 2021;326:137.

109. Boesen AP, Hansen R, Boesen MI, et al. Effect of high-volume injection, platelet-rich plasma, and sham treatment in chronic midportion achilles tendinopathy: a randomized double-blinded prospective study. Am J Sports Med 2017;45:2034–43.
110. Erroi D. Conservative treatment for Insertional Achilles Tendinopathy: platelet-rich plasma and focused shock waves. A retrospective study. Muscle,. Ligaments Tendons J 2017;7:98.
111. Usuelli FG, Grassi M, Maccario C, et al. Intratendinous adipose-derived stromal vascular fraction (SVF) injection provides a safe, efficacious treatment for Achilles tendinopathy: results of a randomized controlled clinical trial at a 6-month follow-up. Knee Surg Sports Traumatol Arthrosc 2018;26:2000–10.
112. Albano D, Messina C, Usuelli FG, et al. Magnetic resonance and ultrasound in achilles tendinopathy: predictive role and response assessment to platelet-rich plasma and adipose-derived stromal vascular fraction injection. Eur J Radiol 2017;95:130–5.
113. Thueakthong W, de Cesar Netto C, Garnjanagoonchorn A, et al. Outcomes of iliac crest bone marrow aspirate injection for the treatment of recalcitrant Achilles tendinopathy. Int Orthop 2021;45:2423–8.
114. Rosenbaum AJ, DiPreta JA, Misener D. Plantar heel pain. Med Clin North Am 2014;98:339–52.
115. Luffy L, Grosel J, Thomas R, et al. Plantar fasciitis: a review of treatments. J Am Acad Physician Assist 2018;31:20–4.
116. Maffulli N, Wong J, Almekinders LC. Types and epidemiology of tendinopathy. Clin Sports Med 2003;22:675–92.
117. Malahias M-A, Cantiller EB, Kadu VV, et al. The clinical outcome of endoscopic plantar fascia release: a current concept review. Foot Ankle Surg 2020;26:19–24.
118. Jain K, Murphy PN, Clough TM. Platelet rich plasma versus corticosteroid injection for plantar fasciitis: a comparative study. The Foot 2015;25:235–7.
119. Monto RR. Platelet-rich plasma efficacy versus corticosteroid injection treatment for chronic severe plantar fasciitis. Foot Ankle Int 2014;35:313–8.
120. Peerbooms JC, Lodder P, den Oudsten BL, et al. Positive effect of platelet-rich plasma on pain in plantar fasciitis: a double-blind multicenter randomized controlled trial. Am J Sports Med 2019;47:3238–46.
121. Jiménez-Pérez AE, Gonzalez-Arabio D, Diaz AS, et al. Clinical and imaging effects of corticosteroids and platelet-rich plasma for the treatment of chronic plantar fasciitis: a comparative non randomized prospective study. Foot Ankle Surg 2019;25:354–60.
122. Fei X, Lang L, Lingjiao H, et al. Platelet-rich plasma has better mid-term clinical results than traditional steroid injection for plantar fasciitis: a systematic review and meta-analysis. Orthop Traumatol Surg Res 2021;107:103007.
123. Hohmann E, Tetsworth K, Glatt V. Platelet-rich plasma versus corticosteroids for the treatment of plantar fasciitis: a systematic review and meta-analysis. Am J Sports Med 2021;49:1381–93.

Protocols and Techniques for Orthobiologic Procedures

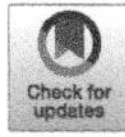

Michael Khadavi, MD, RMSK[a,*], Adam Pourcho, DO, RMSK[b], Luga Podesta, MD[c]

KEYWORDS

• Orthobiologics • PRP • BMC • Stem cell • Technique • Osteoarthritis • Tendonitis

KEY POINTS

- Many procedural techniques have been described and used for orthobiologics procedures with little research on the ideal technique.
- A detailed knowledge of at-risk anatomy and pre-procedural screening is important to any successful procedure.
- Setting expectations is the first step to a successful orthobiologic procedure.
- Local anesthetic or nerve blocks may be used for the more painful orthobiologic techniques, especially intradiscal, intratendinous, and intraosseous procedures.

INTRODUCTION

Although the basic science and clinical research for orthobiologic therapies grows exponentially, outcome data comparing the variety of techniques remain relatively unexamined. Many questions persist such as what is the optimal needle size, method of procedural analgesia, and performance of concomitant procedures such as tendon fenestration for optimal outcomes. This section offers practical guidance in orthobiologic procedural techniques based on both the techniques described in the literature and the authors' own combined anecdotal experience.

This article should be supplemented by formal training and mentorship in orthobiologic procedures. We hope these tips and pearls for orthobiologic procedural techniques will facilitate improved procedural accuracy and patient comfort, enhance the process flow from beginning to end, and encourage further clinical research.

PRE-PROCEDURAL CONSIDERATIONS

The first step of a successful orthobiologic therapy is the in-clinic patient discussion, which will educate the patient, improve compliance, and set realistic expectations. Along with the usual and mandatory explanation of the diagnosis, typical disease

[a] Kansas City Orthopedic Alliance, 10777 Nall Avenue, Suite 300, Overland Park, KS 66211, USA; [b] Elite Sports Performance Medicine, 11545 15th Avenue Northeast, Suite 105, Seattle, WA 98125, USA; [c] Bluetail Medical Group, 1875 Veterans Park Drive, Suite 2201, Naples, FL 34109, USA

* Corresponding author.
E-mail address: mjkhadavi@gmail.com

Phys Med Rehabil Clin N Am 34 (2023) 105–115
https://doi.org/10.1016/j.pmr.2022.08.008

course, and all reasonable treatments for the condition's stage, several discussion points are particularly relevant with a young and often expensive, out-of-pocket therapy.

As with any other rapidly evolving field, when introducing orthobiologic treatments into the discussion, a brief, open discussion of the current knowledge base is necessary to establish a transparent and honest relationship. Explanation of what is not known is as important as what is known. For example, no randomized controlled trials have evaluated platelet-rich plasma (PRP) in distal hamstring tendinosis, and any discussion of outcomes would involve extrapolation of findings from other trials. Similar transparency should occur when knowledge is based on expert opinion or anecdotal data. Transparency builds trust and will benefit the physician in the case of a suboptimal outcome. Furthermore, the experimental nature of such treatments should be discussed upfront with all patients before proceeding with any treatments. Patients ultimately have the autonomy to choose their treatments, and this should be respected. Setting appropriate expectations is the first step to achieving patient satisfaction.

The patient's goals will affect proper treatment selection, and the following questions must be answered:

- What are the functional needs and goals?
- What amount of pain reduction would be tolerable and worthwhile to undergo the procedure?
- What would the patient consider to be a successful outcome?
- What mechanical factors are playing a role in the patient's pain?
- What lifestyle and/or ergonomic factors are playing a role in the patient's complaint?

Expectations of post-procedural pain, rehabilitation, and functional recovery time-periods should also be addressed. As many soft-tissue procedures involve significant pain in the subsequent 3 to 5 days post-procedure, clear expectations must be set and reiterated. Written recovery timeframes with details for return-to-activity and return-to-sport will allow your patient an easier recall of the many details from the clinical discussion and likewise will ease the phone-call burden for you and your staff.

GENERAL PROCEDURAL TECHNIQUES

Although orthobiologic interventions can be learned, all of these techniques rely on a solid subspecialty skillset for musculoskeletal evaluation, expertise in ultrasound and/or fluoroscopic anatomy, and a dedication to continued learning. Although evidence for and training in ultrasound and fluoroscopic guidance techniques have grown to become mainstream, they have not been used in all studies. Nonetheless, image-guidance enhances both accuracy and safety.[1–4] While positioning yourself and the patient, it is important that the target is easily accessible and that the physician is comfortably able to perform the procedure with the image-guidance monitor in easy and close view. The straight-line view places the provider, patient, and monitor all in a line to enhance procedural accuracy and speed (**Fig. 1**). Whether a complete sterile or clean technique is used, great care must be taken during each step of the aspiration, tissue handling and processing, and injection to prevent infection. It has been suggested that needle gauge is another factor that may potentially affect PRP. It has been shown that smaller gauge needles used in blood draws can cause premature activation of platelets.[5] Because platelets release 90% of their GFs within 10 min of activation, needle gauge may therefore affect the timing of GF release and should be considered for harvest and injection.[6] To avoid unintentional activation of PLTs,

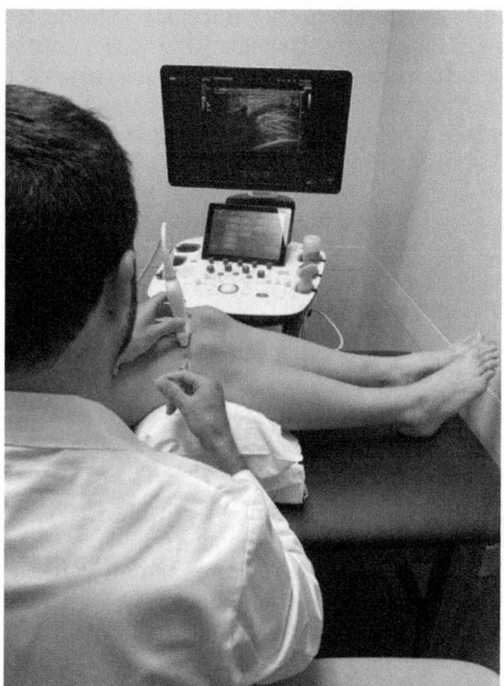

Fig. 1. With a straight line view, the physician can visualize his injection site and ultrasound monitor in a straight line.

clinicians should consider using large bore needles (21-gauge or larger) and slow aspiration during blood harvest. It is unstudied whether needle gauge is an important factor during PRP administration, but this may be a factor. Further research is needed to determine the effects of specific needle gauges on potential pre-mature platelet activation in the context of injection of PRP.

Most orthobiologic solutions can be injected through a small-gauge needle, as even the bore of a 30 gauge needle is over a hundred times the diameter of a platelet, red blood cell (RBC), white blood cell (WBC), or mesenchymal signaling cell (MSC). However, a tiny clot is more likely to clog the thinner needles, and generally a 25-gauge or larger needle is used for basic orthobiologic injections. Larger needles such as a 21 or 18 gauge may be used for tendon fenestration, and in these cases the fenestration may be performed immediately before or during the injection peppering technique.

PROCEDURAL ANESTHESIA

Although including a local anesthetic within a joint capsule is rarely needed, anyone who has injected an orthobiologic into a tendon without some form of anesthesia understands the necessity of local or regional anesthesia. Procedural pain may otherwise be intolerable during these soft-tissue procedures. Because of this need, many researchers have studied the local effects of various anesthetics on platelets, MSCs, chondrocytes, tenocytes and other local cells and tissues.

In summary, of commercially available local anesthetics, all have been shown to negatively affect tenocytes, chondrocytes, and platelets. Among them, bupivacaine appears the most and ropivacaine the least detrimental to platelet function.[7] Similarly, ropivacaine causes the least toxicity to chondrocytes and tenocytes, whereas bupivacaine has the greatest of these negative effects.[7–12] The effects of local anesthetics on outcomes of orthobiologics procedures have not yet been examined. However, based off what we know about the toxicity of anesthetics, it is recommended that the clinician use the minimum necessary local anesthetic dose in the target tissue/structure and consider the type of anesthetic used.

In the case of intratendinous, intra-osseous, and some ligamentous orthobiologic injections and procedures, a nerve block may be considered for procedural regional anesthesia as well as provide several hours of pain relief post-procedure. Although detailed regional anesthesia techniques are beyond the scope of this article, several of these image-guided blocks are worth noting.

- A tibial nerve block at the level of the ankle can be used for plantar fascia procedures (**Fig. 2**).[13]
- A tibial nerve block at the popliteal fossa for Achilles tendon procedures.[14]
- A suprascapular block for rotator cuff procedures.[15]
- A radial nerve block for common extensor tendon procedures.[16]

Bupivicaine 0.5% in a volume of 5 to 20 mL will provide a long blockade of 12 to 24 h of post-procedural anesthesia, and epinephrine may be added to prolong this blockade. Patients should be counseled on rare but potential risks of a nerve block, and cautioned on the anticipated weakness that may follow a nerve block. Post-procedure bracing and ambulatory aids should be considered to prevent inadvertent injury.

Nerve blocks can be used for intra-osseous injections without intravenous sedation. Common blocks for intraosseous orthobiologic procedures include:

- Adductor block or geniculate blocks for the knee.[17]
- Popliteal block for the ankle.[14]
- Femoral nerve branches and obturator nerve branches for the hip.[18]

Regional blocks may not anesthetize the skin, and additional local anesthesia may be necessary to anesthetize the skin and needle track. For tendons without an easily accessible peripheral nerve for regional blockage, 0.5 to 1 mL of 0.5% ropivacaine

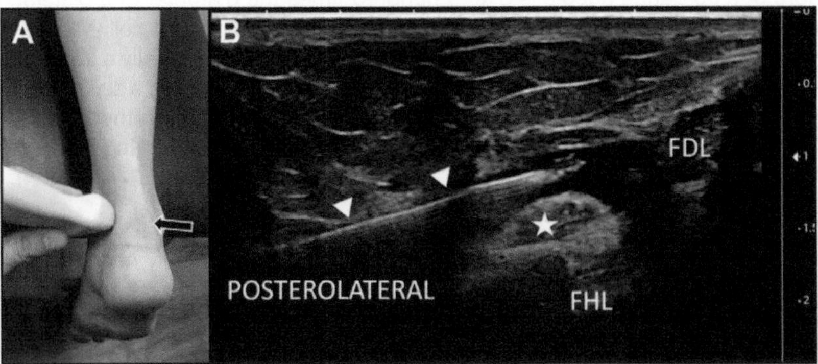

Fig. 2. Probe and needle position (*A*) of a short-axis, in-plane tibial nerve block at the ankle (*B*) with 10 mL 1% lidocaine with surrounding injection "halo." Injection was performed 15 min before a plantar fascia PRP injection. Skin and superficial needle track were also anesthetized with less than 1 mL 0.5% ropivicaine. (*FPL* flexor pollicus longus, *FHL* flexor hallucis longus; tibial nerve; needle).

injected into the target tissue with 10 to 15 min for blockade onset will improve the procedure tolerability. For a patient with anxiety, a small dose of benzodiazepine before the procedure may also be helpful.

POST-PROCEDURAL PAIN MANAGEMENT

Intratendinous, intraosseous, intradiscal, and less frequently intraligamentous orthobiologic procedures and injections will be expected to cause significant post-procedure pain during the subsequent 3 to 5 days. This should be clearly counseled during the preceding clinic visit and again immediately before the procedure to set appropriate expectations.

Although higher levels of pain typically last for 3 to 5 days, pain for longer periods is not uncommon. Several techniques may be used to lessen the pain during this painful timeframe including relative rest, superficial heat, and pain medications. Rest involves load reduction through decreased weight-bearing or immobilization of the affected body part. For example, a knee immobilizer for patellar and quadriceps tendon procedures or a wrist splint for elbow common flexor and common extensor tendon or wrist procedures may be recommended. A heat pack applied consistently throughout the day and night can lessen the intensity of pain. Lastly, medication management for this short period of time with opioid analgesia is often necessary and may be prescribed before the procedure.

This immediate 3- to 5-day post-procedural period of increased pain is often followed by a 2- to 4-week timeframe of moderate, tolerable pain. Although pain persists at an above-baseline level during these several weeks, opioids are rarely necessary after the acute post-procedural period, and acetaminophen is the preferred drug if medication management is needed. Many specialists recommend avoiding nonsteroidal anti-inflammatory drugs (NSAIDs) before

and after PRP treatment secondary to the negative effect on platelet function and, theoretically, reduction of growth factor release.[19] Previous publications have shown that NSAIDs slow the healing rate of various tissues, and therefore may be detrimental in general for healing tissues.[20] Despite the lack of data specifically examining NSAID use with PRP and considering the pharmacokinetics of most NSAIDs, it seems prudent to recommend avoiding NSAIDs at least 5 days before and for 2 weeks after PRP injection.[21]

ASPIRATION TECHNIQUES

Although some variety occurs with adipose harvesting and blood draw techniques, the most discussed and studied orthobiologic harvesting technique is for the aspiration of bone marrow. For outpatient procedures, the posterior iliac crest is most commonly preferred due to its safety and ease of access,[22] response to local anesthesia, and large reservoir of bone marrow.[23] Specifically, the posterior 4 cm of iliac crest may be preferred due to its greater width and safety, although caution must still be taken to avoid injury to the sciatic nerve, gluteal vessels, or breaching the medial or lateral boney table.[22] Frequently debated variants within the aspiration technique include the number of aspiration sites for an ideal bone marrow harvest, the depth or number of different locations of depth at each side of harvest, the volume drawn at each depth and site of bone marrow harvest, and the size of syringe used to aspirate the bone marrow. Thus far, the strongest evidence suggests higher MSC concentrations are obtained with use of multiple bone marrow aspiration sites, multiple depths at each site, with aspiration of 1 to 2 mL of bone marrow at each depth, and drawn from a 10-mL syringe in comparison to a larger syringe. Doctor Hernigou and colleagues[24] showed that the further one strays from these parameters, MSC counts decrease and the bone marrow that is aspirated during the initial draw becomes “contaminated” with blood. Moreover, other factors such as patient comfort and time necessary to complete the bone marrow harvest do play a role in this discussion. Additionally, there is growing evidence that other components of bone marrow besides MSCs contribute significantly to the regenerative and anti-inflammatory effect of our final bone marrow concentrate (BMC).[25] Even among the authors of this article, differences in technique exist. Further research to validate technique is needed to establish an optimal approach.

JOINT TECHNIQUES

A joint may be considered an “organ,” considering the extensive interplay between its many components. From this perspective, biomechanical interplay within the multiple components and compartments of the joint becomes relevant in the process of improving its function and decreasing pain.[26] For osteoarthritis of a joint, in which the whole target of orthobiologics is within the joint capsule, a simple injection into the joint capsule from a single approach may be sufficient. If, however, multiple targets are involved—either directly as a pain generator or indirectly through downstream biomechanical alterations—multiple orthobiologic injection targets may be preferred. Using the knee as an example, as injury to the knee progresses, weakening and tearing of the deep medial collateral ligament components may further destabilize the meniscus and joint as a whole.[27,28] Similarly, a subchondral injury may lead to osteoarthritis[29,30] with a negative feedback cycle that has been shown to leave the subchondral bone as both a victim and culprit. This feedback cycle can result in a cartilaginous wear and tear process of joint space narrowing often leading to subchondral edema and eventual limited nutrition to the articulate cartilage itself.[30–34] This subchondral bone plays both a structural and biomechanical role in a healthy joint function as well as contributing as a pain generator itself.[35] As discussed in prior articles (chapter 4), subchondral injection of orthobiologics has shown improved outcomes compared with intra-articular only injection in severe knee arthritis, with similar, early case series evidence in hips and other joints.[36–39] For this reason, it is increasingly common to evaluate subchondral bone with an MRI in the planning of a more precise orthobiologic procedures.

If an effusion is present, aspirating as much synovial fluid as possible will remove the inflammatory cellular and acellular components and prevent dilution of your orthobiologic treatment. Recent research has shown that there are resident stem cells within the knee joint aspiration.[40,41] However, utilization of these resident stem cells has yet to be investigated.

TENDON AND LIGAMENT TECHNIQUES

Injecting an orthobiologic solution into and around a tendon or ligament involves several considerations. As previously discussed, the utilization of local or regional anesthesia is necessary for the tolerability of most intratendinous orthobiologic procedures. Similarly, ultrasound guidance is recommended for maximal accuracy and safety during these injections.

Continued debate exists on whether tendon fenestration, often called percutaneous tenotomy, should be performed.[42,43] Although various techniques have been described, this procedure may be performed with a needle of between 17 and 23 gauge, either during or just before the orthobiologic injection, and with multiple through the site of pathology, essentially creating a new injury. Platelet concentration may also be tailored to the patient's age for maximal tenocyte proliferation,[44] and with a total volume proportional to the size of the tendon and area of pathology. Use of activators such as autologous thrombin may decrease runoff,[45] particularly in cases of tendon tearing; however, outcomes with these techniques have yet to be evaluated.

Unlike intratendinous injections, injecting into a ligament is generally less painful and requires less anesthesia and tissue fenestration. Small needle sizes such a 25 or 27 gauge can be used, and again image guidance is recommended to improve accuracy of injectate.

SPINE TECHNIQUES

As discussed in chapter 7, intradiscal therapies are supported by the most robust data of spinal orthobiologic procedures.[46,47] Secondary to the risk of iatrogenic infectious discitis,[48] particular emphasis on sterility is necessary for these procedures. In addition to sterile technique and a wide sterile field, several techniques to minimize the risk of discitis may be taken in concert, including:

- sterilization twice with chlorhexidine, allowing each to completely dry before the next step,
- the double needle technique, most commonly an 18 gauge needle placed just past the facet joint before a slightly curved and longer 22-gauge needle is then inserted until central disc placement is confirmed,
- and intradiscal injection of an antibiotic such as gentamycin.

A small dose of ropivacaine injected into the disc before or during orthobiologic injection may be considered as this procedure usually causes immediate, severe pain and stiffness. The authors have found that between 0.2 and 0.5 mL of 0.5% ropivacaine per disc is usually sufficient. Patients should be cautioned of a 3- to 5-day period of severe pain following intradiscal injection, and opioid medications may be considered.

INTRA-OSSEOUS TECHNIQUE

Intraosseous orthobiologic injection techniques have been described several times in the literature.[36–39,49] Although all studies use fluoroscopic guidance, IV sedation, and a needle of 13 gauge or larger, technique advancements have allowed these procedures to be performed in a clinic setting and without sedation.

The aforementioned regional anesthesia may replace the need for IV anesthesia for most intraosseous patients. In our experience, an 18-gauge needle with a metal stylet and centimeter markings is sufficient. For locations with thicker cortical bone such as the anterior patella and medial tibial plateau, a Tuohy needle with a metal stylet may allow for greater ease of cortical penetration without dulling the tip of the needle in the process, a phenomenon that occurs more frequently with a Quincke-type needle.

Although fluoroscopic guidance is the only type of image-guidance that has been researched for intra-osseous orthobiologic procedures, the experienced intraosseous physician may be able to target a large and shallow bone marrow lesion with pre-procedural ultrasound marking, ultrasound guidance, and a needle with measurement markings. As the portion of the needle deep to the cortex is unable to be visualized with ultrasound, small and deep lesions may be better targeted with fluoroscopic or even CT guidance (**Fig. 3**). Although studies on accuracy of intra-osseous lesion targeting with fluoroscopic guidance have not yet been performed, published outcome data are promising.[36–39,49]

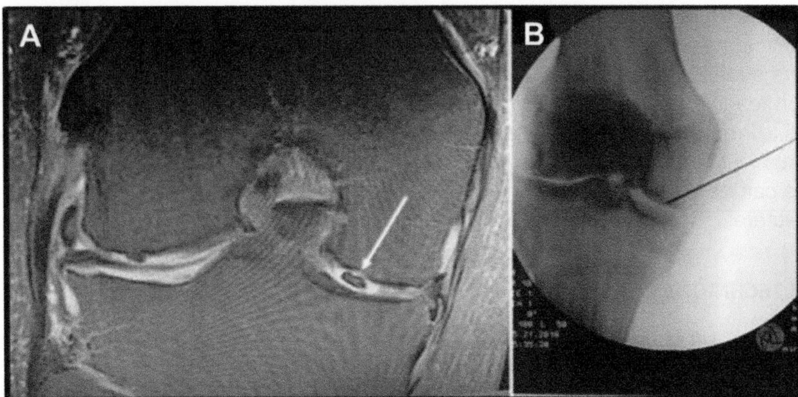

Fig. 3. T2-weighted coronal MRI knee (*A*) showing osteochondritis dissecans of the medial femoral condyle that was treated with fluoroscopically guided intraosseous, subchondral injection of BMC (*B*).

In the above-referenced intraosseous studies, between 2 and 10 mL of orthobiologic solution was injected at each subchondral site. As the approach creates an easy tunnel for our treatment solution to escape, we recommend leaving the needle in place for 5 to 10 min before withdrawal if an activator such as autologous thrombin is not subsequently injected into the tract.

SUMMARY

Orthobiologic procedures have experienced a rapid increase in evidence base in recent years, and technique standardization is yet to be achieved. As with any procedure, an extensive understanding of the regional anatomy and potential risks is essential. Local and regional anesthesia is often necessary to ensure patient comfort during the more painful procedures, such as intratendinous and intradiscal orthobiologic injections. Future outcome studies comparing aspiration techniques, needle gauge, performance of fenestration, and other technique variables are needed.

CLINICS CARE POINTS

- Set realistic expectations and define the patient's functional goals before the procedure.
- Image-guidance will enhance accuracy and safety.
- An extensive knowledge of regional at-risk anatomy is required to perform any procedure safely.
- Regional nerve blocks and local anesthetic injection into the target tissue allow most intratendinous, intradiscal, and intraosseous injections to performed in a clinic setting with minimal pain.
- When injected directly into the target tissue, ropivacaine is the least harmful of available anesthetics to tenocytes, chondrocytes, and platelets.
- Future outcome studies comparing aspiration techniques, needle gauge, performance of fenestration, and other technique variables are needed.
- Great care to prevent infectious discitis should be taken with intradiscal injections.

DISCLOSURE

M. Khadavi: consultant for Arthrex. L. Podesta: Editorial Board, Biologics Journal.

ACKNOWLEDGMENTS

The authors would like to thank Alex Roney for his assistance in the review and preparation of this article.

REFERENCES

1. Deng X, Zhu S, Li D, et al. Effectiveness of ultrasound-guided versus anatomic landmark-guided corticosteroid injection on pain, physical function and safety in patients with subacromial impingement syndrome: A systematic review and meta-analysis. Am J Phys Med Rehabil 2021. Available at. https://doi.org/10.1097/PHM.0000000000001940.
2. Fang WH, Chen XT, Vangsness CT Jr. Ultrasound-guided knee injections are more accurate than blind injections: a systematic review of randomized controlled trials. Arthrosc Sports Med Rehabil 2021;3(4):e1177–87.
3. Pourcho AM, Colio SW, Hall MM. Ultrasound-guided interventional procedures about the shoulder: anatomy, indications, and techniques. Phys Med Rehabil Clin N Am 2016;27(3):555–72.
4. Daniels EW, Cole D, Jacobs B, et al. Existing evidence on ultrasound-guided injections in sports medicine. Orthop J Sports Med 2018;6(2). 2325967118756576.
5. Lippi G, Salvagno GL, Montagnana M, et al. Influence of the needle bore size on platelet count and routine coagulation testing. Blood Coagul Fibrinolysis 2006; 17(7):557–61.
6. Andia I, Sanchez M, Maffulli N. Tendon healing and platelet-rich plasma therapies. Expert Opin Biol Ther 2010;10(10):1415–26.
7. Dregalla RC, Uribe Y, Bodor M. Effect of local anesthetics on platelet physiology and function. J Orthop Res 2021;39(12):2744–54.
8. Durant TJ, Dwyer CR, McCarthy MB, et al. Protective nature of platelet-rich plasma against chondrocyte death when combined with corticosteroids or local anesthetics. Am J Sports Med 2017;45(1):218–25.
9. Bedi A, Trinh TQ, Olszewski AM, et al. Nonbiologic injections in sports medicine. JBJS Rev 2020;8(2):e0052.
10. Piper SL, Laron D, Manzano G, et al. A comparison of lidocaine, ropivacaine and dexamethasone toxicity on bovine tenocytes in culture. J Bone Joint Surg Br 2012;94(6):856–62.
11. Zhang AZ, Ficklscherer A, Gülecyüz MF, et al. Cell toxicity in fibroblasts, tenocytes, and human mesenchymal stem cells-a comparison of necrosis and apoptosis-inducing ability in ropivacaine, bupivacaine, and triamcinolone. Arthroscopy 2017;33(4):840–8, published correction appears in Arthroscopy. 2021 Apr;37(4):1357.
12. Jayaram P, Kennedy DJ, Yeh P, et al. Chondrotoxic effects of local anesthetics on human knee articular cartilage: a systematic review. PM R 2019;11(4):379–400.
13. Redborg KE, Antonakakis JG, Beach ML, et al. Ultrasound improves the success rate of a tibial nerve block at the ankle. Reg Anesth Pain Med 2009;34(3):256–60.
14. Delbos A, Philippe M, Clément C, et al. Ultrasound-guided ankle block. History revisited. Best Pract Res Clin Anaesthesiol 2019;33(1):79–93.
15. Harmon D, Hearty C. Ultrasound-guided suprascapular nerve block technique. Pain Physician 2007;10(6):743–6.

16. Sehmbi H, Madjdpour C, Shah UJ, et al. Ultrasound guided distal peripheral nerve block of the upper limb: a technical review. J Anaesthesiol Clin Pharmacol 2015;31(3):296–307.
17. Vora MU, Nicholas TA, Kassel CA, et al. Adductor canal block for knee surgical procedures: review article. J Clin Anesth 2016;35:295–303.
18. Short AJ, Barnett JJG, Gofeld M, et al. Anatomic study of innervation of the anterior hip capsule: implication for image-guided intervention. Reg Anesth Pain Med 2018;43(2):186–92.
19. Scharf RE. Drugs that affect platelet function. Semin Thromb Hemost 2012;38(8): 865–83.
20. Su B, O'Connor JP. NSAID therapy effects on healing of bone, tendon, and the enthesis. J Appl Physiol (1985) 2013;115(6):892–9.
21. Shi S, Klotz U. Clinical use and pharmacological properties of selective COX-2 inhibitors. Eur J Clin Pharmacol 2008;64(3):233–52.
22. Hernigou J, Picard L, Alves A, et al. Understanding bone safety zones during bone marrow aspiration from the iliac crest: the sector rule. Int Orthop 2014; 38(11):2377–84.
23. Hirahara AM, Panero A, Andersen WJ. An MRI Analysis of the Pelvis to Determine the Ideal Method for Ultrasound-Guided Bone Marrow Aspiration from the Iliac Crest. Am J Orthop (Belle Mead NJ) 2018;47(5). https://doi.org/10.12788/ajo.2018.0038.
24. Hernigou P, Homma Y, Flouzat Lachaniette CH, et al. Benefits of small volume and small syringe for bone marrow aspirations of mesenchymal stem cells. Int Orthop 2013;37(11):2279–87.
25. Ziegler CG, Van Sloun R, Gonzalez S, et al. Characterization of growth factors, cytokines, and chemokines in bone marrow concentrate and platelet-rich plasma: a prospective analysis. Am J Sports Med 2019;47(9):2174–87.
26. Tucker JD, Goetz LL, Duncan MB, et al. Randomized, placebo-controlled analysis of the knee synovial environment following platelet-rich plasma treatment for knee osteoarthritis. PM R 2021;13(7):707–19.
27. Paletta GA Jr, Crane DM, Konicek J, et al. Surgical treatment of meniscal extrusion: a biomechanical study on the role of the medial meniscotibial ligaments with early clinical validation. Orthop J Sports Med 2020;8(7). 2325967120936672.
28. Smith PA, Humpherys JL, Stannard JP, et al. Impact of medial meniscotibial ligament disruption compared to peripheral medial meniscal tear on knee biomechanics. J Knee Surg 2021;34(7):784–92.
29. Linden B. Osteochondritis dissecans of the femoral condyles: a long-term follow-up study. J Bone Joint Surg Am 1977;59(6):769–76.
30. Kon E, Ronga M, Filardo G, et al. Bone marrow lesions and subchondral bone pathology of the knee. Knee Surg Sports Traumatol Arthrosc 2016;24(6): 1797–814.
31. Madry H, van Dijk CN, Mueller-Gerbl M. The basic science of the subchondral bone. Knee Surg Sports Traumatol Arthrosc 2010;18(4):419–33.
32. Johnson DL, Urban WP Jr, Caborn DN, et al. Articular cartilage changes seen with magnetic resonance imaging-detected bone bruises associated with acute anterior cruciate ligament rupture. Am J Sports Med 1998;26(3):409–14.
33. Johnson TC, Evans JA, Gilley JA, et al. Osteonecrosis of the knee after arthroscopic surgery for meniscal tears and chondral lesions. Arthroscopy 2000; 16(3):254–61.
34. Muscolo DL, Costa-Paz M, Ayerza M, et al. Medial meniscal tears and spontaneous osteonecrosis of the knee. Arthroscopy 2006;22(4):457–60.

35. Li G, Yin J, Gao J, et al. Subchondral bone in osteoarthritis: insight into risk factors and microstructural changes. Arthritis Res Ther 2013;15(6):223.
36. Sánchez M, Delgado D, Pompei O, et al. Treating severe knee osteoarthritis with combination of intra-osseous and intra-articular infiltrations of platelet-rich plasma: an observational study. Cartilage 2019;10(2):245–53.
37. Hernigou P, Auregan JC, Dubory A, et al. Subchondral stem cell therapy versus contralateral total knee arthroplasty for osteoarthritis following secondary osteonecrosis of the knee. Int Orthop 2018;42(11):2563–71.
38. Muiños-López E, Delgado D, Sánchez P, et al. Modulation of synovial fluid-derived mesenchymal stem cells by intra-articular and intraosseous platelet rich plasma administration. Stem Cells Int 2016;2016:1247950.
39. Fiz N, Delgado D, Garate A, et al. Intraosseous infiltrations of platelet-rich plasma for severe hip osteoarthritis: a pilot study. J Clin Orthop Trauma 2020;11(Suppl 4):S585–90.
40. Fellows CR, Matta C, Zakany R, et al. Adipose, bone marrow and synovial joint-derived mesenchymal stem cells for cartilage repair. Front Genet 2016;7:213.
41. McGonagle D, Baboolal TG, Jones E. Native joint-resident mesenchymal stem cells for cartilage repair in osteoarthritis. Nat Rev Rheumatol 2017;13(12):719–30.
42. Finnoff JT, Fowler SP, Lai JK, et al. Treatment of chronic tendinopathy with ultrasound-guided needle tenotomy and platelet-rich plasma injection. PM R 2011;3(10):900–11.
43. Krey D, Borchers J, McCamey K. Tendon needling for treatment of tendinopathy: a systematic review. Phys Sportsmed 2015;43(1):80–6.
44. Berger DR, Centeno CJ, Steinmetz NJ. Platelet lysates from aged donors promote human tenocyte proliferation and migration in a concentration-dependent manner. Bone Joint Res 2019;8(1):32–40.
45. Matuska AM, Klimovich MK, Chapman JR. An ethanol-free autologous thrombin system. J Extra Corpor Technol 2018;50(4):237–43.
46. Tuakli-Wosornu YA, Terry A, Boachie-Adjei K, et al. Lumbar intradiskal platelet-rich plasma (PRP) injections: a prospective, double-blind, randomized controlled study. PM R 2016;8(1):1–10.
47. Navani A, Manchikanti L, Albers SL, et al. Responsible, safe, and effective use of biologics in the management of low back pain: american society of interventional pain physicians (ASIPP) guidelines. Pain Physician 2019;22(1S):S1–74.
48. Jerome MA, Lutz C, Lutz GE. Risks of intradiscal orthobiologic injections: a review of the literature and case series presentation. Int J Spine Surg 2021;15(s1):26–39.
49. Nevalainen MT, Repo JP, Pesola M, et al. Successful treatment of early talar osteonecrosis by core decompression combined with intraosseous stem cell injection: a case report. J Orthop Case Rep 2018;8(1):23–6.

Intradiscal Leukocyte Rich Platelet Rich Plasma for Degenerative Disc Disease

Gregory E. Lutz, MD

KEYWORDS

- Degenerative disc disease • Chronic low back pain • Intradiscal Leukocyte-rich PRP
- Intradiscal PRP

KEY POINTS

- CLBP is an unhealed wound.
- Bacteria play a role in degenerative disc disease.
- Leukocyte-rich PRP is a root cause treatment.

INTRODUCTION

If we could choose a single non-fatal medical condition to find a better solution that would make the greatest impact on global health it would be a solution for degenerative disc disease (DDD) - the number one cause of chronic low back pain (CLBP).

According to the numbers, low back pain is a pandemic; a condition that is prevalent globally, affecting millions of people throughout the world. In 2017 the *Global Burden of Disease* (GBD) study reported that the point prevalence (the number of people in the world at one point in time) of activity-limiting lower back pain about 580 million people worldwide—and chronic, low back pain is now regarded as the number one cause of disability globally.[1] This is the most comprehensive analysis of 354 medical conditions from 195 countries for over nearly three decades from 1990 to 2017. Not only was CLBP the number one cause of Years Lived with Disability (YLDs) recently, it has been the number one cause every year since 1990 and its incidence is only increasing with time.

The numbers reported are staggering in the US: as many as seventy million Americans have chronic lower back pain today. An estimated 80% of all Americans will experience disabling lower back pain at some point in their lifetime. What was thought of as a benign condition, really is not. Many patients have chronic recurrent episodes of LBP that just keep getting worse over time. In one study from 2012, researchers

Hospital for Special Surgery, Weill Medical College of Cornell University, Regenerative SportsCare Institute, 62 East 88th Street, New York, NY 10128, USA
E-mail address: lutzg@regensportscare.com

Phys Med Rehabil Clin N Am 34 (2023) 117–133
https://doi.org/10.1016/j.pmr.2022.08.009

published a study in *Physical Medicine and Rehabilitation* that tried to study this issue by surveying thirty different practitioners from a variety of specialties including physical therapists, chiropractors, and surgeons to look at the disease progression of CLBP in 600 new patients.[2] Here's what they found:

35% said their back pain required more than 3 months to improve.
54% reported more than ten episodes of severe, disabling back pain.
20% reported more than fifty episodes of severe, disabling back pain.

An epidemic is a condition that affects a large number of people within a region, and we have been dealing with an opioid epidemic here in the United States (US). Our mismanagement of LBP has only contributed to this problem; in the US, opioids are the most commonly prescribed drug class for patients with LBP and the rates of opioid prescribing is two to three times higher than in most European countries.[3] This is despite evidence that opioids, if they are to be used for managing LBP, should only be used for acute pain and for a short duration of time (a few days at most). There are no studies that support the long-term use of opioids for managing LBP.

Complications of addiction and overdose have risen in parallel with increased prescription rates for LBP. According to the CDC, from 1999 to 2019, nearly 500,000 people have died from opioid overdose involving both illicit and prescription uses.[4] More than 11.5 million Americans reported misusing prescription opioids in 2016.[5] In 2019, more than half of all global overdose deaths occurred in the US.[6] Unfortunately, this trend has only increased; last year overdose deaths from drug overdoses hit an all time high at over 100,000 from both illicit and prescription-based causes. While there are many factors that contributed to these numbers, the liberal prescribing of opioids for patients with CLBP has contributed greatly to this public health crisis. The need for opioid-sparing treatments for patients with CLBP has never been greater.

Having spent a large portion of my professional career at one of the busiest orthopedic hospitals in the world, I have unfortunately seen many patients with complications from spinal surgery. Many of these patients never had taken opioids but were started on them at the time of their surgery to manage their post-operative pain. Failing to achieve adequate pain relief from their surgery, their providers just kept prescribing opioid medications month after month. In a recent meta-analysis of patients after lumbar fusion surgery, investigators found that up to 63% of these patients were on long-term opioids (for > 3 months).[7]

This study also showed that opioid-naive patients were at increased risk for long-term opioids after their fusion surgery. What is equally concerning is, despite these poor outcomes, that the number of these types of lumbar fusions for degenerative conditions has increased according to one study 276% from 2002 to 2014.[8] Think about the millions of people suffering from their CLBP who then become dependent on opioids because we have either mismanaged their treatment with ineffectual nonsurgical treatments or potentially made them worse with surgery.

Drugs and surgery have not been the cure we have been seeking for the majority of patients with CLBP. The economic consequences are not just significant for the individual who fails to get back to gainful employment, but also for our healthcare system as a whole. In 2011 the respected National Academcy of Medicine estimated that just in the US the total direct and indirect costs of managing chronic pain, from all musculoskeletal conditions, to our economy ranges between $560 and $630 billion annually.[9]

Unfortunately, there has been low investment in research to find a cure for CLBP because many are unaware of its severity as most people do not die from it. The US National Institute of Health budget for research on cardiovascular diseases and cancer is dramatically larger than its budget for musculoskeletal conditions ($8.6

Billion combined vs only $754 million in 2018). In 2016 MSK disorders were the largest health expenditures in the US at $380 billion.[10] We spend more money treating MSK conditions than heart disease, diabetes, or cancer, but less than 10% of our research dollars are allocated to finding a cure for them?

The economic consequences of this irrational strategy are significant not just for the US, but for other countries around the world. The increased burden of non-fatal diseases such as CLBP on healthcare systems worldwide is posing considerable challenges to all healthcare systems not equipped to care for such complex and expensive conditions. While healthcare systems have made advancements in the management of fatal diseases, we have not made meaningful advancements in managing "non-fatal" conditions such as CLBP.

We need to reframe our thinking about the root causes of CLBP, and target our treatments directly at them if we want to truly find a cure. We need simple, safe, cost-effective, scalable treatments that are durable in their effect. Healthcare systems need to shift their approach to musculoskeletal diseases away from volume-based palliative treatments to value-based root cause treatments that create sustained improvements. Intradiscal leukocyte-rich platelet-rich plasma (LR-PRP) has the potential to be a value-based root cause treatment for many patients with symptomatic lumbar disc disease.

Getting to the Root Causes of Degenerative Disc Disease

There is mounting scientific evidence that chronic low back pain is nothing more than an unhealed wound inside the disc that frequently gets infected. When the disc tears it can become infected with a certain type of bacteria that impedes the healing process further called *Cutibacterium Acnes (C. Acnes).*[11] Proper wound healing requires the migration of cells to the wound. Since the disc is the largest avascular structure in the body, its inherent capacity to heal after injury is poor.

The low blood supply to the disc is also why most medical and surgical treatments for it fail to provide sustained relief. They are not addressing the underlying root causes of DDD.[12] When a disc develops a tear that doesn't heal the wound can continue to propagate causing the disc to bulge. The bulge then begins to protrude if not addressed, the protrusion then can go on to a disc extrusion or even a disc fragment in the spinal canal. By this stage, the disc has degenerated and that segment of the spine can no longer function properly. Loading of that spinal segment begins to shift elsewhere.

The downward spiral can continue to get worse from here, and this is what we refer to as the "degenerative disc cascade" (**Fig. 1**).[13] The degenerative cascade demonstrates the importance of acting early with a regenerative treatment that heals the disc so that this downward spiral can be avoided. As you can see, wound healing is a necessary and dynamic process for restoring the normal architecture and functionality of tissue.

The downward spiral can continue to get worse from here, and this is what we refer to as the "degenerative disc cascade."[14] The degenerative disc cascade demonstrates the importance of acting early with a regenerative treatment that heals the disc so that this downward spiral can potentially be prevented.

The Role Bacteria Play in Degenerative Disc Disease

A microbiome is an environment of trillions of microorganisms also called microbiota or microbes.[15] These can be a collection of thousands of different species of bacteria, fungi, parasites, and/or viruses that live in harmony when you are healthy, but when out of balance can be harmful. This is referred to as "dysbiosis." Scientists are just

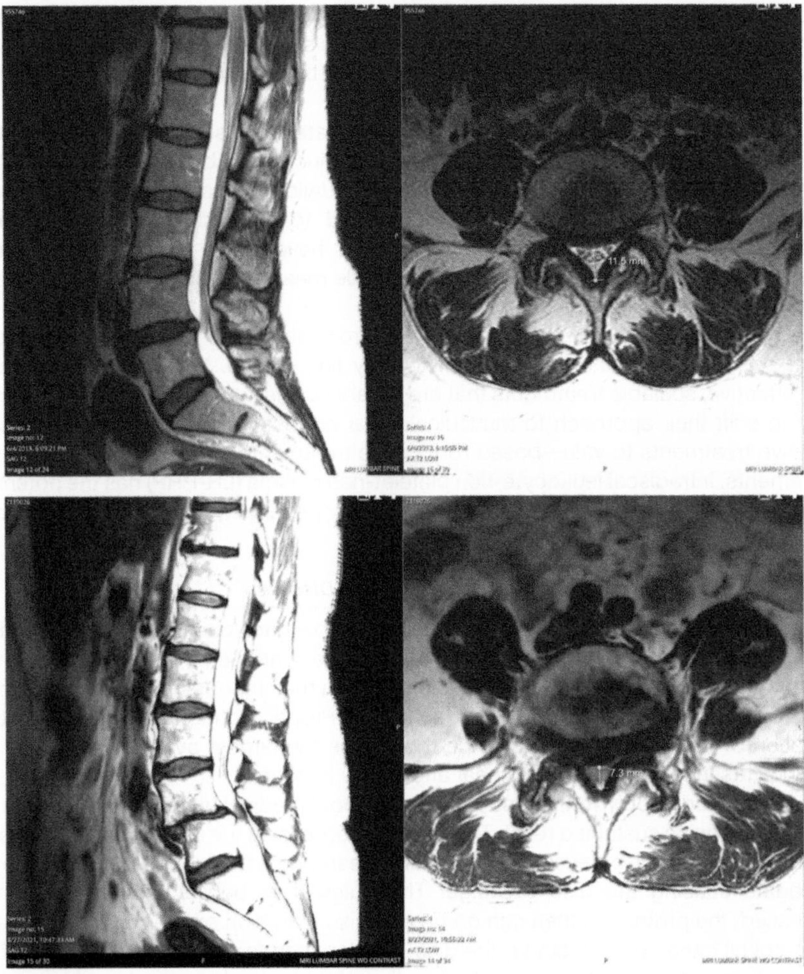

Fig. 1. These are MRI images of a patient of mine demonstraiting the "degenerative cascade." The MRI images on the left are T2- sagittal images of the lumbar spine and on the right are T2-axial images through the L4-5 level. The two MRI images on the top are from 2013. The two MRI images on the bottom are from 2021. Notice how the L4-5 disc has completely degenerated over timecausing progressive narrowing of the spinal canal (spinal stenosis).

realizing the importance of the microbiome not only for your overall health but also with regard to DDD.

A recent study out of Sweden looked at the role the intradiscal microbiome might play in degenerative disc disease.[16] The study examined 162 patients who experienced chronic, low back pain and had particular changes in their MRI (referred to as Modic Type 1 changes (MC1)). In a double-blind randomized controlled study (DB RCT), they separated the patients into two groups and gave one group a 6-month course of oral antibiotics and the other group a placebo. The subset of patients that received the antibiotics improved to a greater degree than the control group. Their findings suggested bacteria may be playing a greater role in the pain caused by degenerative disc disease than we have previously realized.

This issue was also studied in patients having spinal surgery where they harvested disc material, whether from a herniation or degeneration and cultured that material to see if any bacteria would grow. Sure enough, study after study showed that bacteria grew on the disc material and the most common bacteria was *C. Acnes.* At first investigators thought that this was from contamination, but that has later been refuted. The presence of *C. Acnes* infecting extruded and degenerative discs has been unequivocally demonstrated now by more sophisticated testing measures.

In 2016, a group of researchers in China, actually took bacteria (*C. Acnes)* harvested from human disc surgical samples and injected it into rabbit discs to see its effects.[17] When they examined the discs by MRI and under the microscope weeks later, these injected discs demonstrated exactly the same findings you see with degenerative disc disease and MC1.

So why not treat CLBP patients with oral antibiotics? There are a number of valid reasons:

1. The question of whether or not bacteria in the disc represents infection or contamination?
2. Contradictory reports on the efficacy of antibiotics to treat CLBP patients.
3. The potential that widespread use of systemic antibiotics would result in emerging global antimicrobial resistance and the perceived risk of propagating superbugs.
4. Systemic antibiotics can adversely affect your gut's microbiome creating other negative health consequences. Patients in these studies had to take the antibiotic for 100 days.
5. The penetration of oral antibiotics that rely on blood flow to get to the disc is unreliable.

If we view CLBP as an unhealed wound inside the disc that often becomes contaminated with bacteria, you can see how our previous treatments have been off the mark. With LR-PRP we are injecting billions of platelets with thousands of healing growth factors into the disc tissue to stimulate the wound healing process. We are also injecting millions of white blood cells that may also be suppressing the overgrowth of harmful *C. Acnes* or other bacteria that have penetrated those tears.

A Potential Regenerative Medicine Solution for Degenerative Disc Disease

What is regenerative medicine? According to the National Institutes of Health (NIH) it is an emerging area of science that holds great promise for treating and even curing a variety of injuries and diseases by using stem cells and other technologies to repair or replace damaged cells, tissues, or organs. However, it's not just about stem cells. There are many healing cells and proteins in your body that can stimulate your natural healing processes. Regenerative medicine offers not only the hope of a cure for degenerative disc disease, but also a potentially sustainable solution to the most common, most expensive, and most disabling condition globally: DDD. While there are many clinicians investigating a variety of intradiscal biologics, LR-PRP has the most compelling scientific evidence. It has also been the safest and most effective intradiscal biologic we have used in our CLBP patients.

In 2006, researchers at Rush Medical College in Chicago were the first to show that PRP had a beneficial effect on stimulating disc cells.[18] Scientists made PRP from pig's blood and then took their disc cells and cultured them in the lab in a broth of PRP where they measured its effects on cell metabolism. They demonstrated that PRP could stimulate the cells of the disc to turn on and produce collagen. The effect of the PRP was greater on the cells of the annulus fibrosus (AF) than the nucleus pulposus (NP).

At Tapei Medical University in Taiwan,[19] researchers also studied the effects of PRP on human disc cells taken from healthy volunteers. They cultured these cells in PRP and again measured its potential beneficial effects in the lab. Not only were these researchers the first to show the beneficial effects PRP could have on human disc cell metabolism, but they also demonstrated that PRP could decrease the rate of apoptosis. These promising studies showed that PRP caused beneficial effects on cell proliferation (coming to the wound), increased cell metabolism (producing proteins to repair the wound), and decreased cell death (keeping the disc healthy). In addition, researchers also showed that PRP could reduce the number of harmful pro-inflammatory cytokines in the disc that was responsible for pain and degeneration.

Pre-clinical studies like these gave us the support needed to embark on a clinical outcome study. We knew that PRP was not a treatment for every type of CLBP, so we set up very strict inclusion and exclusion criteria for our clinical study. We wanted to specifically study patients suffering from chronic, low back pain as a result of painful annular tears—internal disc disruption (IDD).

Severe disabling back pain that was unresponsive to conservative treatment.

Patients who otherwise would be candidates for a spinal fusion.

Once selected, we performed a discogram to confirm that their disc was the source of their pain and then randomized them into one of two groups: patients who received PRP after the contrast in the discogram and patients who received a placebo, which was just more contrast alone (**Fig. 2**). Then over an initial period of 2 months, we tracked their responses with an independent observer: degree of pain relief, functional improvement, and patient satisfaction. In total, we tracked forty-nine patients. For every two patients who received the PRP one patient was in the control group.

We also added a crossover group, after 2 months if the patient did not see improvement, we unblinded them. If they had received the control and had not improved, we then offered them the intradiscal PRP treatment.[20] In the first 2 months, patients who received the PRP were showing significant improvements in pain and function,

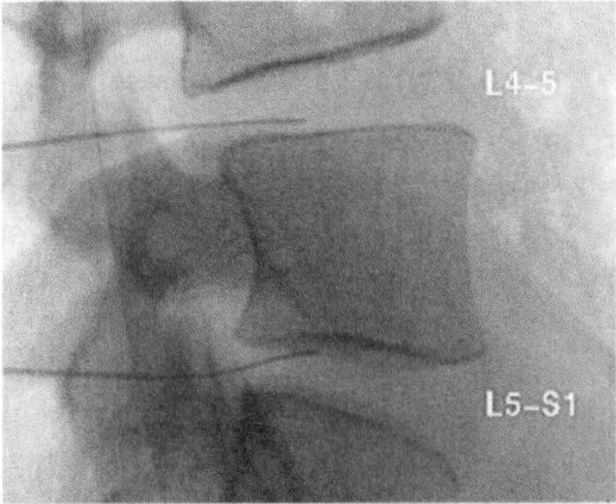

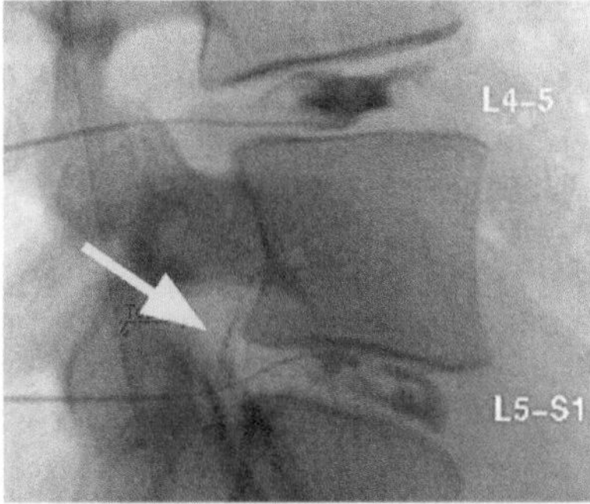

Fig. 2. The fluoroscopic images on the left are the needles placed into the two lower discs(L4-5 and L5-S1) without contrast injection. The images on the right are after contrast injection (black fluid inside the disc).In a normal discogram the contrast should stay in the center of the disc (the nucleus pulposus) and not leak out (L4-5 is normal). If you look closely at the lower disc there is a faint black line of contrast (arrow) outlining the back of the disc that represents a tear of that disc (L5-S1). If the patient experiences similar pain to what they normally have (what is referred to as concordant pain) when we see that tear fill with contrast then that is an abnormal discogram. The discogram helps us confirm the diagnosis of what is referred to as internal disc disruption when the MRI is inconclusive. In our study patients were then randomized to receive either mmore contrast or LR-PRP.

whereas the control group was not. Further, our patients who had been in the control group and then unblinded also saw significant improvement when they crossed over into the treatment group and received the PRP. We then followed the treated patients for years and surprisingly the majority of patients continued to do well from a single intradiscal injection of their PRP.[21,22]

We frequently analyze the MRIs of patients that we have treated. In many of the PRP-treated patients the tears improved significantly or disappeared within months of treatment (**Figs. 3** and **4**). Out of the 49 patients enrolled in the study, only six went on to a spinal fusion. So intradiscal LR-PRP effectively decreased the fusion rate by roughly 80% in this group of patients.

Since our initial DB RCT study in 2016, it has been encouraging to witness other investigators from around the world publishing similar encouraging results.[23–25] Akeda and colleagues recently published another DB RCT comparing intradiscal platelet release to corticosteroid injections in patients with degenerative disc disease. While there are several limitations to this study (no control, only 16 patients, corticosteroid injected with 2 mL saline, not an LR-PRP, no statistical difference in outcome), they found that over a 60-week period the PRP group did experience a greater degree of pain relief and functional improvement. This makes intradiscal PRP the only orthobiologic treatment option with two supportive DB RCT studies.

There was, however, a very recent single-blind randomized controlled study of intradiscal PRP that did not show a significant difference between the treatment group and the control group. If wecritically analyze this study, there were some serious flaws in their methodology that I believe confounded their conclusion that intradiscal PRP was no better than their control: they used a leukocyte- poor PRP, they injected only a small amount (1 cc) of a low platelet concentration PRP, they did not quantify what they injected, they did not use contrast to demonstrate flow into the annular tears, they used saline and antibiotics as the control, and they excluded a very important subset of patients (Modic 1 changes) from their study.

In our experience, it is exactly that subset of patients that have responded the best to intradiscal LR-PRP. In addition, using saline and antibiotics really are not a negative control. These agents have an antibacterial effect that may have improved some of the patients in the control group thereby confounding their results. The type of PRP used to treat degenerative disc disease really does matter. There continues to be a need for more rigorous research on intradiscal PRP for patients with degenerative disc disease.

While overall, the results we were achieving with intradiscal LR-PRP were impressive, there were still a fair number of patients that did not improve—roughly 40%.

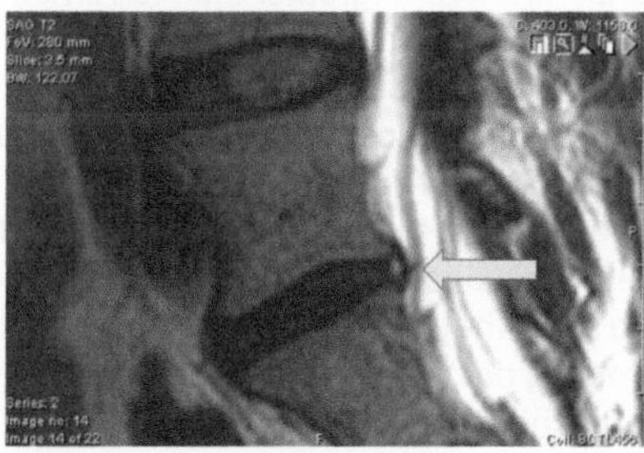

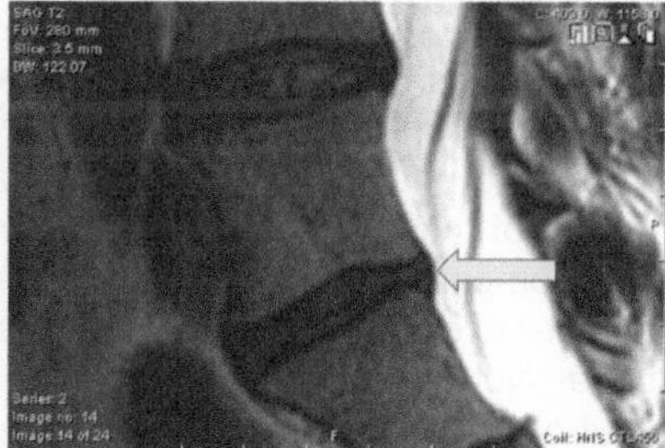

Fig. 3. These are magnified MRI images of lumbar spine from a side view (T2-sagittal images). The image on the left is before PRP treatment and shows a white line in the back of the disc (called a high-intensity zone (HIZ)). The HIZ on the MIR represents a tear inside the disc. The image on the right shows the HIZ healed 3 months after PRP treatment.

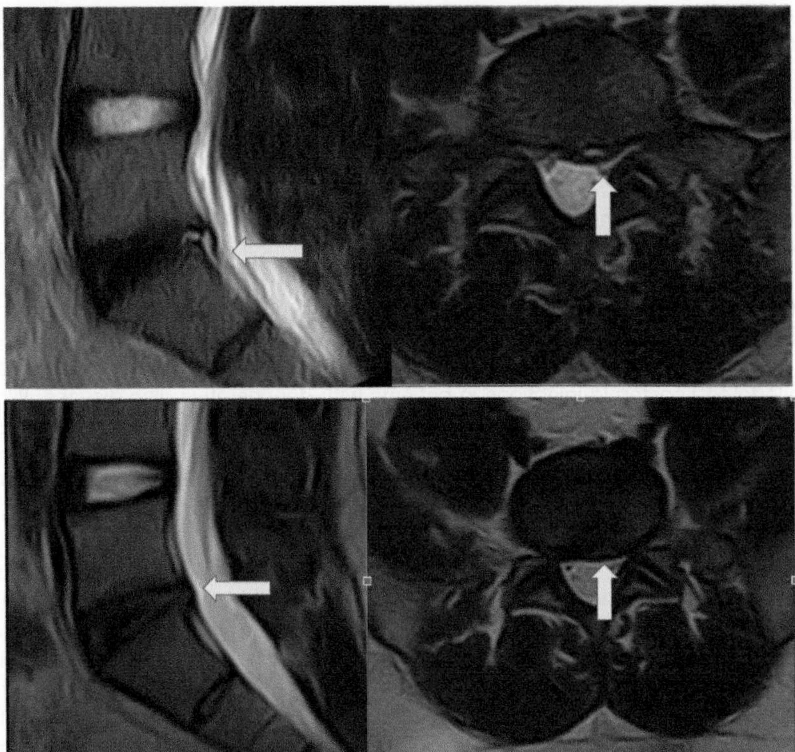

Fig. 4. These are magnified T2 sagittal and axial MRI images of lumbar spine from a patient who received intradiscal LR-PRP treatment. The images on top are before treatment and the images on the bottom are from 3 months after LR-PRP treatment. The images reveal structural improvement in the large annular fissure and a reduction in the size of the left-sided protrusion

During our first clinical study, we concentrated the platelets in our PRP preparation to approximately five times the normal baseline concentration. It seemed logical that more platelets would translate into a higher delivery of healing growth factors, but we needed to test that hypothesis: Could patients with more severe disc disease just require a greater degree of growth factors to obtain pain relief?

We found that we could achieve platelet concentrations of greater than ten times the patients' baseline—sometimes even higher—on a consistent basis by simply lowering the volume of plasma.[26] We then looked retrospectively at the number of patients we had treated over the past few years with this higher concentration PRP and found about forty-five patients who were over a year out. We were able to get data on thirty-seven of those patients, which is an acceptable follow-up rate of over 80%. Then we compared their results—pain relief, functional improvement, and patient satisfaction—to our historic DB RCT results to see if they were equal, worse, or potentially better. Not only did we see greater degrees of pain relief and functional improvement, but our patient satisfaction rates now reached over 80%.[27]

Unfortunately one of the patients in the study had a complication of a spinal infection.[28] She was infected with the same bacteria that you have already learned about - *C. Acnes.* In our attempt to concentrate the platelets to higher levels some patients received a leukocyte-poor PRP, and this is what happened in that patient. She had to be treated with a prolonged course of intravenous antibiotics to recover and the infection destroyed that disc. So her case prompted us to go even further in our research to see what type of PRP is the safest.

Leukocyte-Rich PRP: Are We Killing Two Birds with One Stone?

We wanted to see what more we could do to reduce the risk so that the potential benefits of this promising new procedure would significantly outweigh the potential risks. We already knew from the literature and our own personal experience that *C. Acnes* was the culprit in many of the infections associated with intradiscal biologic procedures.[29] So we went back to the lab and cultured the *C. Acnes* bacteria in different types of PRP - leukocyte rich versus leukocyte poor. We cultured the bacteria for up to 48 hours and found that indeed the LR-PRP created greater kill rates than the LP-PRP (**Fig. 5**).[28] Now we have more evidence for what we believe to be not only the most effective type of PRP for degenerative disc disease but also potentially the safest. Our clinical experience reflects this finding. In more than 1000 disc injection procedures, we have not had any infections thus far using an LR-PRP inside the disc.

I believe we may actually be killing two birds with one stone with our intradiscal LR-PRP. Not only are we igniting the body's natural healing response in the disc, but the high levels of white blood cells in the PRP may also be suppressing the overgrowth of certain types of bacteria associated with disc degeneration.

A 32-year-old woman who presented to my office with severe LBP that had not responded to traditional treatments. What was unusual about her history was that she couldn't attribute the onset of her pain to any specific event. She rated the pain as an 8 out of 10. She had a 2-year-old daughter that she was having a difficult time caring for because she couldn't lift her. So we obtained an MRI of her lumbar spine to see what was going on. It revealed two degenerative discs with significant Modic Type I changes (MC1).

She had already failed oral medications, chiropractic care, acupuncture, and an epidural steroid injection gave only short-term pain relief. Spinal surgery she said

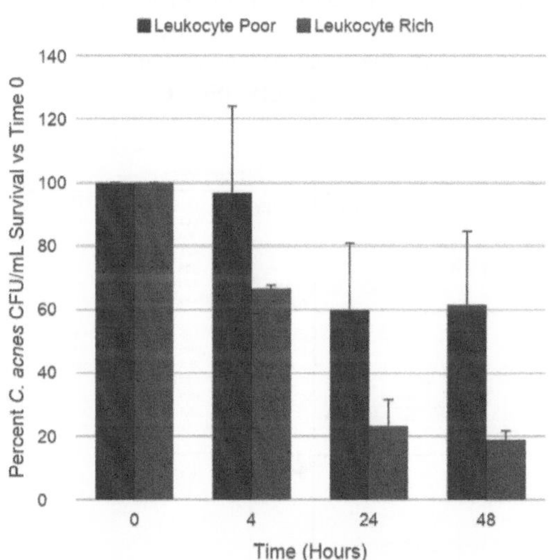

Fig. 5. Graph representing the change in C. Acnes survival over time in LR-PRP vs LP-PRP. LR-PRP creating a greater degree of suppression of C. Acnes growth in-vitro.

was a last resort. So we discussed the pros and cons of intradiscal LR-PRP in her case and she agreed to the procedure.

Working with an industry partner we have been able to develop a new PRP system that is now able to concentrate the platelets and white blood cells to higher levels than the best available commercial PRP system on the market. So to give you an idea of the powerful cocktail we are injecting, we injected over 5 billion platelets and 100 million white blood cells (WBCs) into each of her discs. Think about the 1000s of healing proteins in the platelets and the antibacterial power of the WBCs exactly where they are needed. Finally, a root cause treatment for so many patients with CLBP looking for a better alternative than spinal fusion surgery (**Fig. 6**).

At first, her pain was worse from the pressure of the injection into a painful structure and the inflammatory response these cells cause in the first few days, but within weeks she started to improve. When we repeated the MRI 3 months later and not only was the majority of her pain gone, so were those MC1 changes (**Fig. 7**).

We have treated many patients with Modic 1 changes. I do believe we may be killing two birds with one stone and that is why an intradiscal injection of an LR-PRP is the potential solution we have been searching for to treat DDD. So now that we've identified what we believe to be the safest, most effective intradiscal biologic - how else can we potentially improve patient outcomes?

Precision Cell Delivery

One of the things I have learned over the past three decades of performing interventional spinal procedures is that you need to deliver the therapeutic agent as close to the problem as possible to create the greatest benefit. Even with an epidural steroid injection, the best effects are when it is placed precisely between the inflamed disc and nerve root.

The problem when we perform an intradiscal injection is that we are placing a straight needle into a round structure. When we think about where most of the painful tears are, they are in the periphery of the disc. So we are often unable to get a straight needle into that area consistently. Most of the time the needle is placed in the middle of the disc and then we inject and hope that the LR-PRP flows into these tears. Hope is not a strategy we like in medicine. We prefer to have a reliable means of precisely placing the cells as closely into the tears as possible so with an industry partner we developed the first intradiscal curved catheter (**Fig. 8**).

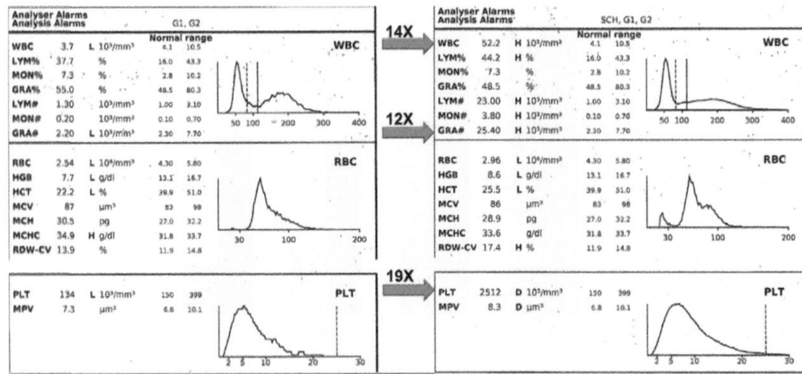

Fig. 6. Hemocytometer measurements of baseline peripheral blood and final LR-PRP concentrations.

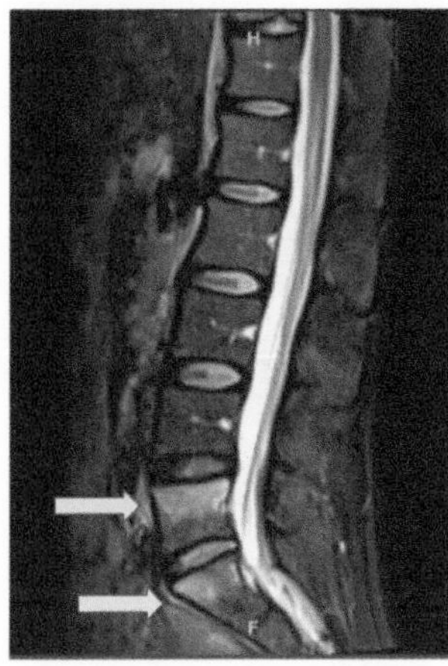

SIGNIFICANT
IMPROVEMENT
IN MC1
CHANGES AND
CLINICAL
SYMPTOMS
AFTER
INTRADISCAL
LR-PRP L4-5 &
L5-S1

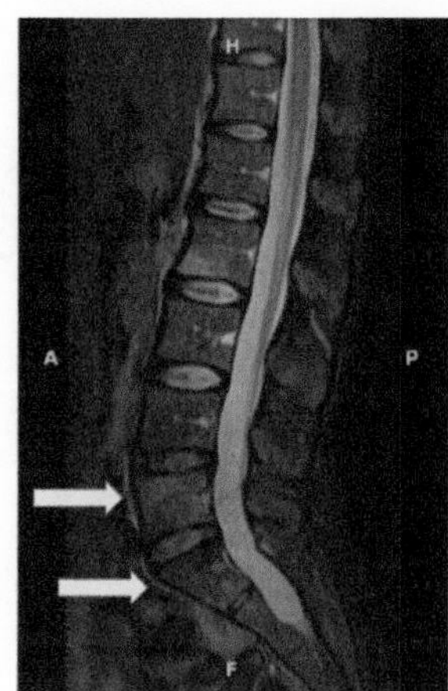

Fig. 7. T2 sagittal MRI images pre and postintradiscal LR-PRP demonstrating improvement in the Modic 1 changes

In our first in-human test, we used it on a 62-year-old gentleman with an 8 year history of low back pain in his right leg who failed conservative treatments. His MRI from 2013 revealed a right foraminal HIZ at L4-5 which was unchanged in his most recent MRI from 2022 (**Fig. 9**). Three months posttreatment not only were his symptoms completely resolved, but there were documented structural changes in his MRI that showed the resolution of the HIZ (**Fig. 10**). What was so interesting about this case were the almost immediate annular changes that occurred within 4 weeks of the intradiscal injection (**Fig. 11**).

A Promising Future

Chronic back pain is usually nothing more than an unhealed wound that can be colonized with a certain types of bacteria that can further contribute to degeneration of the disc. Intradiscal LR-PRP is one of our first treatment options that actually targets directly the root causes of CLBP for many. Treatments that just relieve pain and do not create healing structural changes are only palliative, not curative. This is a complete paradigm shift in how we are managing CLBP patients in our clinical practice.

There are many different types of autologous orthobiologics clinicians are injecting into the disc. There is bone marrow aspirate, bone marrow concentrate, leukocyte

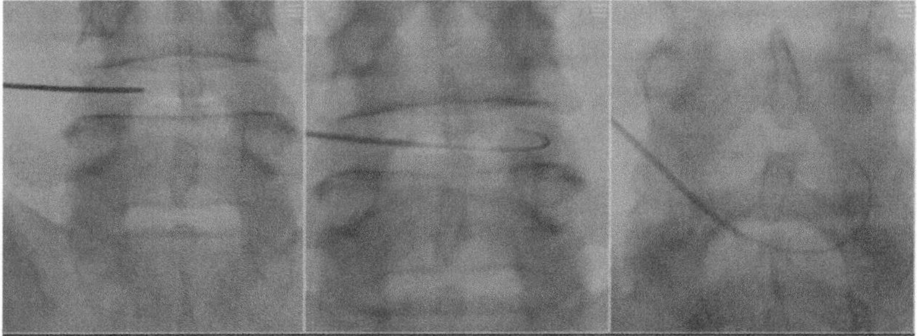

Fig. 8. Fluoroscopic images of the intradiscal insertion of a curved catheter to precisely deliver LR-PRP into the right posterolateral corner of the L4-5 disc.

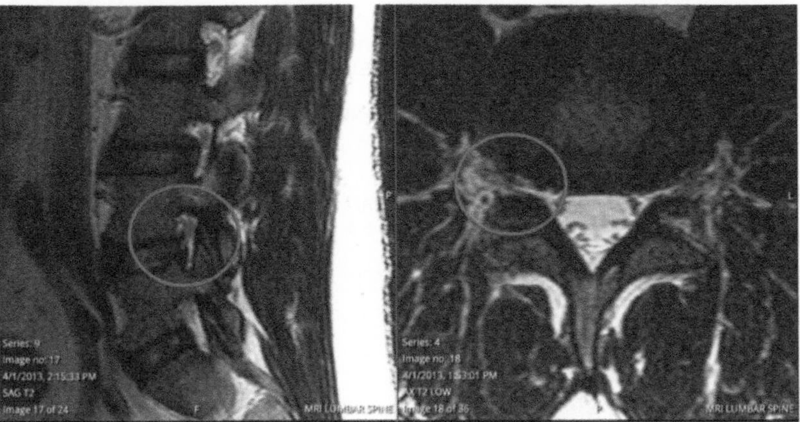

Fig. 9. T2 sagittal and axial MRI images from 2013 revealing an HIZ and a small protrusion effacing the right L4 nerve root.

poor PRP, platelet lysate, etc….I believe based on over a decade of clinical experience performing these procedures, that the infection risk is the least with LR-PRP. LR-PRP is also the only orthobiologic option that has DB RCT support and long-term outcomes data. We have used intradiscal bone marrow concentrate in the past, but have concerns regarding an increased rate of spondylodiscitis for reasons we do not fully understand.[30]

For intradiscal LR-PRP to become the standard of care for patients we will now need multi-center studies demonstrating its efficacy for specific subsets of patients with DDD.[25] We will also need a quality control system that can provide a range of consistency with the LR-PRP preparation method. PRP is relatively easy to quantify quickly on-site when compared to other types of cell therapies. With the use of a hemocytometer one can easily calculate the delivered dose of platelets, white blood

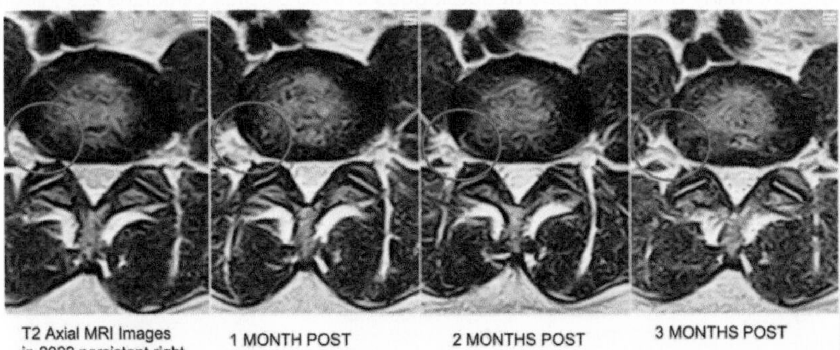

Fig. 10. Serial T2 axial MRI images over time demonstrating structural changes of the right-sided annular fissure and protrusion post-intradiscal LR-PRP precisely delivered with a curved catheter.

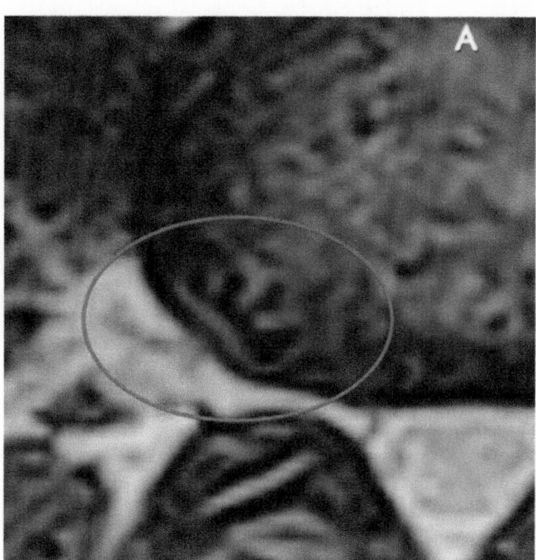

Fig. 11. Magnified T2 Axial MRI image of right foraminal HIZ demonstrating structural changes 1-month postintradiscal LR-PRP delivered precisely into the region with acurved intradiscal catheter.

cells, etc... by simply taking small aliquots of the baseline peripheral blood and the PRP.[25] This is important to also establish a dosing range that can ultimately be linked to clinical outcomes for optimization. What gets measured gets managed.

The power of regenerative medicine is real, and we are in the early stages of a paradigm shift in how we can better manage this global condition. It's going to take time, but this shift is already beginning to happen. We do not yet know for sure if our regenerative treatments halt the progression of degeneration, but it is my belief based on the patients we have treated that it certainly has the potential. Time will tell. Wouldn't that be remarkable if these treatments not only provide substantial pain relief - but also halt or even reverse disc degeneration (**Fig. 12**).

No single drug can come close to mimicking what your body already does so well. The healing process is not a solo, it's a symphony of cells and proteins that are distinctly yours. Our capacity to heal is so much greater than we ever imagined. Our cells are "naturally intelligent" and are perfectly designed to heal each of us.

However, for this paradigm shift to really gain momentum, it is going to be so important for physicians to collaborate not only with the patient, but also with each other, with researchers, with the FDA, hospitals, insurance payors, politicians, and industry to better improve the safety and clinical outcomes of these regenerative procedures.

These procedures need to be democratized so that anyone suffering from CLBP can have this treatment option before crossing the rubicon into the surgical maze. We will need to overcome the reimbursement challenges and provide payors with convincing data on the potential benefit of intradiscal LR-PRP over the current standards of care.

Our healthcare system has over-complicated the CLBP problem and mismanaged patients for decades. It has placed patients at unnecessary risk with poorly conceived, ineffectual treatments that have wasted precious healthcare resources. Drugs and surgery have a very limited role in the management of CLBP. It's been rare to see in my 30 years of practice a patient totally cured from these types of therapeutics. While

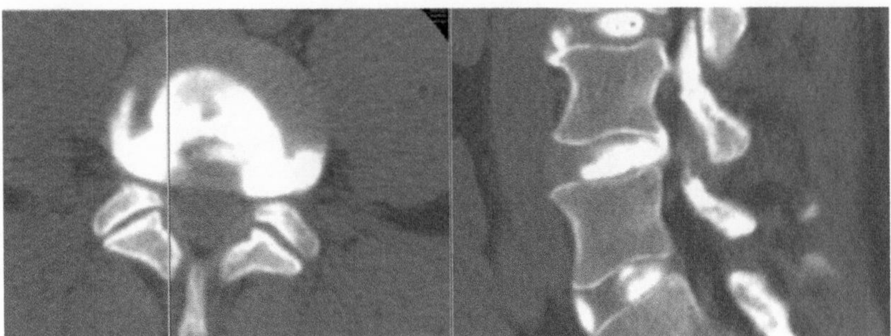
CT DISCOGRAM AT L4-5 REVEALED SIGNIFICANT ANNULAR DISRUPTION IN 2010

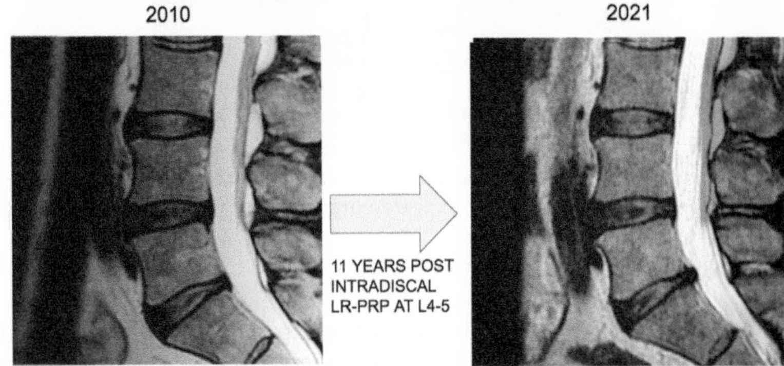
2010
2021
11 YEARS POST
INTRADISCAL
LR-PRP AT L4-5

Fig. 12. Images on top are CT-discogram axial and sagittal images of the first patient I ever treated with intradiscal LR-PRP revealing significant annular disruption of the L4-5 disc. Images below are T2 sagittal MRI images from the same patient treated from before and 11 years after treatment showing no signs of disc degeneration at the treated L4-5 level.

the opposite is now true with the patients we've treated with intradiscal LR-PRP. Many of these patients have had no further treatments, and their MRIs have demonstrated healing of their degenerated discs for years. Further studies are necessary to analyze structural changes in the MRIs of patients treated with intradiscal LR-PRP.

My prediction is that regenerative medicine is going to change how we manage patients with CLBP in the years to come for the better. Think about the millions of lives improved and the billions of healthcare dollars saved when a simple outpatient injection of your own cells replaces many of those costly hospital-based spinal surgeries. Spinal surgery will still be needed for some patients with more severe later stage degenerative disc disease that has associated spinal deformity, but nowhere near how many are currently being performed. Think about how intradiscal LR-PRP kills two birds with one stone, finally offering patients an opioid-sparing treatment option that is readily available and scalable. This is value-based musculoskeletal care.

Low back pain should be nothing more than a hiccup in life, rather than the wrecking ball it is for so many. Unfortunately, our traditional treatments have failed to "fix" low back pain. Mainly because only recently have we really begun to understand the underlying mechanisms that stop a disc from healing. Our understanding of why LBP becomes chronic has been rudimentary at best. So it's exciting to finally identify new and potentially reversible factors contributing to degenerative disc disease that we can target with regenerative medicine. If there is a cure for LBP, it lies within this realm of regenerative medicine.

The Regenerative Medicine Revolution is already underway and it is better for patients if we all collaborate to make these treatments as simple, safe, and effective as we can. While many companies are searching for proprietary cell preparations or pharmaceuticals to stimulate disc healing, it will be difficult to mimic what the body has evolved to do so well on its own over thousands of years. In the time of personalized and precision medicine, what could be more personalized and precise than the use of your own cells to heal your disc?

When you look at the risk/reward comparison with our historical surgical treatments, there really is no comparison. These treatments in the skilled hands of an interventional spine specialist are extremely safe and effective. While there are numerous promising regenerative strategies in development LR-PRP is FDA compliant and available for our patients now. As molecular therapies, biomaterials-based tissue engineering, and other cell therapies evolve - these novel therapies will have to demonstrate better results than what we have already shown with LR-PRP to gain adoption by key opinion leaders.

Finally, we need to think of the disc as the "heart" of the spine. It should not be cut out or fused, it should be healed and preserved. Maybe if we begin to treat it as such, we will have a chance to preserve the spine and end back pain for many. We are on the cusp of an exciting new era in regenerative medicine that will change the way we manage LBP so that it doesn't have to become chronic. Intradiscal LR-PRP is a promising initial regenerative treatment choice to start this paradigm shift. It is currently the safest orthobiologic intradiscal choice with the most supportive pre-clinical and clinical data.

CLIONICS CARE POINTS

- Intradiscal orthobiologics are a promising new treatment for degenerative disc disease.Intradiscal LR-PRP is our preferred orthobiologic because of its safety, efficacy, and pre-clinical support.Further research is needed to optimize cell concentrations and delivery to improve clinical outcomes.

DISCLOSURE

The Authors have nothing to disclose.

Research support from the Regenerative Sportscare Foundation a 501(c) (3).Dr. Gregory Lutz is the inventor of DiscCathTM.

REFERENCES

1. GBD 2017 Disease and Injury Incidence and Prevalence Collaborators. Global, regional, and national incidence, prevalence, and years lived with disability for 354 diseases and injuries for 195 countries and territories, 1990-2017: a systematic analysis for the Global Burden of Disease Study 2017. Lancet 2018; 392(10159):1789–858.
2. Donelson R, McIntosh G, Hall H. Is it time to rethink the typical course of low back pain? PM R 2012;4(6):394–401. Epub 2012 Mar 3. PMID: 22381638.
3. Deyo RA, Von Korff M, Duhrkoop D. Opioids for low back pain. BMJ 2015;350: g6380. PMID: 25561513; PMCID: PMC6882374.

4. Scholl L, Seth P, Kariisa M, et al. Drug and Opioid-Involved Overdose Deaths - United States, 2013-2017, MMWR Morb Mortal Wkly Rep, 67(5152);2018:1419-1427.
5. Centers for Disease Control and Prevention. 2018 annual surveillance report of drug-related risks and outcomes — United States. Surveillance special report 2 pdf icon centers for disease control and prevention. Washington, DC: U.S. Department of Health and Human Services; 2018.
6. GBD 2019 Diseases, Injuries Collaborators. Global burden of 369 diseases and injuries in 204 countries and territories, 1990-2019: a systematic analysis for the Global Burden of Disease Study 2019. Lancet (London, England) 2020; 396(10258):1204–22.
7. Lo YT, Lim-Watson M, Seo Y, et al. Long-Term Opioid Prescriptions After Spine Surgery: A Meta-Analysis of Prevalence and Risk Factors. World Neurosurg 2020;141:e894–920.
8. Deng H, Yue JK, Ordaz A, et al. Elective lumbar fusion in the United States: national trends in inpatient complications and cost from 2002-2014. J Neurosurg Sci 2021;65(5):503–12.
9. Institute of Medicine of the National Academy of Science. Relieving pain in America: a blueprint for transforming prevention, care, Jamesucation, and research. Washington, DC, USA: Institute of Medicine; 2011. p. 5.
10. Dieleman JL, Cao J, Chapin A, et al. US health care spending by payer and health condition, 1996-2016. JAMA 2020;323:863–84.
11. Gilligan CJ, Cohen SP, Fischetti VA, et al. Chronic low back pain, bacterial infection and treatment with antibiotics. Spine J 2021;21(6):903–14. Epub 2021 Feb 19. PMID: 33610802.
12. Grunhagen T, Wilde G, Soukane DM, et al. Nutrient supply and intervertebral disc metabolism. J Bone Joint Surg Am 2006;88(Suppl 2):30–5. PMID: 16595440.
13. Kirkaldy-Willis WH, Wedge JH, Yong-Hing K, et al. Pathology and pathogenesis of lumbar spondylosis and stenosis. Spine (Phila Pa 1976) 1978;3(4):319–28. PMID: 741238.
14. Kho ZY, Lal SK. The human gut microbiome—a potential controller of wellness and disease. Front Microbiol 2018. https://doi.org/10.3389/fmicb.2018.01835.
15. Albert HB, Sorensen JS, Christensen BS, et al. Antibiotic treatment in patients with chronic low back pain and vertebral bone edema (Modic type 1 changes): a double-blind randomized clinical controlled trial of efficacy. Eur Spine J 2013; 22(4):697–707. Epub 2013 Feb 13. PMID: 23404353; PMCID: PMC3631045.
16. Chen Z, Zheng Y, Yuan Y, et al. Modic Changes and Disc Degeneration Caused by Inoculation of Propionibacterium acnes inside Intervertebral Discs of Rabbits: A Pilot Study. Biomed Res Int 2016;2016:9612437.
17. Akeda K, An HS, Pichika R, et al. Platelet-rich plasma (PRP) stimulates the extracellular matrix metabolism of porcine nucleus pulposus and annulus fibrosus cells cultured in alginate beads. Spine (Phila Pa 1976 2006;31(9):959–66.
18. Chen WH, Lo WC, Lee JJ, et al. Tissue-engineered intervertebral disc and chondrogenesis using human nucleus pulposus regulated through TGF-beta1 in platelet-rich plasma. J Cell Physiol 2006;209(3):744–54.
19. Tuakli-Wosornu YA, Terry A, Boachie-Adjei K, et al. Lumbar Intradiskal Platelet-Rich Plasma (PRP) Injections: A Prospective, Double-Blind, Randomized Controlled Study. PM R 2016;8(1):1–10. Epub 2015 Aug 24. PMID: 26314234.
20. Monfett M, Harrison J, Boachie-Adjei K, et al. Intradiscal platelet-rich plasma (PRP) injections for discogenic low back pain: an update. Int Orthop 2016 Jun; 40(6):1321–8. Epub 2016 Apr 12. PMID: 27073034.

21. Cheng J, Santiago KA, Nguyen JT, et al. Treatment of symptomatic degenerative intervertebral discs with autologous platelet-rich plasma: follow-up at 5-9 years. Regen Med 2019;14(9):831–40. Epub 2019 Aug 29. PMID: 31464577; PMCID: PMC6770415.
22. Akeda K, Yamada J, Linn ET, et al. Platelet-Rich Plasma in the Management of Chronic Low Back Pain: A Critical Review. J Pain Res 2019;12:753–67.
23. Akeda K, Takegami N, Yamada J, et al. Platelet-Rich Plasma-Releasate (PRPr) for the Treatment of Discogenic Low Back Pain Patients: Long-Term Follow-Up Survey. Medicina (Kaunas) 2022;58(3):428. PMCID: PMC8952290.
24. Akeda K, Ohishi K, Takegami N, et al. Platelet-Rich Plasma Releasate versus Corticosteroid for the Treatment of Discogenic Low Back Pain: A Double-Blind Randomized Controlled Trial. J Clin Med 2022;11(2):304. PMID: 35053999; PMCID: PMC8777786.
25. Prysak MH, Kyriakides CP, Zukofsky TA, et al. A retrospective analysis of a commercially available platelet-rich plasma kit during clinical use. PM R 2021; 13(12):1410–7. Epub 2021 Apr 12. PMID: 33543595.
26. Lutz C, Cheng J, Prysak M, et al. Clinical outcomes following intradiscal injections of higher-concentration platelet-rich plasma in patients with chronic lumbar discogenic pain. Int Orthop 2022. https://doi.org/10.1007/s00264-022-05389-y. Epub ahead of print. PMID: 35344055.
27. Beatty NR, Lutz C, Boachie-Adjei K, et al. Spondylodiscitis due to *Cutibacterium acnes* following lumbosacral intradiscal biologic therapy: a case report. Regen Med 2019;14(9):823–9. Epub 2019 Aug 19. PMID: 31423905.
28. Jerome MA, Lutz C, Lutz GE. Risks of Intradiscal Orthobiologic Injections: A Review of the Literature and Case Series Presentation. Int J Spine Surg 2021;15(s1): 26–39. Apr 21. PMID: 34376494; PMCID: PMC8092939.
29. Prysak MH, Lutz CG, Zukofsky TA, et al. Optimizing the safety of intradiscal platelet-rich plasma: an *in vitro* study with *Cutibacterium acnes*. Regen Med 2019;14(10):955–67. Epub 2019 Oct 7. PMID: 31587600.
30. Muthu S, Jeyaraman M, Chellamuthu G, et al. Does the Intradiscal Injection of Platelet Rich Plasma Have Any Beneficial Role in the Management of Lumbar Disc Disease? Glob Spine J 2022;12(3):503–14. PMID: 33840260.

Orthobiologic Treatment of Ligament Injuries

Luga Podesta, MD[a,b,*], Eric S. Honbo, PT, DPT, OCS, Cert. DN[c], Raymond Mattfeld, PT, DPT, OCS, ATC[d], Michael Khadavi, MD, RMSK[e,f]

KEYWORDS

- Healing cascade • Orthobiologics • Cell-based treatment
- Leukocyte-rich platelet-rich plasma • LR-PRP • Bone marrow concentrate (BMC)
- Tissue healing • Ligaments

INTRODUCTION

Ligament injuries are common causes of joint pain, dysfunction, and disability and result in disruption of joint homeostasis, leading to the imbalance of joint mobility and stability. Ligaments are the most frequently injured tissues within a joint. Ankle sprains and anterior cruciate ligament (ACL) injuries are the leading causes of injury in college athletes.[1] During the past decade, there has also been a significant increase in injuries to the medial elbow, ulnar collateral ligament (UCL) in younger throwing athletes.[1]

Ligament injuries can lead to abnormal force transmission within the joint, resulting in damage to other supporting structures such as articular cartilage, menisci, tendons, and subchondral bone, eventually resulting in arthrosis.

Currently, literature regarding clinical outcomes using orthobiologic or cell-based therapies for ligament injuries is limited. Although clinical results are very promising, variability and conflicting results observed in clinical studies, may be explained by the reporting of inconsistent procedural technique, preparation methods, heterogenicity of the platelet-rich plasma (PRP) or bone marrow concentrate (BMC) compositions and posttreatment rehabilitation.[2] Due to these inconsistencies in the current literature, several orthobiologic reporting guidelines have been created to minimize heterogenicity in reporting and biologic preparation.[3,4] Successful outcomes will depend on developing a better understanding a ligament healing, the anatomy, physiologic differences in healing of specific injury location, for instance intra-articular versus extra-articular ligaments and the biology of the specific cellular therapies used.

[a] Regenerative Sports Medicine, Bluetail Medical Group Naples, FL, USA; [b] Podesta Orthopedic & Sports Medicine Institute, Florida Everblades, 1875 Veterans Park Drive, Suite 2201, Naples, FL 34109, USA; [c] Advanced Physical Therapy & Sports Medicine- Spine & Sport PT, USC Department of Biokinesiology & Physical Therapy, 101 Hodencamp Road Suite #102, Thousand Oaks, CA 91360, USA; [d] Sports Rehab Consultants & Bright Bay Physical Therapy, 160 Orinoco Drive, Brightwaters, NY 11718, USA; [e] Kansas City Orthopedic Alliance, Leawood, KS, USA; [f] Kansas City Ballet, Sporting Kansas City, 4504 West 139th Street, Leawood, KS 66224, USA
* Corresponding author.
E-mail address: lugamd13@gmail.com

Phys Med Rehabil Clin N Am 34 (2023) 135–163
https://doi.org/10.1016/j.pmr.2022.08.010

LIGAMENT HEALING

When ligaments are exposed to physiologic loads overtime, they increase in mass, stiffness, and load to failure.[5] However, when ligaments are overloaded or exposed to loads greater than they structurally can sustain, tissue failure occurs, resulting in partial or complete ligament disruption.[1]

A ligament healing response begins when normal healthy tissue sustains an injury. Injuries can occur by different mechanisms and occur in different locations, which may initiate distinct and different healing responses specific to the tissue and location of the injury (intra-articular vs extra-articular environments). Bleeding in vascular tissue initiates the healing cascade.[6–10] In normal circumstances, the healing cascade that ensues is a choreographed, highly regulated series of 4 interdependent phases.[6–9] Depending on the severity and magnitude of the injury, this phase can transpire over weeks to months. The phases of the healing cascade include the following (**Fig. 1** Healing Cascade):

1. Hemostasis—clot formation.
2. Inflammatory phase—platelet activation and immune system mobilization.
3. Proliferative phase—cell multiplication and matrix deposition.
4. Remodeling phase—scar formation and tissue restoration.

Each distinct phase is dominated by a particular cell type, which prepares the injured tissue for the physiologic events that occur in the next phase.[1,6–11] It is extremely important that each phase is executed efficiently to ensure the proper transition between phases. If the phases of healing do not properly transition, the repair process may be disturbed leading to the development of chronic or potentially degenerative pathologic tissue.[10,11]

Hemostasis

Hemostasis is the first and shortest phase of the healing cascade occurring within seconds to minutes, and this is the process of forming a blood clot to stop bleeding. Platelets are vital to hemostasis, also functioning as the physiological trigger to activate acute inflammation and program tissue repair.[8]

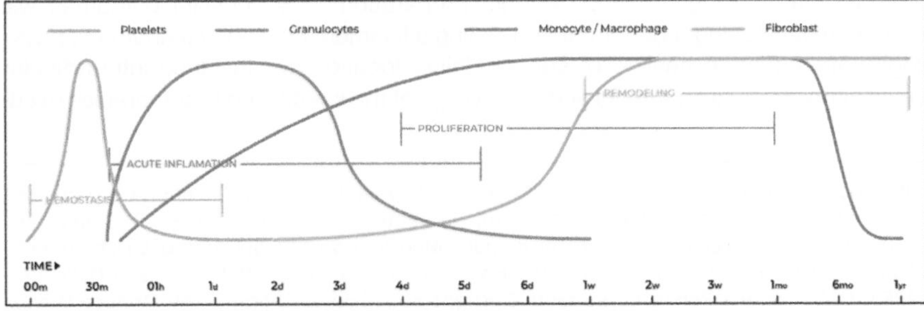

Fig. 1. Healing cascade. The 4 stages of the healing cascade consisting of 4 partially overlapping stages, hemostasis, acute inflammation, proliferation, and remodeling. The particular cell type activity within each phase is crucial for the progression and successful execution of the healing cascade leading to tissue repair. (*Adapted from* Parrish WR, Roides B. Physiology of Blood Components in Wound Healing: an Appreciation of Cellular Co-Operativity in Platelet Rich Plasma Action. J Exec Sports Orthop.4(2):1-14. https://doi.org/10.15226/2374-6904/4/2/00156.)

Platelets contain large numbers of alpha granules that store various growth factors, cytokines, and hormones necessary for wound healing.[8] Platelet activation is a highly regulated process that culminates in degranulation, or the release of granule contents.[10] The process of degranulation is a key step in wound healing because the growth factors and other mediators that platelets release program damaged tissue for repair.[10] In pathological states, such as an injury resulting in bleeding, platelets become activated by contact with components of the extravascular connective tissues including collagen that are exposed at the site of injury.[10] Platelets and leukocytes become activated together in a physiological context for wound repair.[10] Together they have coordinated and cooperative activities in normal would healing that trigger wound repair and limit acute inflammation.[10]

Activated red blood cells (RBCs) influence 3 important actions that contribute critically to the healing cascade: platelet recruitment, thrombin generation, and platelet activation and represents a critical axis between hemostasis and inflammation. The biochemistry and cellular content of the clot is determined by the communication between platelets and red blood cells, to activate thrombin generation during the hemostasis phase.[10,12–14] Activated RBCs play a critical role in amplifying thrombin generation to ensure effective and efficient execution of wound healing.[10,15]

Thrombin is the most powerful natural platelet activation signal and deficiencies at this stage of the healing cascade can lead to chronic inflammation and prolonged healing. Platelet activation in turn will help determine the biochemistry and cellular content of the fibrin clot establishing the potential for tissue regeneration.[10,15]

INFLAMMATORY PHASE

The *inflammatory phase* begins immediately following the injury and continues for 48 to 72 hours. When platelets aggregate and adhere to the injury site,[1,10,11,16] platelet granules are stimulated to degranulate, releasing inflammatory mediators and growth factors.[6,10,17–20] The largest and most the prevalent of these, the alpha granules, release platelet-derived growth factor-AB (PDGF-AB), transforming growth factor beta (TGF-β), vascular endothelial growth factor (VEGF), and fibroblast growth factor (FGF), among others. Each of which has a specific role in the inflammatory process such as stimulating local tissue growth including angiogenesis and collagen synthesis, initiate cellular differentiation and are crucial to the progression of the healing process[1][**Table 1** GFs].

Acute inflammation in response to injury is a completely dependent reaction triggered simultaneously with the activation of hemostasis.[10,11,17,21–25] However, unlike hemostasis that occurs to completion within minutes, acute inflammation typically lasts from 4 to 14 days.[7,8,10,11,26] The duration and magnitude of the acute inflammation phase is thought to be dependent on the extent of injury and whether the wound has been significantly contaminated.[26] The physiology of leukocytes is different in the presence of microbial or foreign body contamination than in sterile inflammation such as a contusion, overuse injury, closed traumatic injury, or uncomplicated surgical wound.[10]

The pairing of hemostasis and acute inflammation occurs through the action of thrombin, which helps to ensure the acute inflammatory response is proportional to the magnitude of injury.[10,27,28] A balanced wound healing physiology is important in determining poor or delayed healing.

During the acute inflammatory phase of healing, mobilization of innate immune cells such as granulocytes occurs functioning to debride and decontaminate the wound. Granulocyte activity is tightly regulated, requiring multiple activation steps to drive an inflammatory reaction. Neutrophils require separate priming and activation signals

Table 1
Growth factors in platelet-rich plasma

Growth Factor	Cell Source	Function
PDGF	Platelets, endothelial cells, macrophages, smooth muscle	Stimulates cell proliferation; promotes angiogenesis; promotes epithelialization, potent fibroblast, and immune cell recruitment factor
VEGF	Platelets	Stimulates endothelial cell proliferation, promotes angiogenesis
TGF-β1	Platelets	Promotes extracellular matrix synthesis, potent immune suppressor
FGF	Platelets	Stimulates proliferation of myoblasts, angiogenesis
EGF	Platelets	Proliferation of mesenchymal and epithelial cells, potentiation of other growth factors
Hepatocyte growth factor	Plasma	Angiogenesis, mitogen for endothelial cells, antifibrotic
Insulin-like growth factor	Plasma	Stimulates myoblasts in fibroblasts, mediates growth and repair of skeletal muscle

to elicit an inflammatory response. The first, or "priming signal," wakes up the resting neutrophil. In the case of a sterile injury, activated platelets can provide that priming signal.[10,29] Leukocytes develop the ability to communicate with their environment and gain the ability to generate and release an array of cytokines and growth factors with the ability to modulate the activity of other cells.[6,10,21,30–39] This is of importance because platelet growth factor release is exhausted in the early inflammatory phase, and it is predominantly the activity of white blood cells that guide the healing cascade forward to proliferation and remodeling.[7–11,19,26,40,41] Several authors have also shown that the leukocyte priming reaction is also reversible,[10,42–44] allowing white blood cells greater flexibility responding to signals in the environment driving wound healing. Because priming does not always lead to activation and an inflammatory response, it possibly plays a key role in limiting the nature of platelet-driven acute inflammatory reactions. This may explain the observations that leukocyte-rich PRP (LR-PRP) does not exacerbate inflammatory cytokines in osteoarthritic joints.[10,45]

When leukocytes are primed but not in an activated state, phagocytic activity is enhanced promoting debridement of damaged tissue and the release of anti-inflammatory and immunomodulatory mediators including TGF-b1, IL-1RA, lipoxins (modulators of inflammation) and resolvins, which actively suppress chronic inflammation, preventing the migration and recruitment of new leukocytes into the treated tissue, directing cellular activities toward tissue repair.[10,46–52] Monocytes then differentiate into anti-inflammatory macrophages, specialized for phagocytosis, which in turn helps to guide tissue repair.

PROLIFERATIVE PHASE

Within 2 to 3 days after the injury, the *proliferative phase* begins with the activation of fibroblasts by growth factors and inflammatory mediators released during the acute inflammatory phase.[7,10,11,26,40,53] The proliferative phase is defined by cell proliferation, neovascularization, and matrix synthesis in addition to other metabolic processes that aid and remodeling and organization of the healing ligament tissue.[54] This phase is initiated by macrophage activity that recruits fibroblasts, endothelial cells, and stem cells into the forming granulation tissue and is primarily driven by macrophage-sustained release of growth factors such as TGF-β, endothelial growth factor (EGF), and VEGF. Growth factors, mitogenic agent, and chemoattractants induce native connective tissue progenitors in locally injured and adjacent tissues to proliferate and differentiate into myoblasts.[55] Various growth factors including PDGF, TGF-b1, and FGF, generated by monocyte-derived macrophages stimulate the process of fibroblast migration from wound margins into the fibrin clot matrix.[8,10,11,40,41] Macrophage-driven fibroblast activity replaces the fibrin matrix with a more durable type 3 collagen matrix, which in turn facilitates the budding and growth of new blood vessels (angiogenesis), that is driven by macrophage factors such as VEGF.

The ability of leukocytes to generate new growth factors overtime becomes critical at this point in the healing cascade to replenish the pool of growth factors that were originally released during the inflammatory phase.[7,10,19]

The establishment of healthy granulation tissue marks the culmination of the proliferation phase. Granulation tissue is made up of primarily fibroblasts and new blood vessels.[7–11,40] Provisional matrix deposition working in parallel with the formation of new blood vessels (angiogenesis), drive tissue repair during the proliferation phase.[10,56] Oxygen is critical in the formation of granulation tissue[10,57] and is a key rate-limiting step in the healing cascade. Macrophage-derived growth factors TGF-b1, PDGF, VEGF, and FGF have all been shown to influence developing capillaries and angiogenesis.[7–9,20,40,41,56,57]

Within the wound, type III collagen is produced from fibroblasts, providing a weaker and less extensively cross-linked tissue matrix, then type I collagen is found in uninjured or mature repaired tissue.[10,56] Type III collagen will be replaced in the matrix by type I collagen as healing progresses from proliferation to the remodeling phase.[7,9,20,26,40,56]

Fibroblasts are driven by macrophage signals (TGF-b1) at the end of the proliferation phase to transdifferentiate into myofibroblasts,[10,58–61] which are specialized cells that generate new matrix and become contractile through the expression of smooth muscle actin. Contraction is important because it provides mechanical strength to the granulation tissue reducing wound size.[59–61] The TGF-b1 autocrine signaling augments collagen I production from the myofibroblast. New collagen I fibers are deposited in bundles aligning with the direction of myofibroblast contractile forces, strengthening and reinforcing the tissue to resist mechanical shear stress.[10,59–61] The proliferation phase transitions to the remodeling phase when granulation tissue matures into a scar[59,62,63] after myofibroblasts degrade the provisional type 3 collagen matrix.[10,59,62,63]

REMODELING PHASE

The *remodeling phase* is the longest phase of the healing cascade, beginning several weeks after the initial injury and may last months to more than a year depending on the severity of the initial injury.[7,9,10,41,43,55]

Fibroblasts are responsible for remodeling, replacing the type 3 collagen matrix with the stronger type 1 collagen matrix. Fibroblasts either die through apoptosis or differentiate into myofibroblasts that align to the direction of force within the tissue. Failure to properly transition from the proliferation phase may lead to excessive or hypertrophic scarring.[10,11,54,58,62]

During the modeling phase, collagen is refined, and its associated extracellular matrix is refined. Healing collagen synthesis and destruction both occur at a greater rate compared with normal tissue.[10,59–61,64] Collagen fibers and ligament matrix components undergo nearly continuous remodeling to promote strong ligamentous growth. Ultimately, ligaments heal with fibrovascular scar, which possess inferior biomechanical and mechanical properties compared with native structures.

Ultimately, collagen realignment restores strength and function to the repair tissue, which evolves into a mature and relatively acellular and avascular scar.[10,64] Overall, the normal outcome of the wound healing cascade is a mature scar and functional tissue, with around 80% of the strength of the original tissue.[10,11,58,59,64]

Cellular cooperativity is important for the execution of each phase of the healing cascade. None of the components of whole blood functions alone in the normal physiology of wound healing.[10]

INTRA-ARTICULAR AND EXTRA-ARTICULAR LIGAMENTS

Studies have shown variability in the potential for healing capabilities between intra-articular and extra-articular structures. The differences in repair potential may be related to the differences in the mechanical stabilization and microenvironment surrounding each ligament. In the knee for example, the ACL is surrounded by synovial fluid, whereas the medial collateral ligament (MCL) is an extra-articular structure and not necessarily influenced directly by synovial fluid.[55,65] Synovial fluid has been shown to prevent clot formation at the injury site of ACL injury, restricts the release of growth factors, limiting its ability to form a provisional scaffold to initiate self-repair.[66–68]

Elbow–Ulnar Collateral Ligament

Injury to the UCL in throwing athletes, particular baseball pitchers, are potentially career ending. At one time, injury of the UCL was predominantly diagnosed in high-level collegiate or professional throwing athletes; however, there has been a dramatic increase in the number of elbow UCL injuries diagnosed in younger adolescent, high school and collegiate athletes. In professional baseball, an estimated one-third of professional baseball pitchers have undergone surgical reconstruction of the UCL.[69,70] With modern surgical treatment, athletes can return to play at their previous level of competition or higher with a low rate of complications but it is a season-ending procedure requiring a prolonged period of rehabilitation, with an estimated return to play of 1 to 2 years.[71–74]

The literature has almost exclusively addressed surgical treatment techniques for UCL injuries such as the Tommy John procedure first performed by Dr Frank Jobe in 1974. Since Jobe and colleagues[75] published their original article describing UCL reconstruction in 1986, many surgical techniques for reconstructing, repairing, and now repairing with augmentation have been described.[71,76,77] The UCL reconstruction has been considered the gold standard of surgical repair but unfortunately, requires a prolonged rehabilitation and recovery period ranging from 1 to 2 years with reported return to play rates between 53% and 90%.[78–85] In general, UCL surgery, reconstruction, repair or repair with augmentation has been reserved for patients with complete or partial UCL tears that have failed nonoperative treatment.[86] However, disparity in the literature exists regarding postoperative UCL reconstruction outcomes. It has been reported that 3% to 40% of surgical reconstructions result in complications.[72,78,84]

Nonoperative treatment of UCL injuries historically has not shown optimal long-term outcome. Rettig and colleagues[87] reported on the 31 athletes with UCL insufficiency, treated nonoperatively with 3 months of rest and exercise with 42% returned to throwing. Classically, nonoperative treatment emphasizes activity modification, correcting ROM deficits, muscle imbalances, scapula mobility and stability, and kinetic chain strengthening.

Treatment of UCL injuries with orthobiologic or cell-based regimens that are capable of reliably returning athletes to play, quickly, and without resorting to season-ending reconstruction have become increasingly desirable.

Improvements in diagnostic imaging has led to improved ability to diagnose partial UCL injuries, thus improving our ability to determine who might better respond to nonoperative treatments. With appropriate patient selection in addition to potentially improving the biological characteristics of the injured tissue, cell-based therapies have gained interest by clinicians and investigators. Cell-based therapies have demonstrated promising healing benefits for the treatment of ligament and various other musculoskeletal injuries.[2,86] PRP has been used as a biologic treatment to enhance tissue and ligament repair, with evidence suggesting pain reduction, accelerated ligament repair and quicker return to function.[2,86,88–91] However, other investigators have found minimal to no benefit using PRP specifically to treat ligament healing after ACL reconstruction (ACL-R).[2,92–94]

Understanding the UCL anatomy, vascular supply, kinematics, and location of the UCL injury, assists in predicting outcomes, for example, why proximal injuries heal better and why distal lesions are more likely to do poorly with nonoperative care.[95,96]

Before Podesta and colleagues[86] 2013 publication, there was no literature regarding the application of orthobiologics therapies for the treatment of UCL injuries in throwing athletes. Before 2010, there was significant variability reported in the literature regarding treatment techniques and orthobiologic content used to treat soft tissue injuries including tendons and ligaments.

Podesta and colleagues[86] performed a prospective study evaluating 34 overhead athletes with partial UCL tears diagnosed by physical examination and confirmed by MRI, and dynamic ultrasound examination. They hypothesized that a single treatment with LR-PRP with a higher platelet and leukocyte concentration would be sufficient to treat the UCL in the thrower, stimulate adequate ligament healing to allow safe return to the same level of function and competition or higher. All patients had failed at least 2 months of conservative treatment and failed an attempt to return to play. Each patient underwent a single intraligamentous UCL LR-PRP injection under ultrasound guidance at the site of injury. LR-PRP was chosen for its increased platelet concentration of 5 to 6 times baseline and increased leukocyte and growth factor concentrations. They successfully determined that a single intraligamentous LR-PRP injection (88%) was sufficient to heal the UCL in the thrower, allowing them to return to the same level of competition in 12 to 15 weeks after injection and at 70-week follow-up (**Box 1**).

Several other clinical studies using biologic adjunct therapies for the nonoperative treatment of UCL injuries have been reported with promising but variable results. Dines and colleagues[69] reported on 44 competitive baseball players treated with 1 to 3 autologous conditioned plasma (ACP; Arthrex, Inc.), injections with lower reported platelet and leukocyte concentration. They reported excellent results in 15 of the 44 players (34%), 17 good, 2 fair, and 10 poor outcomes.

Another study by Deal and colleagues[71] performed a series of 2 LR-PRP injections on 23 UCL injured patients, spaced 2 weeks apart, followed by posttreatment unloader bracing, structured entire body kinetic chain physical therapy, and a structured

Box 1
Ten-year platelet-rich plasma follow-up Podesta[86,97–99]

Long-Term Follow-up-UCL Injuries Treated with LR-PRP 2010-2020

- Since the 2013 AJSM publication, questions remain regarding:
  - Treatment efficacy, long-term viability

Reviewed long-term outcomes of our original 30 patients.
- From 2010 to 2020
- No one lost to follow-up

Series of questions:
1. Where you able to continue to play competitively?
   a. For how long?
   b. What level?
2. Any recurrences of medial elbow pain or UCL injury?
3. When did you stop playing or retire from baseball?
   a. For what reason?

94% 29/30 continued to play for a minimum of 4 y.

34.5% 10/29 continued to play for 8 y.

No new UCL tears or pain recurrence

100% continued to play recreationally

1 player sustained a shoulder injury

None stopped playing or retired due to UCL injury

return-to-throwing program. Ninety-six percent of patients were able to return to play and demonstrated MRI evidence of healing at 6 weeks, 2 of 3 patients that failed PRP therapy had previous UCL surgery.

Questions regarding treatment efficacy and viability over time continue to exist regarding the treatment of UCL injuries with cell-based therapies (**Table 2**).

In 2020, Podesta[97–99] reviewed the long-term outcomes of his original 30 patients who had returned to throw competitively following a single, LR-PRP injection from 2010 through 2020, reporting that 94% of patients were able to continue to throw at the same level of play competitively for more than 4 years, without recurrence of medial elbow pain or UCL injury; 38% continued to play for more than 8 years, at the same level of competition or better, none were forced to retire from baseball as a result of their UCL injuries, and 100% continued to play recreationally. One patient sustained a shoulder injury, after returning to play, forcing him to retire from baseball prematurely and concluded these results confirm that a single ultrasound-guided LR-PRP was a viable treatment and will hold up over time in the thrower (**Fig. 2**).

COMBINED THERAPIES

Can we improve nonoperative therapies in higher demand athletes with more severe UCL injuries, complete tears, or distal injuries? Unfortunately, there are no clinical studies published evaluating combined therapies including the addition of medicinal signaling cells (MSC) or autologous scaffolds in addition to high-platelet concentration LR-PRP for these more severe injuries.

We are currently studying the treatment of higher grade and distal UCL injuries in higher demand elite pitchers with a combination of a single high-platelet concentration LR-PRP combined with bone marrow-derived progenitor cells, with and without

Table 2
Key observations important to improve outcomes

LR-PRP vs LP-PRP	• Cellular cooperativity is important for execution of each phase of the healing cascade. (Plasma, plts, RBCs, WBCs all have important roles in tissue repair)
Deliverable platelets	• 1.5 to 4.0 × 10^5 platelets/μL
Treat the entire ligament	• Treat flexor-pronator tendon/flexor, pronator musculature if necessary
Protect the ligament early	• First 2 wk critical • Bracing for grade 2 lesions
Dynamic US examination	• Ligament heals in ~6 wk, joint space closes narrows[71,86]
Posttreatment rehab progression	• Rehab progression based on dynamic US measurements • Begin valgus loaded exercise after humeral-ulnar jt. space narrows and ligament heals

activation with autologous thrombin with greater than 5-year preliminary data showing promising clinical outcomes regarding ligament healing, elbow stabilization and return to sports[98–100] (**Box 2**).

Understanding the patient's specific circumstances and demands allows us to tailor an appropriate biologic graft specific for that injury and situation. Knowing the patient's age, severity, and chronicity of injury and applied demands are important and needs to be considered. **Box 3** describes the authors recommendations for success compiled during the past 22 years treating UCL injuries in overhand throwing athletes. In our opinion, they are also applicable to treatment of most other ligament injuries encountered as well.

KNEE

Anterior Cruciate Ligament and Medial Collateral Ligament

Knee ligament injuries frequently occur in both athletic and nonathletic populations. Injuries to both the anterior cruciate ligament and collateral ligaments of the knee remain a frequent occurrence and burden to the health-care system.[2] Comparisons between the MCL and ACL have revealed differences in healing capabilities and have been reported by several authors. The ACL is an intra-articular, extrasynovial ligament consisting of 2 separate bundles that serve to resist anterior translation of the tibia relative to the femur, it consists primarily of type 1 collagen, has elastic characteristics that assist maintaining its stability, has a poor blood supply, and is covered with synovial tissue and surrounded by synovial fluid.[54]

There has been significant interest in the use of orthobiologic therapies such as PRP, BMC, and adipose tissue to enhance tissue healing and ligament repair. Investigators have reported early evidence suggesting the combination of cellular molecular components of PRP may reduce pain, accelerate tissue repair, and expedite return the function. However, other investigators have found minimal to no benefit, particularly with applications to enhance surgical reconstruction due to the heterogeneity in clinical studies published.[2]

Data on the use of BMC in the treatment of ACL injuries in humans are limited; however, several case series have shown clinical evidence of improvements in ACL integrity and increased function in patients treated with percutaneous PRP and or BMC injection to the ACL to augment surgical repair or as a nonsurgical therapy.[99,101–107]

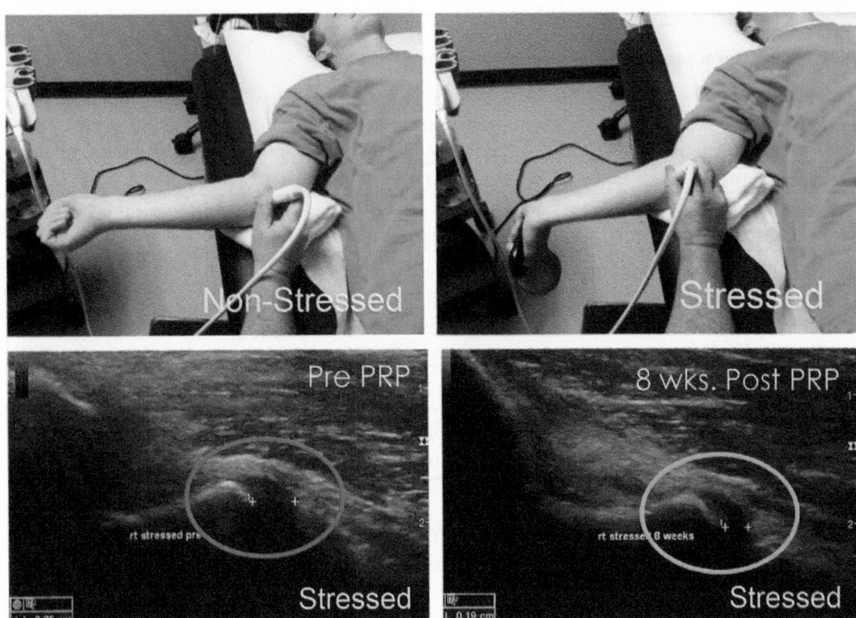

Fig. 2. Dynamic ultrasound imaging. The authors technique of dynamic ultrasound evaluation of the UCL with and without applied valgus stress. Ultrasound images of pretreatment and 8 weeks posttreatment showing normalization of the humeral-ulnar joint space distance secondary to UCL healing and tightening resulting in joint restabilization. (*From* Podesta L, Crow SA, Volkmer D, et al. Treatment of partial ulnar collateral ligament tears in the elbow with platelet-rich plasma. Am J Sports Med 2013;41(7): 1689–94.)

Gobbi and colleagues[101] evaluated 5-year clinical results of 58 athletes treated with ACL suture repair and PRP injection in addition to microfracture of the intercondylar notch. They reported 70% of patients return to sport activities, with a significant difference in anterior translation, in which side-to-side difference decreased from 4.1 mm (SD = 1.6) preoperatively to 1.4 mm (SD = 0.8) postoperatively ($P < .5$). Four players had sports-related retears, undergoing ACL-R within 2 years from the primary surgical repair, concluding that a PRP injection was effective in restoring knee stability and function in young athletes with acute partial ACL tears.[78]

Figueroa and colleagues[108] performed a systematic review of the literature on the use of PRP and ACL-R, finding only 11 clinical articles (516 patients) for inclusion observing different clinical studies showed an enhanced effect over the ligamentization (remodeling) of the intra-articular component of the ACL-R graft, with only 1 study showing improved integration.[104] Most of the investigations reported different PRP volumes and concentrations and failed to have validated methods and scores for measuring graft maturation. Only one study demonstrated a positive correlation with clinical evaluation, showing the PRP-treated patients had significantly better anterior posterior knee stability than patients without PRP.[105]

ACL-R remains the gold standard for treatment of ACL injuries particularly complete tears. There is emerging evidence supporting alternative treatments utilizing orthobiologic therapies alone or while augmenting surgical repairs of partial ACL lesions.[104] Preservation of the native ACL insertion site fibers and proprioceptive function may lead to better physiologic knee biomechanics.[105] Seijas and colleagues[107] reported

Box 2
Combined therapy platelet-rich plasma + bone marrow concentrate

Higher grade tears, higher demand and loads
- Acute and chronic
- Grade 2 partial tears (prox, mid, and distal)
- Calcified ligaments

31 pitchers (HS and College) 2015–present
- Average Age: 18.5 y (16–24 y)

LR-PRP (7% Hct) + BMC (7% Hct)
- ~2 mL, entire ligament, flex pronator fascia
- Single US-guided injection, UCL, FPT

Distal tears, Grade 2+, Grade 3 braced

Same rehabilitation progression

Preliminary results
  Subjective outcome studies
  - KJOC score, DASH, Dash Sports Module
  Objective evaluation
  - Dynamic US–Documented UCL healing and joint stability at 6 wk
  31/31 Return to play 12 to 15 wk
  - Return to play same level of play
  Continue to pitch >5 y s/p tx
  - Same or higher level of play
  1 Failure (2 y, 4 mo out)
  - Grew 6 in in height, increased fastball velocity 10 mph, increased repetitions, and work load

on 19 professional soccer players with partial ACL tears treated with intraligamentous and intra-articular PRP injections under direct arthroscopic guidance, with high return to sports and no complications. MRI evaluation showed complete ligamentization and satisfactory anatomic arrangement of all ACL remnant bundles at 1-year follow-up.

Kunze and colleagues[2] reported a systematic review of the basic science literature with protocol assessment reviewing the efficacy of PRP treatment of ligament injuries. They reviewed 43 articles (31 in vivo and 12 in vitro studies) investigating ACL/cranial cruciate ligament, MCL, suspensory ligament, patella ligament, and Hook ligament. They noted significant reporting variability in PRP regarding platelet concentrations, leukocyte composition, and red blood cell counts. With PRP treatments, 5 of 12 studies demonstrated significant increase in cell viability, 6 of 12 in gene expression, 14 of 32 in vivo studies reported superior ligament repair via histological evaluation, and 13 in vivo studies reported superior mechanical properties. In all articles reviewed, variability in PRP preparation methods was noted. Only 1 study reported all the necessary information to be classified by the 4 schemes used to evaluate reporting. Detection and performance biases were consistently high, although selection, attrition, reporting, and other biases were consistently low in in vivo studies. Concluding the observed conflicting data on the cellular and molecular effects of PRP for ligament injuries was secondary to study heterogenicity, limiting study interpretation and ability to draw meaningful conclusions.

Centeno and colleagues[109] have recently reported on the midterm analysis of their randomized controlled cross-over trial evaluating percutaneous, image-guided injection using a specific protocol of autologous BMC and platelets into partial or full-thickness, nonretracted ACL tears. The results suggest that autologous BMC injection

Box 3
Pearls for success in treating ligament injuries with orthobiologics

Tailor orthobiologic to patients' circumstances, injury severity, chronicity, loads
- Growth factors (GFs) or GF + Progenitor cells (MSCs),
  - Younger, lower demand, small, proximal-mid lig. Lesions–*LR-PRP (5–6+ x plt. conc.),*
  - Older, more demanding, larger or chronic tears–*LR-PRP (incr. plt. conc.); LR-PRP + BMC ± Autologous thrombin.*

Understand the anatomic location of the injury (proximal, mid, distal)?
- Distal lesions do worse, But! – LR-PRP (incr. plt. conc.), (LR-PRP + BMC)
  - Multiple injections
  - + autologous thrombin.

Protect the treated ligament
- Functional/unloader bracing (With ability to control ROM).

Guidance is extremely important!
- Needle guidance is critical,
- Orthobiologic placement needs to be precise for optimal results.

Injection technique
- Treat entire ligament, fenestrate, intraligamentous injection,
  - Flexor/Pronator Fascia-UCL when Perry ligamentous edema is present on imaging or in chronic cases,
  - Multiple treatments if there is no evidence of healing at 6 wk.

Activation with autologous thrombin
- Create a biologic scaffold,
- Stimulates the healing cascade, angiogenesis,
- Prevents run off.

Posttreatment rehabilitation progressions
- Dynamic imaging, MSK US, assists in determining safe rehab progression,
- Guides appropriate valgus exercise progression,
- Safe progression to throwing and athletic activity.

under fluoroscopic guidance into partial or full-thickness, nonretracted ACL tears resulted in improved patient function at 3 months when compared with exercise alone, and this treatment effect was sustained through 24 months across multiple functional outcome measures. MRI analysis was suggestive of interval ligament healing and maturation at 6 months.

Medial Collateral Ligament

The use of PRP for the treatment of knee MCL injuries has focused on enhancing nonoperative management, promoting healing with the goal to obtain a faster rehabilitation, and enabling quicker return to sports. Da Costa and colleagues,[110] and Yoshioka and colleagues,[111] studied the application of PRP to treat MCL injuries in rabbits, reporting accelerated ligament healing and improved structural properties after application of PRP.

The evidence for PRP to treatment of MCL tears is limited mostly to case reports. Zou[112] treated 52 patients with chronic pain for 3 months or greater after low-grade MCL injuries (6.5 ± 1.11 months) with 3 intra-articular PRP injections spaced 1 week apart. They reported superior Visual Analog Scores and International Knee Documentation Committee scores between pretreatment and posttreatment. Posttreatment MRI showed complete healing of proximal ligament injuries. Eirale and colleagues[113] reported on a case study of a professional soccer player with a grade II

Table 3
Ligament injury- exercise progression, goal, clinical rationale

Rehabilitation Phase	Criteria to Progress to This Phase	Anticipated Impairments and Functional Limitations	Intervention	Goal	Rationale
Phase I-II Hemostasis/ Inflammatory Phase Post Injection (0–7 d)	• Post Injection with no signs of infection	• Day 1–2: painful in the tissue/joint • Day 3–6: Diminishing pain and improving significantly • Day 7: Minimal pain, improved quality of ROM	Restrictions: ***Avoid all varus, valgus, A-P & rotational loads or ligament stressing activities/exercises x 7 wk*** • Tissue/joint specific protected bracing & weight bearing • No exercise except for rehab program • UE injections - no lifting > body wt. • Tylenol for pain • Heat pack for 15 min, 4x/day for 1–2 wk. • Avoid ice over treatment site • Shower ok 24 h after procedure • No submersion in water, bath, pool, hot tub or ocean for 1 wk. PT Progression: (Home Based) • Progress PROM to AROM, to point of	• Protect tissue • Allow biologic to absorb • Daily activity as tolerated within provided brace • Avoid excess loading or stress to treated area • Improve tissue vascularity and joint synovialization via gentle movement of extremity to improve • Avoid tissue overload or exercise unless approved by doctor	• Minimizes stress on injection site • Cross link initiation and homeostasis occurring as biologic activating to preparing for cross bridging

(*continued on next page*)

Table 3
(continued)

Rehabilitation Phase	Criteria to Progress to This Phase	Anticipated Impairments and Functional Limitations	Intervention	Goal	Rationale
			initial resistance, within brace restraints, and only within physician ROM restraints • Gentle sub maximum Isometrics (lower to mid-range sub maximal holds) twice a daily		
Phase II Inflammatory Phase (8–14 d)	• No signs of infection *2–4 wk delay/slower progression with ligament injections due to decreased vascularization	• Pain • Limited ROM ○ Pain with light UCL stress tests and ADL's ○ Limited UE strength	Restrictions: • **Avoid all varus, valgus, A-P & rotational loads or ligament stressing activities/exercises x 7 wk** • Tissue/joint specific protected bracing & weight bearing • No exercise except for rehab program • No concentric contractions or exercises to affected tissue except for unloaded ADLs and/or ambulation • For UE procedures, no lifting more than a dinner plate.	• Facilitate collagen deposition • Avoid homeostasis • Avoid disruption of collagen crosslink • Continue Phase 1 Rehabilitation recommendations • Consult physician regarding cross-training and return to exercise options • Improve tissue vascularity and joint synovialization by initiating upper body exercise if you had lower body procedure or LB exercise for UB	• Minimizes stress on injection site • Allow the PRP to absorb at the location • Prepare for cross bridging

			PT Progression: (Home Based) • Gradually progress AROM to point of initial resistance ◦ Obtain > 90% full ROM by end of week 2 ◦ Shoulder-AAROM to point of resistance • Continue Phase 1 exercises, (gentle submax. isometrics) • Gradually progress to full weight bearing with protective brace if applicable • Continue Heat pack as in Phase I		
Phase III Proliferative Phase (3–6 wk)	• Full pain-free ROM • No pain within sagittal plane functional mobility (Flexion/Extension, Dorsiflexion/ Plantarflexion)	• Limited UE/LE strength and cardiovascular endurance • Limited tissue tolerance to tensile loading exercises or functional activities • Pain (diminishing) • Limited tolerance with heavier lifting, pushing, pulling functional activities	Restrictions: ***Avoid all valgus loads or ligament stressing activities/exercises x 7 wk*** • Improve tissue vascularity and joint synovialization by initiating upper body cardiovascular exercise if you had lower body procedure or LB exercise for UB	• Protect tissue • Facilitate collagen deposition • Avoid disruption of collagen cross-link • Minimize deconditioning • *Communication among physician, physical therapist & patient is essential during this key transitional phase*	• Pain threshold significantly reduced • Collagen synthesis occurring, aligning in the longitudinal axis • Cross bridging occurring and matrix integrity improving • Tissue beginning to withstand tensile forces and loads • Use modalities to facilitation collagen formation & remodeling

(*continued on next page*)

Table 3
(*continued*)

Rehabilitation Phase	Criteria to Progress to This Phase	Anticipated Impairments and Functional Limitations	Intervention	Goal	Rationale
			• Continue use of assisted devices as instructed by physician procedures • No over stressing of tissue through exercise or impact activity • No exercises except for supervised rehab program • *(3–6 wk)* PT Progression Overview: • Pain should not increase > 2 points on 10-point VAS Modalities for symptom control: • Moist heat, non-thermal ultrasound, cold laser, Russian stim, ES, Shock Wave Therapy (ESWT) Manual Therapy Techniques: • Gentle Soft Tissue Mobilization along the line of tissue fibers		• Soft tissue mobilization techniques have mechanical, physiological, histological, and neurological effects on the tissue which facilitate the healing mechanism and fiber alignment • Progress toward light ligamentous loading by end of phase III • Ligament tensile strength should be strong enough to initiate stress loading exercises • BFR enables strengthening utilizing a light load and a relatively low volume of work • Cardiovascular training to improve endurance & tissue repair

- Joint Mobilizations to maintain arthrokinematics

Therapeutic Exercises:

- AROM to point of initial resistance sub maximum to
- Max Isometrics
- Emphasize proper postural alignment, distal joint position

Adjust exercise progression based on severity of injury

- Initiate low resistance, high repetition, concentric, open chain exercise
- Initiate Blood Flow Restriction (BFR) exercises
- Initiation and progression of eccentric exercises as concentric strength increases

Neuromuscular Re-education:

- PNF & Rhythmic Stabilization exercises
- Proprioceptive training

(*continued on next page*)

Table 3
(*continued*)

Rehabilitation Phase	Criteria to Progress to This Phase	Anticipated Impairments and Functional Limitations	Intervention	Goal	Rationale
			• Use of taping techniques as indicated for facilitation/ inhibition		
Phase IV Remodeling Phase (6–15 wk)	*Overlap of timelines is based on the patient's condition and severity of injury* • Pain-free ligament provocation & joint stability with stress testing • Demonstrate tissue integrity & joint stability with dynamic imaging • Subjective Functional Index Tool indicates patient is ready to progress through Phase IV to return to play status • Functional Testing performed to determine return to activity	• Limited UE strength • Limited ligament tensile strength during early phase IV • Limited joint proprioception • Altered timing and mechanics with sports specific & functional activities	Diagnostic imaging: • Diagnostic Ultrasound (~6–8 wk) to determine extent of healing and exercise progression and return to activity or sports status PT Progression: (Physical Therapy) Modalities: • Continue as needed Manual Therapy; • Continue Deep transverse friction mobilization/ massage to increase tissue vascularization and break up tissue adhesions Therapeutic Exercise: • Progress exercise and functional mobility integrating UE/LE CKC exercises as appriopriate	• Restore normal tissue integrity & fiber alignment • Maximize tissue vascularity and joint synovialization • Increase tissue tensile strength • Improve joint proprioception • Improve force production, tissue elasticity and ability to withstand tensile stretching ***Critical Decision Making Period- determine if tissue has sufficiently healed via dynamic imaging or if a second injection and/or surgical intervention is warranted* • Prepare for return to activity, sports	• Increased tensile strength of repaired tissue • Improved ability to produce force, withstand tensile stretching and increased elasticity • *Reassess Functional Index Score and dynamic imaging to correlate with objective exam findings to determine ligament healing, joint stability, and if exercise progression can continue or if a second injection and/ or surgical intervention is warranted*

- Progress eccentric exercise
- Progressive plyometric loading from <body weight to full body weight-bilateral to single
- Progress to ballistic, explosive training
- Sport specific training
  - ≤50% effort up to week 8
  - ≤Below 75% effort up to week 10
  - ≤Below 90% effort up to week 12
- Initiate Interval Sport Programs (Throwing, running, on field drills) pending results of Diagnostic US
- Return to sports 10–15 wk depending on the sport/activity

Neuromuscular Reeducation:

- Light concentric resistance pulley or tubing patterns with controlled speed emphasis

(continued on next page)

Table 3
(continued)

Rehabilitation Phase	Criteria to Progress to This Phase	Anticipated Impairments and Functional Limitations	Intervention	Goal	Rationale
			• Light Resistance PNF exercises performed manually using distal hand placements and initiating joint specific motions and adding pulleys or tubing/bands • Progress proprioception exercises to unstable surfaces **Week 6–7 Critical Decision Making Period** ***Dynamic imaging (MSK ultrasound) is utilized to confirm ligament healing, joint stability, and load progression.* • Initiate ligament and joint loading when healing and joint stability are determined, exercise progression is initiated.		

If sufficient healing and stability has not occurred at 6–7 wk, a second injection vs surgical stabilization may be warranted

Week 8–10: Progress to fast twitch and dynamic exercises

- Increase speed, resistance, and functional strengthening
- Add kinetic chain functional and sport specific loading progressions

**Pending repeated US imaging findings progress to return to play phase 4

Week 10–12:

Reassess Objective Exam results, Functional Testing, and Subjective Functional Tool Scores to determine return to higher level activity and/or sport-specific play

(*continued on next page*)

Table 3
(*continued*)

Rehabilitation Phase	Criteria to Progress to This Phase	Anticipated Impairments and Functional Limitations	Intervention	Goal	Rationale
			• Begin interval Return to Sport program. Start interval throwing, batting, tennis serves, volleyball hitting programs pending repeat US imaging findings, *Weeks 12–16*: Progress from 75-90+ % in controlled setting. Gradual return to sport at 12–15 wk		

MCL tear treated conservatively with multiple PRP injections and rehabilitation. They reported symptom free return to play after 18 days with excellent functional outcomes. Radiographic imaging showed incomplete healing of the ligament; however, the athlete had no recurrence of injury or further complications at 16 months follow-up.

SUMMARY

Ligament integrity is extremely important in maintaining joint stability and homeostasis. Chronic ligament instability can lead to chronic pain, osteochondral injury, eventually leading to osteoarthritis. Ligament injuries have historically been treated surgically. However, for more than a decade, there has been increased interest in orthobiologic and cell-based therapies such as PRP and bone marrow–derived progenitor cells to treat ligament injuries particularly in the athlete, supported by promising preclinical and clinical data. Unfortunately, due to lack of reporting standardization in the current literature, conflicting data on the cellular and molecular effects of orthobiologic therapies for the treatment of ligament injuries exists, making it extremely difficult interpret or compare findings. The autologous orthobiologic or cell-based preparation used for treatment can influence the varying results reported in the literature. Therefore, to truly understand and compare results of these powerful therapies, reporting standardization, such as harvesting techniques, concentration techniques, a quantification of the delivered product (platelets, progenitor cells), formulations (leukocyte content), number of injections performed, activation, how injections are performed (guided vs unguided), in addition to the posttreatment rehabilitation process, are all important and necessary to evaluate and compare efficacy of future studies (**Table 3**).

DISCLOSURE

L. Podesta, Editor, Biologic Orthopedic Journal. E.S. Honbo, The Authors have nothing to disclose. R. Mattfeld, The Authors have nothing to disclose. M. Khadavi: Consultant for Arthrex.

REFERENCES

1. Hauser RA, Dolan EE, Phillips HJ, et al. Ligament injury and healing: a review of current clinical diagnostics and therapeutics. Open Rehabil J 2013;6:1–20.
2. Kunze KN, Pakanati MS, Vadhera BS, et al. The efficacy of platelet rich plasma for ligament injuries, A systematic review of basic science literature with protocol quality assessment. Orthop J Sports Med 2022;10(2):1–25.
3. Mautner K, Malanga GA, Smith J, et al. A call for a standard classification system for future biologic research: the rationale for new PRP nomenclature. Pm r 2015;7(4 Suppl):S53–9.
4. Murray IR, Geeslin AG, Goudie EB, et al. Minimum information for studies evaluating biologics in orthopaedics (MIBO). J Bone Joint Surg 2017;99:809–19.
5. West RV, Fu FH. Soft -tissue physiology and repair. In: Vaccaro AR, editor. Orthopedic knowledge update 8. Rosemont, IL: American Academy of Orthopedic Surgeons; 2005. p. 15–27. Chapter 2.
6. Anitua E, Andia I, Ardanzanz B, et al. Autologous platelets as a source of proteins for healing and tissue regeneration. Thronb Heamost 2004;91(1):4–15.
7. Monaco JL, Lawrence WT. Acute wound healing an overview. Clin Plast Surg 2003;30(1):1–12.

8. Broughton G 2nd, Janis JE, Attinger CE. The basic science of wound healing. Plast Reconstr Surg 2006;117(7 Suppl):12S–34S.
9. Singer AJ, Clark RA. Cutaneous wound healing. N Engl J Med 1999;341(10): 738746.
10. Parrish WR, Roides B. Physiology of blood components in wound healing: an appreciation of cellular co-operativity in platelet rich plasma action. J Exec Sports Orthop.4(2):1-14. DOI:10.15226/2374-6904/4/2/00156.
11. Enoch S, Leaper DJ. Basic science of wound healing. Surgery (Oxford) 2008; 26(2):31–7.
12. Santos MT, Valles J, Aznar J, et al. Role of red blood cells in the early stages of platelet activation by collagen. Thromb Haemost 1986;56(3):376381.
13. Whelihan MF, Zachary V, Orfeo T, et al. Prothrombin activation in blood coagulation: the erythrocyte contribution to thrombin generation. Blood 2012; 120(18):3837–45.
14. Wolberg AS. Thrombin generation and fibrin clot structure. Blood Rev 2007; 21(3):131–42.
15. Dohan Ehrenfest DM, Bielecki T, Mishra A, et al. In search of a consensus terminology in the field of platelet concentrates for surgical use: platelet-rich plasma (PRP), platelet-rich fibrin (PRF), fibrin gel polymerization and leukocytes. Curr Pharm Biotechnol 2012;13(7):1131–7.
16. de Witt SM, Verdoold R, Cosemans JM, et al. Insights into platelet-based control of coagulation. Thromb Res 2014;133(Suppl 2):S139–48.
17. Blair P, Flaumenhaft R. Platelet alpha-granules: basic biology and clinical correlates. Blood Rev 2009;23(4):177–89.
18. Rendu F, Brohard-Bohn B. The platelet release reaction: granules' constituents, secretion, and functions. Platelets 2001;12(5):261–73.
19. Golebiewska EM, Poole AW. Platelet secretion: From haemostasis to wound healing and beyond. Blood Rev 2015;29(3):153–62.
20. Italiano JE Jr, Battinelli EM. Selective sorting of alpha-granule proteins. J Thromb Haemost 2009;7(Suppl 1):173–6.
21. Zarbock A, Polanowska-Grabowska RK, Ley K. Platelet-neutrophil-interactions: linking hemostasis and inflammation. Blood Rev 2007;21(2):99–111.
22. Cerletti C, de GG, Lorenzet R. Platelet - leukocyte interactions: multiple links between inflammation, blood coagulation and vascular risk. Mediterr J Hematol Infect Dis 2010;2(3):e2010023.
23. Weyrich AS, Zimmerman GA. Platelets: signaling cells in the immune continuum. Trends Immunol 2004;25(9):489–95.
24. Nurden AT. Platelets, inflammation, and tissue regeneration. Thromb Haemost 2011;105(Suppl 1):S13–33.
25. Gear AR, Camerini D. Platelet chemokines and chemokine receptors: linking hemostasis, inflammation, and host defense. Microcirculation 2003;10(3–4): 335350.
26. Demidova-Rice TN, Hamblin MR, Herman IM. Acute and impaired wound healing: pathophysiology and current methods for drug delivery, part 1: normal and chronic wounds: biology, causes, and approaches to care. Adv Skin Wound Care 2012;25(7):304–14.
27. Strukova SM. Thrombin as a regulator of inflammation and reparative processes in tissues. Biochemistry (Mosc) 2001;66(1):8–18.
28. Suo Z, Citron BA, Festoff BW. Thrombin: a potential proinflammatory mediator in neurotrauma and neurodegenerative disorders. Curr Drug Targets Inflamm Allergy 2004;3(1):105–14.

29. Condliffe AM, Kitchen E, Chilvers ER. Neutrophil priming: pathophysiological consequences and underlying mechanisms. Clin Sci (Lond) 1998;94(5):461–71.
30. Marcus AJ. Neutrophils inhibit platelet reactivity by multiple mechanisms: relevance to thromboregulation. J Lab Clin Med 1990;116(2):138–9.
31. Mocsai A. Diverse novel functions of neutrophils in immunity, inflammation, and beyond. J Exp Med 2013;210(7):1283–99.
32. Bazzoni G, Dejana E, Del Maschio A. Platelet-neutrophil interactions. Possible relevance in the pathogenesis of thrombosis and inflammation. Haematologica 1991;76(6):491–9.
33. Hallett MB, Lloyds D. Neutrophil priming: the cellular signals that say 'amber' but not 'green. Immunol Today 1995;16(6):264–8.
34. Shen L, Smith JM, Shen Z, et al. Inhibition of human neutrophil degranulation by transforming growth factor-beta1. Clin Exp Immunol 2007;149(1):155–61.
35. Spisani S, Giuliani AL, Cavalletti T, et al. Modulation of neutrophil functions by activated platelet release factors. Inflammation 1992;16(2):147–58.
36. Del MA, Dejana E, Bazzoni G. Bidirectional modulation of platelet and polymorphonuclear leukocyte activities. Ann Hematol 1993;67(1):23–31.
37. Della Corte A, Maugeri N, Pampuch A, et al. Application of 2-dimensional difference gel electrophoresis (2D-DIGE) to the study of thrombin-activated human platelet secretome. Platelets 2008;19(1):43–50.
38. Rex S, Beaulieu LM, Perlman DH, et al. Immune versus thrombotic stimulation of platelets differentially regulates signaling pathways, intracellular protein-protein interactions, and alpha-granule release. Thromb Haemost 2009;102(1):97–110.
39. Halpern BC, Chaudhury S, Rodeo SA. The role of platelet-rich plasma in inducing musculoskeletal tissue healing. HSS J 2012;8(2):137–45.
40. Schaffer CJ, Nanney LB. Cell biology of wound healing. Int Rev Cytol 1996;169:151–81.
41. Bielecki T, Dohan Ehrenfest DM, Everts PA, et al. The role of leukocytes from L-PRP/L-PRF in wound healing and immune defense: new perspectives. Curr Pharm Biotechnol 2012;13(7):1153–62.
42. Ekpenyong AE, Toepfner N, Chilvers ER, et al. Mechanotransduction in neutrophil activation and deactivation. Biochim Biophys Acta 2015;1853(11 PtB):3105–16.
43. Singh NR, Johnson A, Peters AM, et al. Acute lung injury results from failure of neutrophil de-priming: a new hypothesis. Eur J Clin Invest 2012;42(12):1342–9.
44. Aquino EN, Neves AC, Santos KC, et al. Proteomic Analysis of Neutrophil Priming by PAF. Protein Pept Lett 2016;23(2):142–51.
45. Mariani E, Canella V, Cattini L, et al. Leukocyte-Rich Platelet-Rich Plasma Injections Do Not Up-Modulate Intra-Articular Pro-Inflammatory Cytokines in the Osteoarthritic Knee. PLoS One 2016;11(6):e0156137.
46. Serhan CN, Savill J. Resolution of inflammation: the beginning programs the end. Nat Immunol 2005;6(12):1191–7.
47. Serhan CN. Novel omega – 3-derived local mediators in anti-inflammation and resolution. Pharmacol Ther 2005;105(1):7–21.
48. Xing L, Remick DG. Neutrophils as firemen, production of anti-inflammatory mediators by neutrophils in a mixed cell environment. Cell Immunol 2004;231(1–2):126–32.
49. Sugimoto MA, Sousa LP, Pinho V, et al. Resolution of Inflammation: What Controls Its Onset? Front Immunol 2016;7:160.
50. Soehnlein O, Lindbom L. Phagocyte partnership during the onset and resolution of inflammation. Nat Rev Immunol 2010;10(6):427–39.

51. Ortega-Gomez A, Perretti M, Soehnlein O. Resolution of inflammation: an integrated view. EMBO Mol Med 2013;5(5):661–74.
52. Gilroy D, De Maeyer R. New insights into the resolution of inflammation. Semin Immunol 2015;27(3):161–8.
53. Andia I, Sanchez M, Maffulli N. Tendon healing and platelet-rich plasma therapies. Expert Opin Biol Ther 2010;10(10):1415–26.
54. Dean R, DePhillipo N, LaPrade R. Ligament Lesions: Cell Therapy. *In* G. Filardo et al. (eds.), Orthobiologics, Chap 20, 245-255, https://doi.org.org/10.1007/978-3-084744-9_20.
55. Nguyen D, Ramwadhdoebe T, et al. Intrinsic healing response of the human anterior cruciate ligament: a historical study of reattached ACL remnants. J Orthop Res 2014;132:296–301.
56. Li J, Chen J, Kirsner R. Pathophysiology of acute wound healing. Clin Dermatol 2007;25(1):9–18.
57. Thackham JA, McElwain DL, Long RJ. The use of hyperbaric oxygen therapy to treat chronic wounds: a review. Wound Repair Regen 2008;16(3):321–30.
58. Ariel A, Timor O. Hanging in the balance: endogenous anti-inflammatory mechanisms in tissue repair and fibrosis. J Pathol 2013;229(2):250–63.
59. Darby IA, Laverdet B, Bonte F, et al. Fibroblasts and myofibroblasts in wound healing. Clin Cosmet Investig Dermatol 2014;7:301–11.
60. Desmouliere A, Chaponnier C, Gabbiani G. Tissue repair, contraction, and the myofibroblast. Wound Repair Regen 2005;13(1):7–12.
61. Hinz B. Formation and function of the myofibroblast during tissue repair. J Invest Dermatol 2007;127(3):526–37.
62. Xue M, Le NT, Jackson CJ. Targeting matrix metalloproteases to improve cutaneous wound healing. Expert Opin Ther Targets 2006;10(1):143–55.
63. McCawley LJ, Matrisian LM. Matrix metalloproteinases: they're not just for matrix anymore. Curr Opin Cell Biol 2001;13(5):534–40.
64. Hardy MA. The biology of scar formation. Phys Ther 1989;69(12):1014–24.
65. Bray RC, Leonard CA, Salo PT. Vascular Physiology and long-term healing of partial ligament tears. J Orthop Res 2002;20:984–9.
66. Murray MM, Fleming BC. Biology of anterior cruciate ligament injury and repair: kappa delta anndoner vaughn award paper 2013. J Orthop Res 2013;31: 1509 -6.
67. Murray MM, Spindler KP, Ballard P, et al. Enhanced histologic repair in a central wound of the anterior cruciate ligament with a collagen-platelet-rich plasma scaffold. J Orthop Res 2007;25:1007–17.
68. Murray MM, Martin SD, Martin TL, et al. Histological changes in the human anterior cruciate ligament after rupture. J Bone Jt Surg Am 2000;82:1387–97.
69. Dines J, Williams P, ElAttrache N, et al. Platelet-rich plasma can be used to successfully treat elbow ulnar collateral ligament insufficiency in high-level throwers. Am J Orthop 2016;45(5):296–300.
70. Keller RA, Steffes MJ, Zhuo D, et al. The effects of medial ulnar collateral ligament reconstruction on Major League pitching performance. J Shoulder Elbow Surg 2014;23(11):1591–8.
71. Deal J, Smith E, Heard W, et al. Platelet-rich plasma for primary treatment of partial ulnar collateral ligament tears: MRI correlation with results. Orthop J Sports Med 2017;5(11):1, 6D 2325967117738238.
72. Azar FM, Andrews JR, Wilk KE, et al. Operative treatment of ulnar collateral ligament injuries of the elbow in athletes. Am J Sports Med 2000;28(1):16–23.

73. Cain EL Jr, Andrews JR, Dugas JR, et al. Outcome of ulnar collateral ligament reconstruction of the elbow in 1281 athletes: results in 743 athletes with minimum 2-year follow-up. Am J Sports Med 2010;38(12):2426–34.
74. Vitale MA, Ahmad CS. The outcome of elbow ulnar collateral ligament reconstruction in overhead athletes: a systematic review. Am J Sports Med 2008; 36(6):1193–205.
75. Jobe FW, Stark H, Lombardo SJ. Reconstruction of the ulnar collateral ligament in athletes. J Bone Joint Surg Am 1986;68(8):1158–63.
76. Savoie FH III, Morgan C, Yaste J, et al. Medial ulnar collateral ligament reconstruction using hamstring allograft in overhead throwing athletes. J Bone Joint Surg Am 2013;95(12):1062–6.
77. Savoie FH III, Trenhaile SW, Roberts J, et al. Primary repair of ulnar collateral ligament injuries of the elbow in young athletes: a case series of injuries to the proximal and distal ends of the ligament. Am J Sports Med 2008;36(6):1066–72.
78. Chahla J, Kennedy M, Aman Z. the prod R. Orthobiologics for ligament repair and reconstruction. Clin Sports Med 2019;38:97–107.
79. Erickson BJ, Gupta AK, Harris JD, et al. Rate of return to pitching and performance after Tommy John surgery in Major League Baseball pitchers. Am J Sports Med 2014;42(3):536–43.
80. Makhni EC, Lee RW, Morrow ZS, et al. Performance, return to competition, and reinjury after Tommy John surgery in major league baseball pitchers: a review of 147 cases. Am J Sports Med 2014;42(6):1323–32.
81. Osbahr DC, Cain EL Jr, Raines BT, et al. Long-term outcomes after ulnar collateral ligament reconstruction in competitive baseball players: minimum 10-year follow-up. Am J Sports Med 2014;42(6):1333–42.
82. Park JY, Oh KS, Bahng SC, et al. Does well-maintained graft provide consistent return to play after medial ulnar collateral ligament reconstruction of the elbow joint in elite baseball players? Clin Orthop Surg 2014;6(2):190–5.
83. Rohrbough JT, Altchek DW, Hyman J, et al. Medial collateral ligament reconstruction of the elbow using the docking technique. Am J Sports Med 2002; 30(4):541–8.
84. Conway JE, Jobe FW, Glousman RE, et al. Medial instability of the elbow in throwing athletes. Treatment by repair or reconstruction of the ulnar collateral lig10(2), ament. J Bone Joint Surg Am 1992;74(1):67–83.
85. Dodson CC, Thomas A, Dines JS, et al. Medial ulnar collateral ligament reconstruction of the elbow in throwing athletes. Am J Sports Med 2006;34(12): 1926–32.
86. Podesta L, Crow SA, Volkmer D, et al. Treatment of partial ulnar collateral ligament tears in the elbow with platelet-rich plasma. Am J Sports Med 2013; 41(7):1689–94.
87. Rettig AC, Sherrill C, Snead DS, et al. Nonoperative treatment of ulnar collateral ligament injuries in throwing athletes. Am J Sports Med 2001;29(1):15–7.
88. Chen X, Jones IA, Park C, et al. The efficacy of platelet-rich plasma on tendon and ligament healing: a systematic review and meta- analysis with bias assessment. Am J Sports Med 2018;46(8):2020–32.
89. Filardo G, Di Matteo B, Kon E, et al. Platelet-rich plasma in tendon-related disorders: results and indications. Knee Surg Sports Traumatol Arthrosc 2018; 26(7):1984–99.
90. Del Torto M, Enea D, Panfoli N, et al. Hamstrings anterior cruciate ligament reconstruction with and without platelet rich fibrin matrix. Knee Surg Sports Traumatol Arthrosc 2015;23(12):3614–22.

91. Boswell SG, Cole BJ, Sundman EA, et al. Platelet-rich plasma: a milieu of bioactive factors. Arthroscopy 2012;28(3):429–39, 2019;100(2):336-349.
92. Magnussen RA, Flanigan DC, Pedroza AD, et al. Platelet-rich plasma use in allograft ACL reconstructions: two-year clinical results of a MOON cohort study. Knee 2013;20(4):277–80.
93. Mirzatolooei F, Alamdari MT, Khalkhali HR. The impact of platelet-rich plasma on the prevention of tunnel widening in anterior cruciate ligament reconstruction using quadrupled autologous hamstring tendon: a randomised clinical trial. Bone Joint J 2013;95(1):65–9.
94. Valenti Azcarate A, Lamo-Espinosa J, Aquerreta Beola JD, et al. Comparison between two different platelet-rich plasma preparations and control applied during anterior cruciate ligament reconstruction: is there any evidence to support their use? Injury 2014;45(suppl 4):S36–41.
95. Buckely P, Morris E, Robbins C, et al. Variations in blood supply from proximal to distal in the ulnar collateral ligament of the elbow: a qualitative descriptive cadaveric study. Am J Sports Med 2019;47(5):1117–23.
96. Frangiamore SJ, Lynch TS, Vaughn MD, et al. Magnetic resonance imaging predictors of failure in the nonoperative management of ulnar collateral ligament injuries in professional baseball pitchers. Am J Sports Med 2017;45(8):1783–9.
97. Podesta L. Orthobiologics and the UCL: Treatment or delaying surgical treatment: The Overhead Athlete, Annual Assembly of the American Academy of Physical Medicine and Rehabilitation 2019, San Antonio, TX, November 14, 2019.
98. Podesta L. Ulnar Collateral Ligament (UCL) Treatment with PRP & BMC in the Throwing Athlete, TOBI Virtual, 11th Annual Orthobiologics Symposium, June 13, 2020.
99. Podesta L. Orthobiologics and the UCL: Treatment or delaying surgical intervention? 34th Annual Kerlan-Jobe Alumni Research Conference, July 8, 2020.
100. Lopez-Vidriero E, Goulding KA, Simon DA, et al. The use of platelet-rich plasma in arthroscopy and sports medicine: optimizing the healing environment. Arthroscopy 2010;26(2):269–78.
101. Gobbi A, Karnatzikos G, Sankineani SR, et al. Biological augmentation of ACL re-fixation in partial lesions in a group of athletes: results at the 5-year follow-up. Tech Orthop 2013;28(2):180–4.
102. Centeno CJ, Pitts J, Al-Sayegh H, et al. Anterior cruciate ligament tears treated with percutaneous injection of autologous bone marrow nucleated cells: A case series. J Pain Res 2015;8:437–47.
103. Centeno C, Markle J, Dodson E, et al. Symptomatic anterior cruciate ligament tears treated with percutaneous injection of autologous bone marrow concentrate and platelet products: a non-controlled registry study. J Transl Med 2018;16(1):246.
104. Figueroa D, Figueroa F, Calvo R, et al. Platelet-rich plasma used in anterior cruciate ligament surgery: Systematic review of the literature. Art Ther 2015;31: 981–8.
105. Vogrin M, Rupreht M, Crnjac A, et al. The effect of platelet-derived growth factors on the stability after anterior cruciate ligament reconstruction: a prospective randomized clinical study. Wien Klin Wochenschr 2010;122:91–5.
106. Dallo I, Chahla J, Mithchel J, et al. Biologic approaches for the treatment of partial tears of the anterior cruciate ligament: a current concepts review. Orthop J Sports Med 2017;5:1–9.

107. Seijas R, Ares O, Cusco X, et al. Partial anterior cruciate ligament tears treated with intraligamentary plasma rich in growth factors. World J Orthop 2014;5:373–8.
108. Figueroa D, Guiloff R, Figueroa F. Ligament lesions: biologics. *In* Filardo G. et al. (eds.), Orthobiologics, Chap 21, 257-263, doi.org.org/10.1007/978-3-030-84744-9_21
109. Centeno C, Matthew L, Stemper I, et al. Image-guided injection of anterior cruciate ligament tears with autologous bone marrow concentrate and platelets: mid-term analysis from a randomized controlled trial. Ortho J 2022;3(SP2):e7–20, 2.
110. da Costa EL, Teixeira LEM, Padua BJ, et al. Biomechanical study of the effect of platelet-rich plasma on the treatment of medial collateral ligament injuries in rabbits. Acta Cir Bras 2017;32:827–35.
111. Yoshioka T, Kanamori A, Washio T, et al. The effects of plasma rich in growth factors (PRGF-Endoret) on healing of medial collateral ligament of the knee. Knee Surg Sports Traumatol Arthrosc 2013;21:1763–9.
112. Zou G, Zheng M, Chen W, et al. Autologous platelet-rich plasma therapy for refractory pain after low-grade medial collateral ligament injury. J Int Med Res 2020;48:1–7.
113. Eirale C, Mauri E, Hamilton B. Use of platelet rich plasma in an isolated complete medial collateral ligament lesion in a professional football (soccer) player: a case report. Asian J Sports Med 2013 2006;4(2):158–62.

Prolotherapy

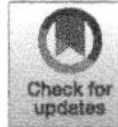

A Narrative Review of Mechanisms, Techniques, and Protocols, and Evidence for Common Musculoskeletal Conditions

Connie Hsu, MD[a], Kevin Vu, MD[a], Joanne Borg-Stein, MD[a,b,*]

KEYWORDS

- Prolotherapy • Prolotherapy techniques • Dextrose prolotherapy • Orthobiologics
- Tendinopathy • Treatment

KEY POINTS

- Current hypotheses suggest that prolotherapy stimulates growth factors via a multimodal mechanism of action to resume or initiate connective tissue repair, potentially strengthening attachments, and reducing or eliminating pain.
- The injection technique is focused on the regional treatment of connective tissue disease with an emphasis on fundamental anatomy. The standardization of optimal injectate technique is an active area of research.
- Prolotherapy is most commonly utilized for soft-tissue injuries, primarily tendinopathies and enthesopathies as well as joint osteoarthritis.

INTRODUCTION

In the United States, musculoskeletal disorders are the most common reason for a doctor's visit.[1] Musculoskeletal conditions are not only distressing to patients burdened by significant pain, but they may also result in significant disability. In the United States, 55% of adults with joint pain have difficulty with basic functioning, frequently limiting their participation in social, occupational, and household situations.[2] The increasing burden of musculoskeletal conditions has led to an interest in effective nonsurgical treatment strategies, including but not limited to corticosteroids, platelet-rich plasma injections, stem cell injections, and prolotherapy. In this article, we will be discussing a nonoperative, practical, and efficacious treatment for many common musculoskeletal conditions: prolotherapy.

[a] Department of Physical Medicine and Rehabilitation, Spaulding Rehabilitation Hospital, 300 1st Avenue, Charlestown, MA 02129, USA; [b] Harvard Medical School, Boston, MA, USA
* Corresponding author. 300 1st Avenue, 2nd Floor, Charlestown, MA 02129.
E-mail address: jborgstein@mgh.harvard.edu

Phys Med Rehabil Clin N Am 34 (2023) 165–180
https://doi.org/10.1016/j.pmr.2022.08.011
pmr.theclinics.com

Prolotherapy is defined as a nonsurgical regenerative injection technique that introduces small amounts of an irritant solution to the site of painful and degenerated tendon insertions, joints, and ligaments to promote the growth of normal cells and tissues.[3] A major goal of prolotherapy is the stimulation of regenerative processes in the joint that help facilitate the restoration of joint stability through the strengthening and stabilization of ligaments, tendons, joint capsules, menisci, and labral tissue.[4]

Prolotherapy as a treatment for musculoskeletal pain has gained a significant amount of visibility and traction over the past two decades among both physicians and patients.[5] This is, in part, due to an increase in the amount and quality of recent clinical trials that have shown strong evidence in support of prolotherapy for the treatment of chronic musculoskeletal pain. In addition, prolotherapy has been proven to be a relatively safe therapy, with few adverse effects reported across the board in the reviewed studies discussed below.

In this review, we will give a broad overview of the basic science behind prolotherapy as well as the currently utilized techniques and protocols for prolotherapy injections. Finally, we will discuss the evidence for the use of prolotherapy in common and uncommon musculoskeletal conditions.

MECHANISM OF ACTION

Prolotherapy, a portmanteau of "proliferative" and "therapy," was initially developed by surgeon George Hackett, who used these injections on soft-tissue injuries.[6] Prolotherapy, inaccurately described as sclerotherapy before its mechanism of action was investigated, refers to a nonbiologic injection of the solution proposed to repair connective tissues.[7]

The current proposed mechanisms of action are focused on the generation of low-grade inflammation related to the injection of hyperosmolar solutions. One proposed pathway is the transportation of glucose via GLUT 1-4 channels that occurs in surrounding cells following localized injection.[8] This transport, as well as the osmotic effect of solutions leading to release of water and lipids from nearby cells, is related to the generation of a temporary low-grade inflammation at the site of injury.[9] This process is primarily mediated by the production of cytokines. At the fibro-osseus junction of ligaments and tendons, this inflammation leads to a healing cascade of various paracrine pathways relating to cell growth and repair.[10,11] Cells that are activated in this pathway include fibroblasts, chondrocytes, and nerve cells.[12,13] One notable study noted chondrogenesis on articular surfaces that had been injected with 12.5% dextrose.[14] Direct needling of the tissue may also stimulate repair, with disruption of cellular membranes and local blood supply resulting in the release of healing and inflammatory blood factors such as calcitonin gene-related protein (CGRP), bradykinin, and prostaglandins.[15] The direct injection of hyperosmotic solutions such as dextrose may also promote the activation of pain receptors, such as the capsaicin pain receptor. Upregulation of these channels results in an increase in substance P, CGRP, and nitric oxide, thought to have a downregulating effect on receptors.[16] In addition, the transmission of pain via the alpha-delta nerve fiber may result in endogenous opioid-mediated pain suppression, as described in the gate-control theory.[17]

TECHNIQUES AND PROTOCOL

When considering the use of prolotherapy to treat a soft-tissue disorder, there are basic principles of needle technique and application that must be kept in mind. There are two general approaches to prolotherapy that are largely utilized, and physicians commonly combine the aspects of both methods. The first method was named after the approach used by George Hackett, named the Hackett method. With the Hackett method, dextrose is the preferred proliferant, with a frequency of treatment lasting months with sessions every 6 to 12 weeks. The West Coast method predominantly uses a mixture of phenol, dextrose, and glycerin or sodium morrhuate with weekly treatments and larger bore needles than the Hackett method. This section will detail the most important techniques and protocols involved in prolotherapy as well as information for patients to ensure proper selection of their prolotherapy treatment.

Solution Preparation

Before the injection, the provider must have the required equipment on hand. Prolotherapy is primarily done with dextrose injections ranging from 10% to 25%, although animal models have noted improvement with as little as 5% dextrose.[18] Uncommonly used injectates include phenol and sodium morrhuate, with variable results.[19] Syringes can be prepared using ¼ or ½ of 50% dextrose to create 12.5% or 25% soft-tissue solutions, respectively. If using xylocaine, the percentages of xylocaine can range between 0.4% and 0.075%. Alternatively, concentrations of 0.5% to 0.75% phenol may also be utilized or combined with dextrose. In addition, sodium morrhuate, which is available as a 5% solution, can be added to a 10 mL syringe to create a 0.5% to 1% concentration. Providers should ensure that normal saline for titration of injectate, syringes appropriate to the amount of prolotherapy needed, needles, and disinfectant swabs are on hand for the injection. When considering prolotherapy for soft tissues surrounding the joints, consider a sterile office procedure similar to intraarticular joint injection: chlorhexidine/iodine prep, draping, and sterile gloves and instruments may be required. Anesthetic gel and anesthetic blebs are commonly applied to diminish skin sensation with lidocaine before injection.

Guidance

Prolotherapy is generally a region-based intervention, versus comparable tender or trigger point injections, and thus requires a thorough physical examination before and immediately following an injection. Strong anatomic knowledge and fundamentals are vital to performing prolotherapy injections successfully, particularly regarding ligament and tendon referral patterns of pain. Like trigger point injections, twitch contractions may be elicited. However, unlike trigger points, reflex twitch contractions are likely a secondary phenomenon secondary to irritation of the muscles overlying the tendon or ligament in question, reproducing the connective tissue pain referral pattern.

Prolotherapy can be palpation- or ultrasound-guided. Palpation-guided prolotherapy injections have been successfully performed for decades and require a strong understanding of anatomy. However, ultrasound-guided injections have become increasingly more popular due to improvements in accuracy and visualization of the needle during injection. The use of ultrasound injections, in general, MSK injections, has been shown to improve both efficacy and accuracy.[20] However, there has been minimal investigation on the use of ultrasound concerning outcomes from prolotherapy injections, and there is no conclusive evidence in this field.[21]

Needling

The needling technique can be summarized with the "ABCs" of prolotherapy injection: anatomy, bony endpoint, and compression (**Fig. 1**). A technique called peppering is commonly utilized with prolotherapy injections. Peppering is a technique where a small amount of solution (around 0.5 cc) is injected into the injured structure multiple

The ABC's

Anatomy: know your entheses, vasculature, and nerves

Bony Endpoint: make sure to always touch bone with the needle tip before injecting

Compression: compress the superficial tissues while injecting to maximize accuracy of the injection

Fig. 1. The ABCs of prolotherapy technique.

times with the needle partially withdrawn, redirected, and reinserted around the injured area between the small injections.[22]

Patient Education

With any orthobiologic injection, patient education and setting expectations are vital. The risks of prolotherapy are typically rare but can be serious due to the injury of internal organs if caution is not used. Anecdotal risks of injection include infection, bleeding, nerve damage (as a result of irritation), and pneumothorax and are usually associated with peri-spinal or cervical injections.[23] The more common adverse effects include immediate pain, soreness, and mild bleeding as a result of needle trauma. Post-injection pain flares are common during the first 72 hours after and can be treated with acetaminophen or non-steroidal anti-inflammatory drugs (NSAIDs).[5] In addition, patients should be counseled that the efficacy of this treatment may require multiple rounds of injection and time until maximal effect.[1] The benefits of this treatment include minimal downtime after injection as well as potential pain reduction and functional improvement as described below in the evidence section for selected pathologies.

Patients should also be informed that prolotherapy is not a standalone treatment, and should be used in conjunction with standard treatment, including physical therapy (PT), adjustment of biomechanics, periprocedural rehabilitation, and consistent follow-up.

Limitations

The major limitation with prolotherapy, like many orthobiologic injections at this time, is the nonstandardization of injection protocol and injectate concentration. In addition, the selection of regional areas, number of injections, and amount of injectate may be provider- and experience-dependent. The following section attempts to highlight the most common musculoskeletal (MSK) applications for prolotherapy as well as typical prolotherapy protocols used for each condition.

EVIDENCE FOR COMMON AND UNCOMMON MUSCULOSKELETAL CONDITIONS

Numerous studies have investigated the use and efficacy of prolotherapy for various musculoskeletal conditions. There has been promising evidence for the use of prolotherapy to treat chronic, painful tendinopathies as well as knee and hand osteoarthritis. There is abundant yet inconsistent evidence for the use of prolotherapy in the treatment of chronic low back pain (LBP) alone, but good evidence to support the treatment of chronic low back pain with prolotherapy when coupled with adjunctive therapies.[24] In addition, there has been promising evidence to support prolotherapy as a treatment for SI joint pain. Finally, there is growing evidence for the use of prolotherapy with more uncommon musculoskeletal diagnoses, such as joint laxity and hypermobility. A general overview of the most common musculoskeletal conditions that have been studied with prolotherapy will be discussed below.

Tendinopathies

Lateral epicondylosis

Chronic lateral epicondylosis or "tennis elbow" pain, is a common, yet debilitating and often refractory condition.[25] There have been multiple studies that suggest a benefit to treating lateral epicondylosis with prolotherapy. One of the earliest studies on the efficacy of prolotherapy in lateral epicondylosis was a small double-blind randomized control trial (RCT) study: the treatment group, treated with 50% dextrose, 5% sodium morrhuate, 4% lidocaine, and 0.5% sensorcaine at 0, 1, and 4 months, showed significant improvement in pain levels compared with the control group.[26] Another RCT study reported similar improvements in the reported pain levels in patients treated exclusively with dextrose prolotherapy compared with the control group.[27] A different study treated patients with lateral epicondylosis (confirmed by ultrasound) with 15% dextrose prolotherapy and found that patients who received prolotherapy showed a significant reduction of pain from baseline as well as evidence of tendon healing on ultrasound imaging at subsequent follow-up appointments.[28] A recent study aimed to compare the clinical effectiveness of prolotherapy monotherapy, physiotherapy monotherapy, and a combination of both prolotherapy and physiotherapy in a single-blinded clinical trial.[29] At 52 weeks, there were significant improvements from baseline status for all outcome groups; however, there were no significant differences between groups.[29] Finally, a different triple-blinded RCT compared the effect of dextrose prolotherapy with saline in chronic epicondylopathy and reported that both groups demonstrated improvement in their outcome measures of Patient-Rated Tennis Elbow Evaluation, disability, handgrip strength, pain, with the dextrose prolotherapy group showing significantly higher improvement in pain rating outcomes.[30]

A couple of studies compared prolotherapy with other nonoperative treatments. One such study compared the efficacy of prolotherapy versus corticosteroid injections in the treatment of chronic lateral epicondylosis and reported that while both treatments were well tolerated and provided benefit to the patients' pain and disability scores at the 1 to 6 month follow-up, the sample size was too small to determine whether one therapy was superior to the other.[31,32]

For prolotherapy injections of the lateral epicondyle, it is important to position the patient in a way that optimizes accessibility of the attachment sites of the common extensor tendons. Injection sites are driven by ultrasound and physical examination findings (**Fig. 2**). Common injection sites include the common extensor tendon, the annular ligament, the supracondylar ridge over the radial collateral ligament, joint capsule, and the medial and lateral condyle (**Table 1**).

Rotator cuff tendinopathy

Rotator cuff pathology is one of the major causes of shoulder pain and disability.[33] Like other tendinopathies, treatment of chronic rotator cuff pain with prolotherapy has been shown to reduce pain and disability. In one RCT, it was revealed that injections of hypertonic dextrose on painful entheses resulted in improvement in long-term pain

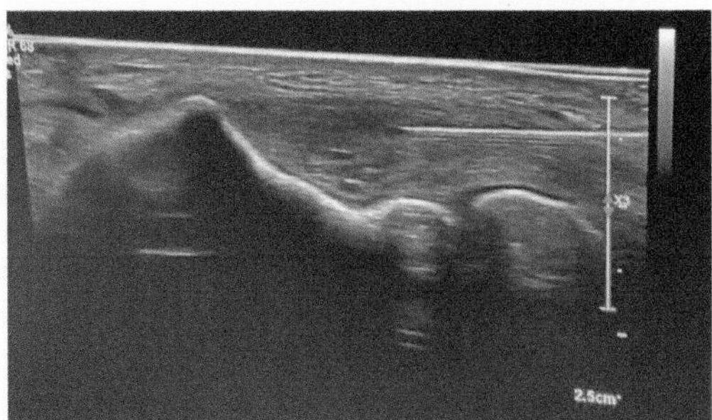

Fig. 2. In plane injection into the elbow for Lateral epicondylosis.

ratings and patient satisfaction compared with saline injections.[34] Seven and colleagues similarly studied the efficacy of dextrose prolotherapy in reducing pain and improving function by dividing patients into a control group that was treated with exercise, and a prolotherapy injection group treated with ultrasound-guided prolotherapy injections. Although both groups reported improved outcomes in all categories, there were significantly more improved scores across the board in the prolotherapy treatment group for pain, function, and shoulder range of motion.[33] A retrospective study measured the outcomes of shoulder pain and disability score in patients who received prolotherapy injections and found significant improvement in pain and disability scales 1 week to 3 months after treatment.[35] A systematic review conducted by Catapano and colleagues[36] that included 5 RCTs concluded that dextrose prolotherapy is a potentially effective adjuvant intervention to physical therapy for patients with rotator cuff tendinopathy.

Several potential injection sites target the shoulder and its supporting rotator cuff muscles. Posterior injection sites include the posterior lateral aspect of the acromion, the infraspinatus and teres minor, and into and around the AC joint. Anteriorly, the subscapularis, pectoralis major, coracoid process, anterior lateral clavicle, and lateral humerus may be injected. Positioning is important in shoulder injections, and small amounts should be peppered into each injection site with time in-between injections to range the shoulder as needed to distribute the solution along the joint (see **Table 1**).

Plantar fasciopathy

Plantar fasciopathy is defined as pain and structural changes at the tendon insertion site of the plantar fascia in the os calcis located at the bottom of the foot.[37] Several studies have studied prolotherapy as a treatment for chronic plantar fasciopathy, many comparing prolotherapy to various other nonsurgical treatments, such as extracorporeal shockwave therapy and platelet-rich plasma (PRP) injections. One RCT conducted by Ersen and colleagues divided patients into either a control group, who were given instructions for stretching exercises, or treatment group, treated with ultrasound-guided prolotherapy injections. This study discovered that while pain and foot and ankle outcome scores were significantly improved in both treatment groups, prolotherapy injections showed significantly greater improvement after 42 days of treatment.[38] Another study evaluated similar outcome measures with the addition of plantar fascia thickness and found improvements in pain and foot function across all subgroups, and significantly higher plantar fascia thickness in the prolotherapy group compared with the control group.[39] Multiple studies comparing prolotherapy and shockwave therapy found comparable and noninferior efficacy in reducing pain and function in patients with plantar fasciopathy with no serious adverse effects from either treatment.[40,41] Finally, Kim and Lee conducted a single-blinded RCT

Table 1
Common prolotherapy complaints and injection sites[a]

Joint	Common Pathologies Treated with Prolotherapy	Needle Size	Common Injection Sites
Shoulder	Rotator cuff tendinopathy	27 gauge	Supraspinatus insertion sites Infraspinatus/teres minor insertion sites Insertions on coracoid process Biceps long head Subscapularis insertion Interior glenohumeral ligament Teres minor origin Teres major origin Posterior inferior glenohumeral ligament
Elbow	Lateral epicondylosis	25 gauge	Common extensor tendon insertion sites Annular ligament and lateral collateral ligament Radial collateral ligament Radial head Supracondylar ridge Joint capsule Medial and lateral condyle
Knee	Knee osteoarthritis Collateral ligament strain	25 gauge, 22 gauge spinal needle	Thigh adductor insertions Vastus medialis insertion Collateral ligament origin and insertions Knee capsule Distal hamstring Anterior tibialis Peroneal muscles
Ankle/Foot	Achilles tendinopathy Plantar fasciitis	25 gauge, 27 gauge 22 gauge spinal needle	Achilles tendon Calcaneonavicular ligament Calcaneocuboid ligament Long plantar ligament Tarsometatarsal ligaments Tibionavicular ligament Tibiotalar ligament Tibiocalcaneal ligament
Low back/ Posterior Hip	SI joint pain Lumbar back pain	25 gauge, 22 gauge spinal needle	Facet ligaments Lumbar intertranverse ligaments Sacroiliac ligament/joint Iliolumbar ligaments Gluteal insertions Sacrospinous ligament Deep articular ligaments External rotator/abductor muscle insertion

[a] Common injection sites are not comprehensive, other tender areas along entheses and adjacent to the joint may also be injected.

comparing autologous platelet-rich plasma (PRP) versus prolotherapy for chronic plantar fasciitis and discovered that while PRP treatment resulted in better initial improvement in function compared with dextrose prolotherapy, sustained improvement was comparable between the two groups at 2 and 6 months follow-up.[42]

There are three primary insertion points for prolotherapy treatment of plantar fasciitis: the calcaneus, mid-arch, and attachments to the metatarsal heads. These sites should be palpated for tenderness before the procedure. Owing to the superficial and specific nature of these targets, these injections are ideally accomplished with ultrasound guidance to ensure therapeutic accuracy. The entry point for the calcaneal attachment is located distal to the heel pad on the medial plantar surface of the foot. A small amount (3 mL) of lidocaine should be injected first at around a 1-inch depth, followed by the insertion of a 2 inch, 25 gauge needle containing the prolotherapy solution. A 2 inch needle is recommended to reach the plantar ligament origin and insertions from the insertion site. A small amount of prolotherapy solution should be peppered into the calcaneal attachment. The second primary injection site is the mid-arch, which is located just plantar to the navicular tubercle. Again, a 25 gauge, 2 inch needle is used to insert across the arch to contact the bone on the lateral side of the arch. Finally, the metatarsal and tarsal bones may be targeted and approximately 3 to 5 mL of prolotherapy solution is injected into the metatarsal and tarsal bone injection sites (see **Table 1**).

Achilles tendinopathy

Achilles tendinopathy is one of the most common overuse injuries in sports and a frequent cause of pain and disability in active patients.[43] Multiple studies have evaluated the efficacy of prolotherapy in treating pain and function secondary to Achilles tendinopathy. In a single-blinded RCT conducted by Yelland and colleagues[43] comparing the effectiveness of eccentric loading exercises used singly and in conjunction with prolotherapy found greater improvements in pain and activity scores in eccentric loading exercises (ELE) and prolotherapy groups (86% improvement) compared with ELE therapy only (73% improvement). In another study, Maxwell and colleagues injected dextrose into patients suffering from chronic Achilles tendinopathy with abnormal areas in the tendon and partial tears on ultrasound. They discovered that on follow-up imaging, there were significant reductions from baseline in the size of the tendinosis and the size of the tear, suggesting that the tendons had become healthier after the course of prolotherapy.[44] Another similar study also recruited patients with Achilles tendon symptoms refractory to all previous therapies and found that participants treated with prolotherapy not only had improvement in pain up to 81% at 14 months posttreatment, but also had significant reductions in the size of hypoechoic regions, intratendinous tears, and neovascularization at the injury site on ultrasound.[45] In conclusion, there is good evidence to suggest a benefit in pain, function, and even tendon regeneration from prolotherapy treatment in patients with Achilles tendinopathy.

Achilles tendinosis injection is completed at multiple points along the medial and lateral aspects surrounding the Achilles tendon. A 25 or 27 gauge needle should be used and inserted gently through the skin until slight resistance is met, indicating the ideal location near the peritendinous areas. Around 3 mL of the prolotherapy solution may be peppered into the injured structure (see **Table 1**).

Osteoarthritis

Hand Osteoarthritis

Several studies have investigated the efficacy of prolotherapy on various hand and finger joints. One RCT study treated patients with chronic thumb or finger pain and radiographic evidence of hand osteoarthritis with either dextrose prolotherapy or lidocaine injections and found that patients treated with dextrose prolotherapy had greater improvements with pain and movement after 6 months.[46] Another study compared dextrose prolotherapy to steroid injections on patients with chronic thumb pain and trapeziometacarpal joint osteoarthritis and reported that pain and function were improved to a greater extent with patients treated with dextrose prolotherapy compared with steroidal injections.[47] Although the existing studies on the treatment of hand osteoarthritis with prolotherapy are promising, more evidence will be needed to determine the efficacy of prolotherapy treatment.

Metacarpophalangeal (MCP) injections are typically performed with the MCP in flexion with the insertion points around the joint, injection from the dorsal surface of the hand, with a 5 to 10 degree distal inclination from vertical. Proximal interphalangeal (PIP) and distal interphalangeal (DIP) joints are performed with a lateral approach with the injection slightly above the midline to minimize the irritation of nerve fibers. Similar to prior discussed small anatomic targets, these injections are ideally done with ultrasound-guided injection to ensure accuracy.

Knee OA

Many studies have shown a positive effect of hypertonic dextrose benefiting patients with knee OA. In one RCT, 90 adults with at least 3 months of painful knee OA were randomized to blinded prolotherapy or saline injections or at-home exercise with follow-up visits at 52 weeks. At follow-up, the patient receiving dextrose prolotherapy showed improved Western Ontario McMaster University Osteoarthritis and knee pain scores than patients receiving saline and exercise with high satisfaction rates.[48] Reeves and colleagues[49] investigated patients with knee laxity treated with dextrose prolotherapy and reported that at 12 month follow-up, the treatment group showed significant improvement in laxity compared with the control group. In a different RCT, Eslamian and colleagues[49] demonstrated significant therapeutic effects of prolotherapy with intraarticular dextrose injection in patients with moderate OA based on outcome measures of pain severity at rest and during activity as well as an articular range of motion.[50] Another study found significant improvement in the reduction of pain, swelling, and range of motion with dextrose compared to lidocaine injections or exercise at a follow-up of 52 weeks and 2.5 years after the initial study.[51]

There have also been a few experimental studies comparing the usage of prolotherapy to other existing injectable treatments for knee OA. One such study compared the effect of dextrose prolotherapy, PRP, and autologous conditioned serum on knee OA and showed no improvement in pain intensity and knee function from dextrose prolotherapy compared to ACS or PRP.[52] However, another study reported improved pain and knee joint functioning scores that were most effective for dextrose prolotherapy and botulinum toxin type A, followed by physical therapy, and lastly, intraarticular hyaluronic acid injection.[53] A systemic review published in 2019 agreed that in terms of pain reduction and functional improvement, prolotherapy was more effective than infiltrations with local anesthetics. In addition, prolotherapy was comparable to infiltrations with hyaluronic acid, ozone, or radiofrequency, but less effective than PRP and erythropoietin in short, medium, and long term based on currently existing studies.[54] There is good evidence to support the use of prolotherapy as a treatment for osteoarthritis with comparable efficacy to other nonsurgical treatment options.

The best positioning for prolotherapy knee injections is with the patient's knee bent and in slight external rotation. The knee ligaments' origins and insertions should be palpated and injected if painful. The knee capsule itself may also be injected inferomedially with prolotherapy. Common muscle attachment sites targeted for injection include the thigh adductors and vastus medialis insertions sites about the medial condyle of the femur and the hamstring insertion site medially (see **Table 1**).

Low Back and Sacroiliac Joint Pain

Low back pain

The use of prolotherapy for low back pain is controversial. Several early studies demonstrated little-to-no improvements to pain and function in patients with chronic low back pain treated with prolotherapy. One RCT investigated the efficacy of prolotherapy on chronic low back pain by dividing patients into groups of prolotherapy with or without cointerventions, and control groups with or without interventions. At 2 to 12 months, there were no significant differences in pain intensity or disability between the groups.[55] Another study had similar findings. After 1 to 6 months, there was no difference between range of motion (ROM) or pain in the prolotherapy experimental group compared with the control group that received saline. However, this study had a significant limitation given that the injector was not able to examine the patient before injection, which is an important technique required for prolotherapy administration.[56] Furthermore, other studies discovered that even in the case where prolotherapy shows a significant benefit in the improvement of pain and function, the presence of many cointerventions confound the aforementioned conclusions.[57] However, more recent prospective case series studies have demonstrated significant improvements in pain from baseline in patients treated with prolotherapy at 12 month follow-ups.[58,59]

In general, there has been conflicting evidence regarding the efficacy of prolotherapy on chronic low back pain, and this is likely the case due to a large number of different mechanisms and pathologies involved in chronic back pain. However, the literature agrees that while there is little evidence that prolotherapy injections alone were more effective than control, there does seem to be a benefit to prolotherapy in conjunction with other cointerventions, namely physical therapy, compared with control groups who are not treated with prolotherapy.[57]

SI joint pain

One subset of low back pain is caused by sacroiliac (SI) joint dysfunction or instability. Several studies have investigated the treatment of prolotherapy for chronic SI or SI joint pain with promising results. One such study found a remarkable decrease in pain levels for dextrose prolotherapy patients compared with patients who received steroid injections. In addition, the effect of prolotherapy lasted longer than steroid injections.[18] A prospective study found significant improvements at 3, 12, and 24 month follow-ups in patients treated with 3 sessions of hypertonic dextrose solution into the dorsal interosseous ligament of the affected SI joint.[60] A similar study found that a large proportion of patients with symptomatic SI joint instability as an etiology of low back pain treated with 3 prolotherapy sessions at approximately 1 month interval showed significant functional gains at follow-up.[61]

For low back and posterior hip injections, before injection, the patient's bony landmarks should be palpated. This includes the iliac crest (L4 lumbar level) and posterior superior iliac spine (PSIS) (S2 sacral level). Common injection sites include the intertransverse and facet ligaments located at L5 just below the iliac crest, and the iliolumbar and SI ligaments superior to the iliac crest. Several injection sites target the posterior hip, including gluteal muscle insertions, sacrospinous ligaments, and deep articular ligaments. These injections are typically completed with a 25 gauge 2 to 3 inch needle or 22 gauge spinal needle (see **Table 1**).

Joint Laxity

Owing to the proposed mechanism of prolotherapy, based on strengthening lax tendons and ligaments through the release of local growth factors, it is hypothesized that prolotherapy may achieve beneficial results in patients with pain secondary to joint laxity. Prolotherapy as a treatment for TMJ has been extensively studied with impressive results. One study treated patients with recurrent TMJ laxity with a modified technique of prolotherapy containing lignocaine and 50% dextrose for 1 to 4 treatment sessions, and discovered that after 6 months, 91% of the patients had no further dislocation or subluxation of their jaw.[62] A recent study investigated the efficacy of dextrose prolotherapy as monotherapy for TMJ hypermobility compared with treatment with dextrose prolotherapy along with arthrocentesis. Although both treatment groups showed significantly improved pain scores and significantly decreased locking of the jaw, treatment with dextrose prolotherapy with arthrocentesis displayed greater improvement in the outcome measures.[63] One other RCT compared the efficacy of dextrose prolotherapy in treating TMJ with that of occlusal splints, another commonly utilized conservative treatment of TMJ. This study discovered that patients receiving prolotherapy showed significantly greater improvements in pain, mouth opening, and clicking compared to treatment with occlusal splints.[64]

In addition to treatment for TMJ, there have been a few studies investigating the effect of prolotherapy on other laxity in other joints. One study examined the effects of prolotherapy on 18 patients with 6 months or more of knee pain plus ACL laxity and found that at the 3 year mark, up to 10 patients no longer had ACL laxity defined by KT1000 anterior displacement. In addition, patients reported improved pain at rest, with walking, and stair use as well as improved range of motion and subjective welling at the 3 year follow-up.[65] Lumbar spine instability due to ligamentous laxity has also been studied, with data to suggest that prolotherapy may be beneficial in restoring spinal stability and resolving chronic low back pain, compared with other mechanisms of chronic back pain.[66] In summary, apart from TMJ laxity, which has been well studied and documented, there are only a few studies to investigate the treatment of prolotherapy on ligamentous laxity in other joints. More data will be required to determine the benefits of prolotherapy for treating joint laxity in joints other than the TMJ.

TMJ prolotherapy injection is directed at the joint capsule and its surrounding supportive ligaments and tendon. With the patient's mouth closed and teeth unclenched, the physician should palpate the zygomatic arch and insert a 1 inch 30 gauge needle or 1 $^{1}/_{4}$ inch 27 gauge needle $^{1}/_{4}$ inch inferior to the palpated zygomatic arch. The needle should be advanced 1 inch and 0.75 mL of the proliferant solution should be injected. It is the authors' opinion that this specialized injection should only be performed by experienced clinicians and ultrasound guidance is recommended.

SUMMARY

The use of prolotherapy continues to be an ongoing research interest for the use of soft tissue and MSK conditions in the body. The mechanism of prolotherapy is thought to be multifactorial in nature and broadly focuses on generating a localized inflammatory response to promote endogenous healing and growth factors. Applications for prolotherapy injection include the above tendinopathy and osteoarthritis, with each of the above areas showing RCTs with significant positive effects.

However, there are limitations to the conclusions of these studies. The use of small sample sizes may limit the generalizability of several published studies. Protocol and injectate concentration and makeup varied across these studies as well as frequency. These studies often use adjunct conservative treatment which may also limit the conclusions on the efficacy of prolotherapy. Therefore, more research on prolotherapy will be important for the field of sports medicine and the many patients who present to their physicians with musculoskeletal pain.

Future areas of research on prolotherapy involve the standardization of injection protocols, exploration of alternative mechanisms of action as well as efficacy and cost-utility in other soft-tissue pathology.

CLINICS CARE POINTS

- Prolotherapy injections have been successfully performed with dextrose solutions ranging from 10% to 25%, with variable results from uncommonly used injectates such as phenol and sodium morrhuate.
- A strong understanding of anatomy and bony landmarks is important for performing prolotherapy injections. Although prolotherapy has historically been performed with palpation guidance, the development of ultrasound guided injections has been shown to improve efficacy and accuracy of joint and soft tissue injections, and is emerging as the new gold standard for joint injection guidance.
- Prolotherapy has been shown to have the most success treating tendinopathies, specifically lateral epicondylosis, and osteoarthritis of the hand and the knee. It is important to keep in mind that most studies involving prolotherapy injections have evaluated the efficacy of prolotherapy on chronic injuries. The efficacy of prolotherapy injections on acute injuries has not yet been investigated in depth.

DISCLOSURE

None of the authors have any financial conflicts of interest to disclose.

REFERENCES

1. Hauser RA, Lackner JB, Steilen-Matias D, et al. A systematic review of dextrose prolotherapy for chronic musculoskeletal pain. Clin Med Insights Arthritis Musculoskelet Disord 2016;9:139–59. CMAMD-S39160.
2. American Academy of Orthopaedic Surgeons. The burden of musculoskeletal diseases in the united states: prevalence, societal, and economic cost. Am Acad Orthopaedic Surgeons 2009;208(1).
3. Goswami A. Prolotherapy. J Pain Palliat Care Pharmacother 2012;26(4):376–8.
4. DeChellis DM, Cortazzo MH. Regenerative medicine in the field of pain medicine: Prolotherapy, platelet-rich plasma therapy, and stem cell therapy—Theory and evidence. Techniques in Regional Anesthesia and Pain. Management 2011; 15(2):74–80.
5. Rabago D, Slattengren A, Zgierska A. Prolotherapy IN PRIMARY CARE PRACTICE. Prim Care Clin Office Pract 2010;37(1):65–80.
6. Hackett GS, Hemwall GA, Montgomery GA. Ligament and tendon relaxation. Charles C Thomas; 1958.
7. Borg-Stein J, Osoria HL, Hayano T. Regenerative sports medicine: past, present, and future (adapted from the PASSOR Legacy Award Presentation; AAPMR; October 2016). PM&R. 2018;10(10):1083–105.
8. Thorens B, Mueckler M. Glucose transporters in the 21st Century. Am J Physiology-Endocrinology Metab 2010;298(2):E141–5.
9. Reeves KD. Prolotherapy: basic science, clinical studies, and technique. Pain Procedures in Clinical Practice. 2nd Ed. Hanley and Belfus Philadelphia; 2000. p. 172–90.
10. Yoshii Y, Zhao C, Schmelzer JD, et al. The effects of hypertonic dextrose injection on connective tissue and nerve conduction through the rabbit carpal tunnel. Arch Phys Med Rehabil 2009;90(2):333–9.

11. Ekwueme EC, Mohiuddin M, Yarborough JA, et al. Prolotherapy induces an inflammatory response in human tenocytes in vitro. Clin Orthopaedics Relat Research® 2017;475(8):2117–27.
12. Mobasheri A. Glucose: an energy currency and structural precursor in articular cartilage and bone with emerging roles as an extracellular signaling molecule and metabolic regulator. Front Endocrinol 2012;3:153.
13. Stecker MM, Stevenson M. Effect of glucose concentration on peripheral nerve and its response to anoxia. Muscle & nerve 2014;49(3):370–7.
14. Topol GA, Podesta LA, Reeves KD, et al. Chondrogenic effect of intra-articular hypertonic-dextrose (prolotherapy) in severe knee osteoarthritis. PM&R. 2016;8(11):1072–82.
15. Dommerholt J. Dry needling—peripheral and central considerations. J Man Manipulative Ther 2011;19(4):223–7.
16. Han DS, Lee CH, Shieh YD, et al. A role for substance P and acid-sensing ion channel 1a in prolotherapy with dextrose-mediated analgesia in a mouse model of chronic muscle pain. Pain 2021;163(5):622–33.
17. Kietrys DM, Palombaro KM, Azzaretto E, et al. Effectiveness of dry needling for upper-quarter myofascial pain: a systematic review and meta-analysis. J Orthop Sports Phys Ther 2013;43(9):620–34.
18. Kim HJ, Jeong TS, Kim WS, et al. Comparison of histological changes in accordance with the level of dextrose-concentration in experimental prolotherapy model. J Korean Acad Rehabil Med 2003;27(6):935–40.
19. Nair LS. Prolotherapy for tissue repair. Translational Res 2011;158(3):129–31.
20. Finnoff JT, Hall MM, Adams E, et al. American Medical Society for Sports Medicine (AMSSM) position statement: interventional musculoskeletal ultrasound in sports medicine. PM&R. 2015;7(2):151–68.
21. Fullerton BD, Reeves KD. Ultrasonography in regenerative injection (prolotherapy) using dextrose, platelet-rich plasma, and other injectants. Phys Med Rehabil Clin 2010;21(3):585–605.
22. Bellapianta J, Swartz F, Lisella J, et al. Randomized prospective evaluation of injection techniques for the treatment of lateral epicondylitis. Orthopedics 2011;34(11):e708–12.
23. Dagenais S, Ogunseitan O, Haldeman S, et al. Side effects and adverse events related to intraligamentous injection of sclerosing solutions (prolotherapy) for back and neck pain: a survey of practitioners. Arch Phys Med Rehabil 2006;87(7):909–13.
24. Distel LM, Best TM. Prolotherapy: a clinical review of its role in treating chronic musculoskeletal pain. PM R 2011;3(6 Suppl 1). https://doi.org/10.1016/j.pmrj.2011.04.003.
25. Rabago D, Lee KS, Ryan M, et al. Hypertonic dextrose and morrhuate sodium injections (prolotherapy) for lateral epicondylosis (tennis elbow): Results of a single-blind, pilot-level, randomized controlled trial. Am J Phys Med Rehabil 2013;92(7):587–96.
26. Scarpone M, Rabago DP, Zgierska A, et al. The efficacy of prolotherapy for lateral epicondylosis: a pilot study. Clin J Sport Med 2008;18(3):248–54. https://doi.org/10.1097/JS.
27. Shin JY, Seo KM, Kim DK, et al. The effect of prolotherapy on lateral epicondylitis of elbow. J Korean Acad Rehabil Med 2002;26(6):764–8.
28. Park JH, Song IS, Lee JB, et al. Ultrasonographic findings of healing of torn tendon in the patients with lateral epicondylitis after prolotherapy. J Korean Soc Med Ultrasound 2003;22(3):177–83.

29. Yelland M, Rabago D, Ryan M, et al. Prolotherapy injections and physiotherapy used singly and in combination for lateral epicondylalgia: a single-blinded randomised clinical trial. BMC Musculoskelet Disord 2019;20(1):509.
30. Akcay S, Gurel Kandemir N, Kaya T, et al. Dextrose prolotherapy versus normal saline injection for the treatment of lateral epicondylopathy: a randomized controlled trial. J Altern Complement Med 2020;26(12):1159–68.
31. Carayannopoulos A, Borg-Stein J, Sokolof J, et al. Prolotherapy versus corticosteroid injections for the treatment of lateral epicondylosis: a randomized controlled trial. PM R 2011;3(8):706–15.
32. Apaydin H, Bazancir Z, Altay Z. Injection therapy in patients with lateral epicondylalgia: hyaluronic acid or dextrose prolotherapy? a single-blind, randomized clinical trial. J Altern Complement Med 2020;26(12):1169–75.
33. Seven MM, Ersen O, Akpancar S, et al. Effectiveness of prolotherapy in the treatment of chronic rotator cuff lesions. Orthopaedics Traumatol Surg Res 2017; 103(3):427–33.
34. Bertrand H, Reeves KD, Bennett CJ, et al. Dextrose prolotherapy versus control injections in painful rotator cuff tendinopathy. Arch Phys Med Rehabil 2016;97: 17–25. W.B. Saunders.
35. Ryu K, Ko D, Lim G, et al. Ultrasound-guided prolotherapy with polydeoxyribonucleotide for painful rotator cuff tendinopathy. Pain Res Manag 2018;2018: 8286190.
36. Catapano M, Zhang K, Mittal N, et al. Effectiveness of dextrose prolotherapy for rotator cuff tendinopathy: a systematic review. PM&R 2020;12(3):288–300.
37. Monteagudo M, de Albornoz PM, Gutierrez B, et al. Plantar fasciopathy: a current concepts review. EFORT Open Rev 2018;3(8):485–93.
38. Ersen Ö, Koca K, Akpancar S, et al. A randomized-controlled trial of prolotherapy injections in the treatment of plantar fasciitis. Turkish J Phys Med Rehabil 2017; 64(1):59–65.
39. Mansiz-Kaplan B, Nacir B, Pervane-Vural S, et al. Effect of dextrose prolotherapy on pain intensity, disability, and plantar fascia thickness in unilateral plantar fasciitis: a randomized, controlled, double-blind study. Am J Phys Med Rehabil 2020;99(4):318–24.
40. Kesikburun S, Uran Şan A, Kesikburun B, et al. Comparison of ultrasound-guided prolotherapy versus extracorporeal shock wave therapy in the treatment of chronic plantar fasciitis: a randomized clinical trial. J Foot Ankle Surg 2021. https://doi.org/10.1053/j.jfas.2021.06.007.
41. Asheghan M, Hashemi SE, Hollisaz MT, et al. Dextrose prolotherapy versus radial extracorporeal shock wave therapy in the treatment of chronic plantar fasciitis: a randomized, controlled clinical trial. Foot Ankle Surg 2021;27(6):643–9.
42. Kim E, Lee JH. Autologous platelet-rich plasma versus dextrose prolotherapy for the treatment of chronic recalcitrant plantar fasciitis. PM R 2014;6(2):152–8.
43. Yelland MJ, Sweeting KR, Lyftogt JA, et al. Prolotherapy injections and eccentric loading exercises for painful Achilles tendinosis: a randomised trial. Br J Sports Med 2011;45(5):421–8.
44. Maxwell NJ, Ryan MB, Taunton JE, et al. Sonographically guided intratendinous injection of hyperosmolar dextrose to treat chronic tendinosis of the Achilles tendon: a pilot study 2007;189:w215–20. AJR Am J Roentgenol 2007;189: 215–20.
45. Ryan M, Wong A, Taunton J. Favorable outcomes after sonographically guided intratendinous injection of hyperosmolar dextrose for chronic insertional and midportion achilles tendinosis. AJR Am J Roentgenol 2010;194(4):1047–53.

46. Reeves KD, Hassanein K. Randomized, prospective, placebo-controlled double-blind study of dextrose prolotherapy for osteoarthritic thumb and finger (DIP, PIP, and Trapeziometacarpal) joints: evidence of clinical efficacy. J Altern Complement Med 2000;6(4):311–20.
47. Jahangiri A, Moghaddam FR, Najafi S. Hypertonic dextrose versus corticosteroid local injection for the treatment of osteoarthritis in the first carpometacarpal joint: a double-blind randomized clinical trial. J Orthop Sci 2014;19(5):737–43.
48. Rabago D, Patterson JJ, Mundt M, et al. Dextrose prolotherapy for knee osteoarthritis: a randomized controlled trial. Ann Fam Med 2013;11(3):229–37.
49. Reeves KD, Hassanein K. Randomized prospective double-blind placebo-controlled study of dextrose prolotherapy for knee osteoarthritis with or without ACL laxity. Altern Ther Health Med 2000;6(2):68–74, 77-80.
50. Eslamian F, Amouzandeh B. Therapeutic effects of prolotherapy with intra-articular dextrose injection in patients with moderate knee osteoarthritis: a single-arm study with 6 months follow up. Ther Adv Musculoskelet Dis 2015; 7(2):35–44.
51. Reeves D, Rabago D. Therapeutic injection of dextrose: Prolotherapy, perineural injection therapy and hydrodissection. PM&R Knowledge Now 2019.
52. Pishgahi A, Abolhasan R, Shakouri SK, et al. Effect of dextrose prolotherapy, platelet rich plasma and autologous conditioned serum on knee osteoarthritis: a randomized clinical trial. Iranian J Allergy Asthma Immunol 2020. https://doi.org/10.18502/ijaai.v19i3.3452.
53. Rezasoltani Z, Azizi S, Najafi S, et al. Physical therapy, intra-articular dextrose prolotherapy, botulinum neurotoxin, and hyaluronic acid for knee osteoarthritis: randomized clinical trial. Int J Rehabil Res 2020;43(3):219–27.
54. Arias-Vázquez PI, Tovilla-Zárate CA, Legorreta-Ramírez BG, et al. Prolotherapy for knee osteoarthritis using hypertonic dextrose vs other interventional treatments: systematic review of clinical trials. Adv Rheumatol 2019;59(1):39.
55. Yelland MJ, Glasziou PP, Bogduk N, et al. Prolotherapy injections, saline injections, and exercises for chronic low-back pain: a randomized trial. Spine 2004; 29(1):9–16.
56. Dechow E, Davies RK, Carr AJ, et al. A randomized, double-blind, placebo-controlled trial of sclerosing injections in patients with chronic low back pain. Rheumatology 1999;38(12):1255–9.
57. Yelland M, del Mar C, Pirozzo S, et al. Prolotherapy injections for chronic low-back pain. In: Yelland M, editor. Cochrane database of systematic reviews. John Wiley & Sons, Ltd; 2004. https://doi.org/10.1002/14651858.CD004059.pub2.
58. Khan S, Kumar A, Varshney M, et al. Dextrose prolotherapy for recalcitrant coccygodynia. J Orthop Surg 2008;16(1):27–9.
59. Miller MR, Mathews RS, Reeves KD. Treatment of painful advanced internal lumbar disc derangement with intradiscal injection of hypertonic dextrose. Pain Physician 2006;9(2):115–21.
60. Cusi M, Saunders J, Hungerford B, et al. The use of prolotherapy in the sacroiliac joint. Br J Sports Med 2010;44(2):100–4.
61. Hoffman MD, Agnish V. Functional outcome from sacroiliac joint prolotherapy in patients with sacroiliac joint instability. Complement Therapies Med 2018; 37:64–8.
62. Zhou H, Hu K, Ding Y. Modified dextrose prolotherapy for recurrent temporomandibular joint dislocation. Br J Oral Maxillofac Surg 2014;52(1):63–6.

63. Taşkesen F, Cezairli B. Efficacy of prolotherapy and arthrocentesis in management of temporomandibular joint hypermobility. CRANIO 2020;1–9. https://doi.org/10.1080/08869634.2020.1861887.
64. Priyadarshini S, Gnanam A, Sasikala B, et al. Evaluation of prolotherapy in comparison with occlusal splints in treating internal derangement of the temporomandibular joint – A randomized controlled trial. J Cranio-Maxillofacial Surg 2021; 49(1):24–8.
65. Reeves K, Hassanein KM. Long-term effects of dextrose prolotherapy for anterior cruciate ligament laxity. Altern Ther Health Med 2003;9(3):58–62.
66. Hauser RA, Matias D, Woznica D, et al. Lumbar instability as an etiology of low back pain and its treatment by prolotherapy: A review. J Back Musculoskeletal Rehabil 2022;1–12. https://doi.org/10.3233/BMR-210097.

Orthobiologic Interventions for Muscle Injuries

Philip M. Stephens, DO, MBA[a], Ryan P. Nussbaum, DO[a], Kentaro Onishi, DO[b,*]

KEYWORDS

• Orthobiologic • Muscle injury • Stem cell • Platelet-rich plasma • Prolotherapy

KEY POINTS

- Basic science research for treating muscle injury with platelet-rich plasma (PRP) or stem cells continues to increase.
- Clinical studies are sparse for treating muscle injuries with stem cells.
- The clinical trials for muscle injuries treated with PRP demonstrate an inconclusive outcome.
- Some evidence supports the use of early aspiration and PRP injection for acute muscle hematomas.
- Local anesthetic has myotoxic properties and should be used sparingly near muscle injuries.

INTRODUCTION

Epidemiology

Muscle injuries are one of the most commonly reported sporting injuries.[1] In 1 study, authors stated 1 soccer team of 25 athletes can expect 15 total muscle injuries per season.[2] Muscle injuries are typically classified into 3 subtypes based on the injury mechanism as detailed under “Muscle injury mechanisms” in later discussion. Indirect muscle tear and contusion injuries make up the majority (90%), while the third type, laceration injuries, ranks a distant third.[3,4] Muscles affected typically span 2 joints, such as the rectus femoris, semitendinosus, and gastrocnemius.[5–7] Financial impact modeled of 1 professional soccer team showed an average of 15 missed matches per club each season representing approximately €500,000 or more than $550,000.[8]

Normal Muscle Architecture

Basic muscle architecture lays the groundwork for the review of muscle injuries, grading classification, and the healing response. The simplest functional element of

[a] Physical Medicine & Rehabilitation, University of Pittsburgh Medical Center, Kaufmann Medical Building Suite 9103471 Fifth Avenue, Pittsburgh, PA 15213, USA; [b] Physical Medicine & Rehabilitation, Orthopedic Surgery, University of Pittsburgh School of Medicine and University of Pittsburgh Medical Center, Kaufmann Medical Building Suite 2013471 Fifth Avenue, Pittsburgh, PA 15213, USA
* Corresponding author.
E-mail address: onishik2@upmc.edu
Twitter: @PhilipStephens1 (P.M.S.); @DrRyanNuss (R.P.N.); @kenonishi0918 (K.O.)

Phys Med Rehabil Clin N Am 34 (2023) 181–198
https://doi.org/10.1016/j.pmr.2022.08.012

a muscle is the myofibril, composed of actin and myosin, which forms the basis for crosslinking required for contraction within a series of sarcomeres (**Fig. 1**). Myofibrils create the first bundle called a muscle fiber that is then covered in endomysium. A group of muscle fibers called a muscle fascicle is surrounded by perimysium, and these fascicles are bundled in a covering of epimysium to form a muscle. Muscle size changes, whether hypertrophy or atrophy, are predominantly attributed to a change in the number/size of actin and myosin within the myofibril in addition to the increased storage of glycogen in the sarcomere depending on the type of activity. Skeletal muscle stem cells, also known as satellite cells, are typically in a quiescent state until they are stimulated by exercise or injury to replicate and differentiate into mature skeletal muscle by fusing to muscle fibers.[9,10] Finally, the neuromuscular junction is the site of electrical stimulation of muscle fibers to induce a contraction, which has been shown to undergo morphologic changes, such as enhanced neurotransmission with increased use, or in muscular injury resulting in decruitment and ultimately impaired muscular performance.[11]

Muscle Injury Mechanisms

Injury to muscles and their underlying components results in the disruption of the meticulous organization described above. Indirect injuries, also commonly referred to as muscle strains or tears, are the most common of the 3 main injury types, as they do not require direct contact for injury and occur in eccentric (lengthening) contraction.[3,12,13] This injury type accounts for 31% of soccer injuries, 31% of baseball injuries, and 21% of basketball injuries, most commonly involving the hamstrings, rectus femoris, and medial head of gastrocnemius.[2,14,15] The second most common mechanism of muscle injuries is known as a muscle contusion. Muscle contusion is defined as a muscle injury that occurs as a result of blunt nonpenetrating trauma.[16] American football and rugby players are at highest risk for contusion owing to the

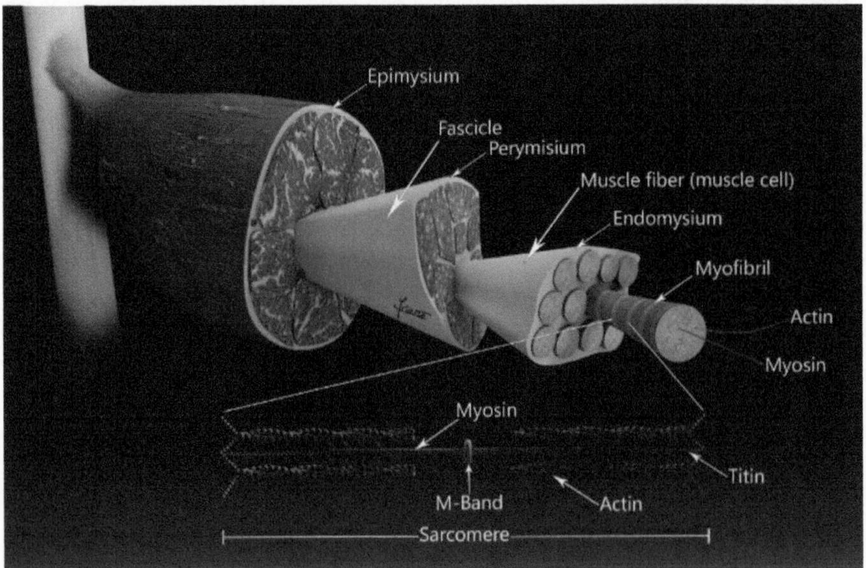

Fig. 1. Structure of a muscle form. (*From* Iriarte I, Pedret C, Balius R, Cerezal L. Ultrasound of the Musculoskeletal System Anatomical exploration and pathology. 1st edition. Bilbao: Msk Room distribution; 2021. P. 15.)

speed and level of contact representing 12% of sports injuries.[1] The least common muscle injury mechanism is laceration, blunt penetrating trauma, representing 5% and 7% of rugby and hockey injuries, respectively.[1,17]

Outside of the typical categorization of muscle injuries that is gaining attention in the field of regenerative rehabilitation is less frequent although potentially more chronically debilitating muscle injury sequela called volumetric muscle loss. This refers to the surgical or traumatic loss of muscle beyond the muscles' inherent regenerative capacity, leading to functional impairments seen in war veterans, for example,[18,19]

Clinical Classification of Muscle Injury

One of earliest muscle injury grading systems was crafted in 1963 by Dr O'Donoghue.[20] His first blueprint for universal grading was based on level of function and level of tear as either complete, moderate, or none. Limitations to this grading system included the inability to describe the injury location, size, or involvement of myotendinous structures. More recent muscle injury assessments currently in use are the Munich and British classifications.[12,13] The Munich classification incorporates type-specific categories (indirect injury types 1–4 and direct injury contusion/laceration).[13] Each category has a definition of the injury, symptoms, clinical signs, location of the injury in reference to the muscle-tendon region, and MRI/ultrasound findings.[13] The British classification aimed to use prognostic factors. Based on MRI findings, injuries were graded 1 to 4.[14] Grade 1 was a small tear; grade 2 was a moderate tear.; grade 3 was an extensive tear, and grade 4 was a complete tear. The site of injury was also included as either (a) myofascial, (b) muscular/musculotendinous, or (c) intratendinous. To date, the British classification has been validated the most in literature and is the recommended tool for utilization in practice.[21,22]

Normal Healing Response

There are 3 phases of normal muscle healing: destruction, repair, and remodeling, as described by Kalimo and colleagues[6] (**Fig. 2**). The destruction phase of the muscle repair process starts with any type of muscle architecture damage: initiating the body's reaction, including the inflammatory cell cascade and a degree of muscle necrosis. Skeletal muscle stem cells are activated as part of this response with an increase of nuclei from approximately 5% up to 15% of total nuclei observed in skeletal muscle. These cells give rise to committed myoblasts that differentiate into new multinucleated myofibers. The skeletal muscle stem cells response is influenced by injury severity, although it can be deranged in severe cases where the response may not compensate completely, or the presence of scar tissue can prevent complete myocyte to myocyte fusion.[23] Hematoma formation, a prominent feature of contusion injuries, is an additional hindrance that can prolong the healing course owing to additional cellular debris. Removal of necrotic cells, production of scar tissue, and revascularization begin the repair phase at approximately day 2 directed by the release of inflammatory mediators. The repair phase will overlap with the remodeling phase as muscle cells mature through scar tissue generally around day 7, eventually leading

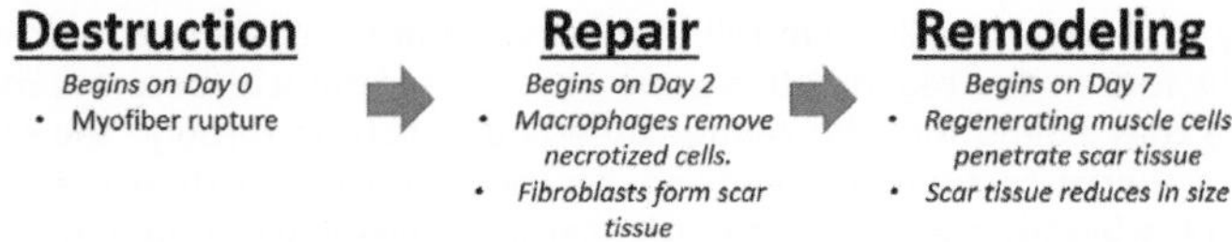
Destruction
Begins on Day 0
• Myofiber rupture
Repair
Begins on Day 2
• Macrophages remove necrotized cells.
• Fibroblasts form scar tissue
Remodeling
Begins on Day 7
• Regenerating muscle cells penetrate scar tissue
• Scar tissue reduces in size

Fig. 2. Three phases of muscle healing.

to functional recovery of the muscle with minimal residue scar tissue and the goal of reaching original structural integrity at day 21 (**Fig. 3**).[5,24]

DISCUSSION

Orthobiologic Therapeutic Options

Prolotherapy

General theory. The name prolotherapy refers to the guiding principle that the injected solution stimulates the proliferation of new cell growth with some of the earliest musculoskeletal clinical applications occurring in the 1930s when Dr Earl Gedney[25] was treating hypermobile joints. An animal study has shown that through a theoretical inflammatory and proliferation mechanism, prolotherapy can increase ligamentous tensile strength and thickness.[26] This has yet to be demonstrated in muscle. Injections can consist of a combination of dextrose (osmotic rupture of local cells), lidocaine (analgesia), sodium morrhuate (inflammatory mediator chemotactic, vascular sclerosant), phenol (vascular sclerosant), and/or glycerin (cellular irritant) in normal saline. Recently, tetradecyl was also used as a prolotherapy to treat hypermobile subjects.[27]

Basic science. One relevant study evaluating murine muscle contusion treatment found dextrose appeared to reduce macrophage reactive oxygen species damage and increase skeletal muscle stem cell regeneration. Lactate dehydrogenase, creatinine, and creatinine kinase were all decreased in prolotherapy treatment groups compared with the nontreatment control group.[28] There are no known clinical studies on muscle injury and prolotherapy.

Stem cells

General theory. Skeletal muscle stem cells are the resident regenerative cell of skeletal muscle located near blood vessels. Their population density is greater at sites

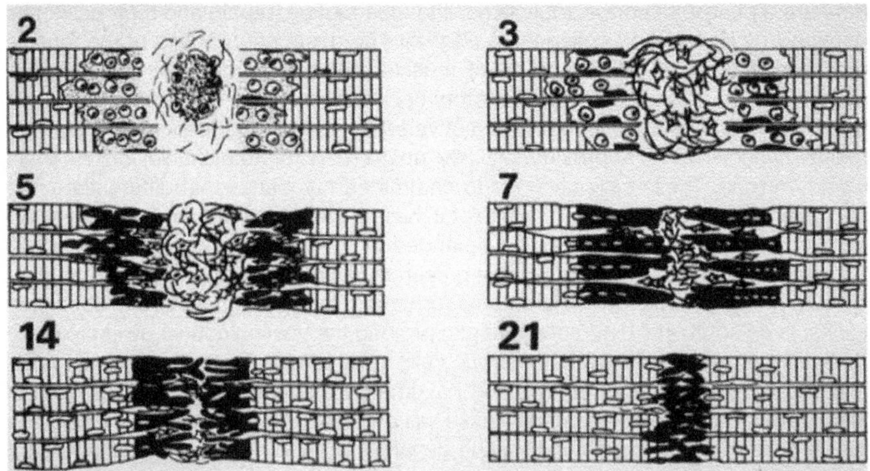

Fig. 3. Day 2: Macrophages remove necrotized muscle cells and scar tissue begins forming centrally. Day 3: Skeletal muscle stem cells are recruited in to regenerate muscle cells. Day 5: Muscle cells fuse in the regeneration zone and the central scar becomes more dense. Day 7: Muscle cells extend into the central zone and penetrate through the scar. Day 14: Central scar continues to condense, and regenerating muscle cells close the central zone gap. Day 21: Muscle cells are fused with little scar in between. (*From* Järvinen, T.A., et al., Muscle injuries: biology and treatment. Am J Sports Med, 2005. 33(5): p. 745-64.)

more likely to be stressed, such as myotendinous and neuromuscular junctions. As the master regulator of muscle remodeling induced by exercise and injury, a major role is to ensure the quiescent stem cell population is maintained to transform into muscle cells.[29] The niche or microenvironment in which these cells reside contains a delicate balance of the appropriate inputs to fuel proliferation. The general theory surrounding the implantation of stem cells, whether from bone-marrow, adipose, or perinatal tissues, is not as much differentiation into muscle cells but rather to enhance relevant environmental factors and immunoregulatory signaling to the resident stem cell population via the cell-free portion called the secretome, which increases the inherent regenerative potential. The secretome is composed of paracrine substances within exosomes and microvesicles. Two observed drawbacks of these therapies include fibrotic tissue deposition (scarring) and persistent inflammation at the site of injection. Given the limited number of clinical studies on stem cell orthobiologic treatments for muscle injuries, the emphasis of the content will be more on 3 stem cell sources, that is, bone-marrow aspirate, adipose tissue, and perinatal tissue.

Basic science

Bone marrow-derived mesenchymal stem cells The mechanism of bone marrow-derived mesenchymal stem cells (BM-MSC) and muscle tissue repair is largely unknown with their capacity for muscle differentiation uncertain because of the paucity of literature in this area. BM-MSC has been evaluated in a rodent crush trauma model with delivery intramuscularly and intra-arterially. The intra-arterial delivery did not show improvement in muscle function, whereas the intramuscular showed improved muscle regeneration and function. It was theorized by the authors that the intra-arterial route allowed stem cells to target the location of injury unlike intramuscular placement, although this was not the case.[30] Similarly, an animal contusion muscle model treated with local intramuscular injection of BM-MSC improved the number of regenerating myofibers and muscle strength.[31]

The investigators suspected that the paracrine functionality of secreted cytokines and growth factors stimulated increased activity of local skeletal muscle stem cells. Multiple recent studies have supported these paracrine effects.[31–33] An additional rat muscle reinjury model showed BM-MSC when paired with a 3-dimensional gel matrix consisting of reconstituted basement membrane allowed cells to remain at the site of injury for a prolonged time period producing increased muscle cross-section, mature muscle fibers, and contractility without a change in scar formation.[34] In summary, there is early basic scientific evidence that BM-MSC helps muscle crush and contusion injuries via paracrine mechanisms.

Adipose-derived mesenchymal stem cell When compared with BM-MSC, adipose-derived mesenchymal stem cells (AD-MSC) can be more easily harvested with minimally invasive procedures typically of the abdomen.[35] Studies have shown the highly inducible myogenic tendency of these cells while in vitro.[36,37]

One concern of these orthobiologic therapies has been the development of more than expected scarring at times likely owing to the incorrect balance of cells, exosomes, and various injectates. Scarring in muscles disrupts contraction force and muscle cell stability potentially attributing to increased reinjury rates. Muscular dystrophy, with its hallmark of muscle fibrosis, was investigated by 2 studies. One study attested to AD-MSC's ability to downregulate transforming growth factor-beta (TGF-B), a fibrosis mediator, by 2.5-fold to decrease excess collagen production.[38] The other muscular dystrophy study combined AD-MSC with Losartan, a medication widely known to have antifibrotic properties commonly prescribed in muscular dystrophy, which found the combination to have lower levels of TGF-B than AD-MSC or Losartan alone.[39] Further controlled clinical trials and in vivo studies must be completed before the true potential of this therapy can be known. Further controlled trials and in vivo studies are necessary to understand the efficacy of the promising treatment of AD-MSC and Losartan for reducing muscle fibrosis.

Perinatal sources As early as 2004, the first studies were completed documenting MSCs derived from fetal tissues could be transplanted without immunologic rejection—opening the door to the study of a variety of applications for these cells with early embryologic origin.[40] **Fig. 4** demonstrates the different perinatal tissues. Umbilical cord blood (UCB) and umbilical cord tissue (UCT) as well as placenta receive less ethical scrutiny in comparison to other fetal cell lines. When it comes to mesenchymal stem cells, with the ability to treat muscular injuries, UCB is the most limited of the 3 owing to low potency and slow rate of replication in vitro when compared with other sources, such as BM-MSC.[40] Although UCB-MSCs may not be first line, they do retain trilineage differentiation into chondrocytes, adipocytes, and osteocytes,[41] UCT-MSCs isolated from Wharton jelly of the umbilical cord are extracted at a much greater rate than from UCB.[42] Wharton jelly is connective tissue in the umbilical cord that exists between the amniotic epithelium and the umbilical vasculature.[43] In addition, Wharton jelly UCT-MSCs have exhibited robust myogenic differentiation when injected into injured murine tibialis anterior muscle.[44] These cells were also shown to reduce

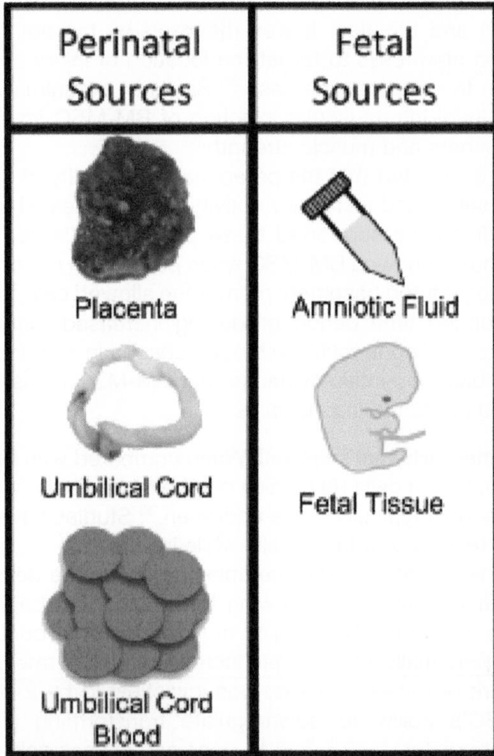

Fig. 4. Different perinatal tissues. (*From* Brown C, McKee C, Bakshi S, et al. Mesenchymal stem cells: Cell therapy and regeneration potential. J Tissue Eng Regen Med. 2019;13(9):1738-1755.)

fibrosis by modulating neutrophil response and improve functional outcomes in a murine quadriceps muscle injury model.[45] In a study comparing placenta with bone-marrow sources, placenta was found to have a better proliferative rate and superior longevity for stem cells.[46] An additional study demonstrated benefits of UCT-MSCs through antifibrotic, proangiogenic, and antiapoptotic properties that also included being immunoprivileged.[44,46,47]

Clinical trials. A specific literature review in PubMed of clinical trials using MSCs for muscle injury in the last 10 years resulted in only 1 study of hip abductor injury sustained during total hip arthroplasty treated with placenta stem cells. This study, using allogeneic placenta-derived, mesenchymal-like adherent cells, represents the first successful treatment of its kind for skeletal muscle injury at the scale of a phase I/IIa randomized, double-blinded, and placebo-controlled trial. Twenty patients were enrolled that were split into 3 groups randomized 1:1:1 into either low-dose stem cells (1.5×10^8), high-dose stem cells (3.0×10^8), or placebo. Overall, the treatment group had significantly improved strength and muscle volume. Histology confirmed accelerated healing with cell injury, and biomarkers revealed the low-dose treatment superiorly reduced the surgery-related immune reaction.[48] Two key findings of this investigation are (1) allogeneic cells serve an important immunoregulatory role in muscle injury that has the ability to improve muscle volume and strength; and (2) substantiation of upper dose-response threshold of cell concentration.

Platelet-rich plasma

General theory. The idea of implanting concentrated platelets to injured tissues relies on the influence of the biologically active microparticles released by these cells that work on all 3 phases of the healing cascade. These microparticles consist of cytokines, chemokines, growth factors, and lysosomes. Muscle injuries appear to benefit from these platelet-rich plasma (PRP) microparticles, which facilitate healing.[32,49]

Basic science. The variations of PRP preparations, including activating agents, platelet counts, centrifugation, and pH, only add to the complexities of interpreting study outcomes on PRP for muscle injuries.[32,33] Mautner and colleagues[50] proposed a standard classification system for PRP that includes platelet cell count, leukocyte cell count, red blood cell count, and use of activation (PLRA) to improve research quality. An in vitro study investigated the effects of 7 LP-PRP fractions; preparations with the lowest platelet concentrations established the greatest myocyte differentiation into muscle tissue and the lowest cell proliferative rates.[51] This important study with side-by-side comparisons of various compositions provides a poignant example of how these treatments must be tailored to the specific indication instead of the one-size-fits-all treatment it has previously been thought to be. As the field continues to delineate the intricacies of these biological approaches, it is imperative while studies are designed and outcomes in the clinic are measured that the terminology evolves with the fund of knowledge to advance collective understanding.[32,50,52–54]

Animal studies that have looked at the optimal time point in the healing response to reduce fibrosis and improve exercise tolerance found it to be day 7, corresponding to the time when mature muscle cells start penetrating through the scar when the repair phase transitions to the remodeling phase.[55] Additional murine studies aimed at decreasing fibrosis and improved skeletal muscle stem cell activation found PRP preparations depleted of TGF-b1, a mediator of fibrosis, enhanced both aspects of the target muscle tissue's regeneration.[56] In addition, when losartan provided orally is combined with PRP to the muscle contusion, there is decreased TGF-b1–mediated fibrosis and increased angiogenesis when compared with PRP alone.[57]

Clinical trials. PRP has the largest number of clinical studies for muscle injuries. Of the 10 total studies, 6 are randomized controlled trials (RCT).[58–63] Four additional studies are a mix of case series, case control, and cohort.[64–67] Overall, hamstring muscle injuries are most commonly evaluated in these studies, and there are mixed results with regards to benefit of PRP for muscle injury (see **Table 1** for a more detailed summary of these research studies). All 10 studies investigated the effect of PRP for acute lower-limb muscle injuries, and 9 studies pertained to muscle injuries sustained by athletic populations. One hundred ninety-five professional athletes were represented out of 483 indexed cases. Nine out of 10 studies used ultrasound guidance for PRP placement. Of 6 RCTs, 4 studies used ultrasound AND revealed PRP formula. Two studies using ultrasound-guided leukocyte-rich platelet-rich plasma (LR-PRP) on 58 athletes showed benefits, whereas 2 studies using ultrasound-guided leukocyte-poor platelet-rich plasma (LP-PRP) showed no clinical benefits. As for safety, no adverse reactions were reported besides 1 athlete experiencing painful dermal hyperaesthesia at injection site, preventing return to play during follow-up.[61]

In summary, clinical benefits are most commonly seen with LR-PRP when it is guided by ultrasound. Generalizability of this statement to the nonathletic population is yet to be studied.

ADDITIONAL CLINICAL CONSIDERATIONS

Improving Rotator Cuff Muscle Atrophy

Two murine research studies focused on supraspinatus muscle strengthening. This is an important avenue owing to the muscle atrophy that can rapidly result following a rotator cuff tear. The first study used BM-MSCs with saline and untreated groups as controls, showing statistically significant muscle mass increase compared with both controls.[68] PRP was the subject of another study on this topic that found suppression of fatty degenerative change, although they did not find an increase in the weight of the supraspinatus, which the authors attributed to TGF-b levels that are known to prevent adipocyte differentiation.[69] Given the limited studies, there is insufficient evidence to support orthobiologic therapies for treating rotator cuff muscle atrophy.

To Aspirate or Not to Aspirate Hematoma

Injuries associated with hematoma increase healing time based on their size owing to the need to reabsorb blood components and debris, which can be mitigated by aspiration of the hematoma before coagulation.[70,71] It could also be hypothesized that limiting blood product–related irritation could reduce scar formation at the site. Ultrasound has been established as an effective tool for evaluating and guiding aspiration with recommendations to follow up initial assessment with a scan at 48 hours to rule out additional hematoma formation.[65,72]

A recent article compared athletes with grade 2 hamstring tear with hematoma formation on MRI within 3 days of injury treated conservatively with physical therapy against treatment with hematoma aspiration and PRP injection, finding a statistically significant reduction of return to play by 9 days and hematoma recurrence of 28.6% to less than 4% in the aspiration + LR-PRP group.[73] Another study compared hematoma evacuation alone with evacuation plus LP-PRP and found the addition of LP-PRP did not significantly change return to play time or hematoma formation.[60] Although more research is needed, clinicians can consider aspirating acute hematomas and injecting PRP for an acute grade 2 hamstring muscle injuries.

Table 1
Summary of research studies treating muscle injuries with platelet-rich plasma

Study	Population	Injury Location & Grade	Chronicity	Study Type	Level of Evidence	Type of PRP	Ultrasound	Control	Outcomes
RCTs									
Hamid, 2014[61]	28 athletes	Hamstring, grade 2	Acute (<7 d)	SB RCT	Level I	LR-PRP (Biomet GPS III)	Yes	Rehabilitation only (PATS protocol)	PRP + PATS rehabilitation sig for reduction of pain & RTP: PRP 42.5 vs control 26.7 PRP group had sig lower pain severity scores at all time points though not stat sig
Hamilton, 2015[59]	90 professional athletes	Hamstring, grade 1 or 2	Acute (<5 d)	DB RCT, 3-arm	Level I	LR-PRP (Biomet GPS III Platelet Separation System)	No, palpation	PPP + rehabilitation; rehabilitation only	Median RTP: PRP 21 d vs PPP 27 d vs control 25 d, no sig of RTP for PRP over rehabilitation only Hazard ratio dem. PRP patient has 2.29 times greater chance of RTP compared with PPP

(*continued on next page*)

Table 1
(continued)

Study	Population	Injury Location & Grade	Chronicity	Study Type	Level of Evidence	Type of PRP	Ultrasound	Control	Outcomes
Reurink, 2014[62]; 2015[63]	80 athletes	Hamstring, grade 1 or 2	Acute	DB RCT	Level I	LP-PRP (Arthrex double syringe ACP system)	Yes	Saline injection + rehabilitation	No sig of PRP over saline in RTP no benefit of PRP injection in acute hamstring injury on RTP and the reinjury rate within 2 mo post RTP
Rossi, 2017[54]	75 athletes	Hamstrings, quadriceps, gastrocnemius, grade 2	Acute (<7 d)	SB RCT	Level I	NR	Yes	Rehabilitation only	Stat sig RTP: PRP 21.1 vs control 25 Stat sig pain improvement at all time points
Bubnov, 2013[58]	30 professional athletes	Thigh, foot/ ankle, shoulder trauma, grade NR	Acute	RCT	Level I	LR-PRP (unknown)	Yes	Rehabilitation only	Stat sig strength improves for first 7 days, pain decreases for first 21 d, and ROM improvement through 28 d

Study	Population	Injury Location	Chronicity	Study Type	Level of Evidence	Type of PRP	Ultrasound	Control	Outcomes
Martinez-Zapata, 2013[60]	71 patients	Hematoma at the gastrocnemius muscle or the lower portion of the rectus femoris, grade NR	Acute	DB RCT	Level I	LP-PRP activated with $CaCl_2$ (MCS+, Haemonetics)	Yes	Hematoma evacuation + sham	No sig of healing time between groups
Non-RCT									
Rettig, 2013[66]	10 NFL players	Hamstring, grade 1 or 2	Acute (<2 d)	Case control	Level III	NR w/bicarb for pain (Biomet GPS III)	Yes	Rehabilitation only	No sig between PRP + rehabilitation and rehabilitation only
Guillodo, 2015[65]	34 athletes	Hamstring, grade 3	Acute (<8 d)	Cohort	Level II	NR (Ortho. Pras 20 kit)	Yes	Rehabilitation only	No sig RTP: PRP 50.9 vs rehabilitation only 52.8 Participants that chose rehabilitation over PRP alone practiced at a sig (P = .01) higher level (ie, international)
Zanon, 2016[67]	25 professional soccer players	Hamstring, grade 2	NR	Case series	Level IV	LR-PRP w/Ca Glu (NR)	Yes	None	MRI of PRP-treated lesions revealed minimal scarring suggestive of the healed tissue

(*continued on next page*)

Table 1
(*continued*)

Study	Population	Injury Location	Chronicity	Study Type	Level of Evidence	Type of PRP	Ultrasound	Control	Outcomes
									Lack of control to quantify change in healing time
Bezuglov, 2019[64]	40 professional soccer players	Hamstring, grade 2	Acute	Case control	Level III	LR-PRP w/$CaCl_2$ (Endoret PRGF System BTI 4)	Yes	Saline injection + rehab	Stat sig RTP: PRP 11.4 vs control 21.3

Abbreviations: Bicarb, Bicarbonate; DB RCT, double-blinded randomized controlled trial; Dem, demonstrated; NR, not reported; PATS, Progressive Agility and Trunk Stabilization; PPP, platelet poor plasma; ROM, Range of Motion; RTP, return to play; SB RCT, single blinded randomized controlled trial; Sig, significant; Stat, statistical.

Local Anesthetic and Muscle Injury

In many instances, pain relief is a main indication patients seek in treatment for their muscle injury, which leads practitioners to consider adding anesthetic to their orthobiologic treatment. An in vitro study showed a decrease in myocyte viability in a concentration-dependent manner of lidocaine exposure with replication arrest at the lowest concentrations.[74] Skeletal muscle stem cells are shown to be spared by anesthetic, although repeat injections can cause fibrous deposition. In addition, when epinephrine is added to the injection, it results in blood vessel constriction, leading to prolonged exposure and increased myotoxic effects with the most severe injury attributed to bupivacaine and lidocaine.[75] A large systematic review of anesthetic use demonstrated necrosis of muscle fiber may consequently increase muscle repair time by 2 to 5 weeks.[63] When performing an injection, clinicians should minimize local anesthetic administration in muscle to prevent myotoxicity. An alternative practice to minimize procedural pain could include use of a larger-gauge needle.

GUIDELINES FROM PROFESSIONAL SPORT ORGANIZATIONS

Sport organizations have published guidelines for use of orthobiologics in sport injuries. One of earliest consensus statements published by a large governing body includes the 2008 International Olympic Committee (IOC) statement addressing the mechanism of muscle injury and the need for high-quality studies to address the knowledge gap in treatment of these injuries.[76] The IOC came together again in 2010 publishing a consensus statement for the use of PRP in sports medicine. Their report acknowledged the theoretical benefits of delivering growth factors and immunoregulators to speed muscle regeneration and minimize scar formation while heeding caution because of the lack of RCTs with clear parameters: clear diagnosis, PRP production, PRP delivery, defined outcome measures/endpoints, standardized posttreatment protocols, and reporting of adverse reactions.[77] Organizations including the American Medical Society for Sports Medicine (AMSSM) and National Basketball Association (NBA) have also published similar guidelines (see **Table 2** for a summary of these guidelines). All 3 organizations recognize there is not enough evidence to endorse the use of orthobiologics for muscle injuries[78–80]

Key Takeaway

Basic science research continues to develop a framework for treating muscle injuries with orthobiologic therapies. There continues to be a void of clinical data to strongly support orthobiologic therapies for muscle injury and the necessary indications for use. LR-PRP injections used in lower-limb muscles of athletic populations under ultrasound guidance seem to result in the best outcomes based on available literature today.

Table 2
Guidelines from professional sport organizations for orthobiologic use in muscle injuries

AMSSM 2021[79]	Currently, the efficacy of PRP injections for muscle injuries is unknown, as this area has not been well studied
NBA 2020[78]	The NBA Team Physicians Society and the National Basketball Players Association (NBPA) do not recommend the routine use of orthobiologic injections for acute muscle injuries at this time
IOC 2010[77]	In summary, at present there is little scientific support for the use of PRP for the management of muscle strain injuries

SUMMARY

Successful treatment of muscle injuries remains a difficult challenge. Fortunately, basic science research in orthobiologics and some clinical studies provide optimism for treating this condition. Specifically, basic science has focused on reducing scar formation during the muscle-healing process by downregulation of TGF-B. To this point, there is not enough research to support the wide utilization of orthobiologics for treating muscle injuries. Regardless, newer studies on acute muscle hematomas treated with aspiration and PRP injection have beneficial outcomes that make this intervention worth considering. Muscle injuries treated with LR-PRP injections, using ultrasound guidance, appear to have the strongest evidence. When performing interventions around injured muscle, medical providers should be aware of the myotoxic properties of local anesthetic and the risk of further injuring the muscle with an intramuscular injection.

CLINICS CARE POINTS

- There is inconclusive evidence to support platelet-rich plasma as an effective treatment option of muscle injuries. Some evidence supports using platelet-rich plasma in combination with aspiration for an acute muscle hematoma.
- There is inconclusive evidence to support stem cells or prolotherapy as effective treatments for muscle injuries.
- Because of the myotoxic property of local anesthetic, consider using the minimal amount in muscle during an injection.
- Scar formation during the muscle-healing process represents one of the major challenges during recovery. Future treatments will likely aim to reduce transforming growth factor-B to prevent scar development, such as losartan.

DISCLOSURE

K. Onishi discloses royalties from Springer Co Ltd for Tendinopathy book. P.M. Stephens & R.P. Nussbaum have nothing to disclose.

REFERENCES

1. Fernandez WG, Yard EE, Comstock RD. Epidemiology of lower extremity injuries among US high school athletes. Acad Emerg Med 2007;14(7):641–5.
2. Ekstrand J, Hägglund M, Waldén M. Epidemiology of muscle injuries in professional football (soccer). Am J Sports Med 2011;39(6):1226–32.
3. Chan O, Del Buono A, Best TM, et al. Acute muscle strain injuries: a proposed new classification system. Knee Surg Sports Traumatol Arthrosc 2012;20(11): 2356–62.
4. Järvinen MJ, Lehto MU. The effects of early mobilisation and immobilisation on the healing process following muscle injuries. Sports Med 1993;15(2):78–89.
5. Järvinen TA, Järvinen M, Kalimo H. Regeneration of injured skeletal muscle after the injury. Muscles Ligaments Tendons J 2013;3(4):337–45.
6. Kalimo H, Rantanen J, Järvinen M. Muscle injuries in sports. Bailliere's Clin Orthopaedics 1996;2:1–24.
7. Kujala UM, Orava S, Järvinen M. Hamstring injuries. Sports Med 1997;23(6): 397–404.

8. Ekstrand J. Keeping your top players on the pitch: the key to football medicine at a professional level. Br J Sports Med 2013;47(12):723–4.
9. Exeter D, Connell DA. Skeletal muscle: functional anatomy and pathophysiology. Semin Musculoskelet Radiol 2010;14(2):97–105.
10. Frontera WR, Ochala J. Skeletal muscle: a brief review of structure and function. Calcif Tissue Int 2015;96(3):183–95.
11. Deschenes MR, Covault J, Kraemer WJ, et al. The neuromuscular junction. Sports Med 1994;17(6):358–72.
12. Mueller-Wohlfahrt H-W, Haensel L, Mithoefer K, et al. Terminology and classification of muscle injuries in sport: the Munich consensus statement. Br J Sports Med 2013;47(6):342–50.
13. Pollock N, James SL, Lee JC, et al. British athletics muscle injury classification: a new grading system. Br J Sports Med 2014;48(18):1347–51.
14. Camp CL, Dines JS, van der List JP, et al. Summative report on time out of play for major and minor league baseball: an analysis of 49,955 injuries from 2011 through 2016. Am J Sports Med 2018;46(7):1727–32.
15. Rodas G, Bove T, Caparrós T, et al. Ankle sprain versus muscle strain injury in professional men's basketball: a 9-year prospective follow-up study. Orthop J Sports Med 2019;7(6). 2325967119849035.
16. Grazier K. The frequency of occurrence, impact, cost of selected musculoskeletal conditions in the United States. Am Acad Orthop Surgeon 1984;1(1):73–5.
17. Anderson GR, Melugin HP, Stuart MJ. Epidemiology of injuries in ice hockey. Sports Health 2019;11(6):514–9.
18. Gentile NE, Stearns KM, Brown EH, et al. Targeted rehabilitation after extracellular matrix scaffold transplantation for the treatment of volumetric muscle loss. Am J Phys Med Rehabil 2014;93(11 Suppl 3):S79–87.
19. Rando TA, Ambrosio F. Regenerative rehabilitation: applied biophysics meets stem cell therapeutics. Cell Stem Cell 2018;22(3):306–9.
20. O'Donoghue DH. Introduction. Treatment of injuries to athletes. 1962. Clin Orthop Relat Res 2002;(402):3–8.
21. Patel A, Chakraverty J, Pollock N, et al. British athletics muscle injury classification: a reliability study for a new grading system. Clin Radiol 2015;70(12): 1414–20.
22. Wangensteen A, Tol JL, Roemer FW, et al. Intra-and interrater reliability of three different MRI grading and classification systems after acute hamstring injuries. Eur J Radiol 2017;89:182–90.
23. Sassoli C, Vallone L, Tani A, et al. Combined use of bone marrow-derived mesenchymal stromal cells (BM-MSCs) and platelet rich plasma (PRP) stimulates proliferation and differentiation of myoblasts in vitro: new therapeutic perspectives for skeletal muscle repair/regeneration. Cell Tissue Res 2018;372(3):549–70.
24. Järvinen TA, Järvinen TL, Kääriäinen M, et al. Muscle injuries: biology and treatment. Am J Sports Med 2005;33(5):745–64.
25. Gedney E. Hypermobile joint: a preliminary report. Osteopath Prof 1937;4:30–1.
26. Liu YK, Tipton CM, Matches RD, et al. An in situ study of a Sclerosing solution in rabbit medial collateral ligaments and its junction strength. Connect Tissue Res 1983;11(2–3):95–102.
27. Burling F. Comparison of tetradecyl sulfate versus polidocanol injections for stabilisation of joints that regularly dislocate in an Ehlers-Danlos population. BMJ Open Sport Exerc Med 2019;5(1):e000481.
28. Tsai S-W, Hsu Y-J, Lee M-C, et al. Effects of dextrose prolotherapy on contusion-induced muscle injuries in mice. Int J Med Sci 2018;15(11):1251.

29. Dunn A, Talovic M, Patel K, et al. Biomaterial and stem cell-based strategies for skeletal muscle regeneration. J Orthop Res 2019;37(6):1246–62.
30. von Roth P, Duda GN, Radojewski P, et al. Intra-arterial MSC transplantation restores functional capacity after skeletal muscle trauma. Open Orthop J 2012;6: 352–6.
31. Chiu CH, Chang TH, Chang SS, et al. Application of bone marrow-derived mesenchymal stem cells for muscle healing after contusion injury in mice. Am J Sports Med 2020;48(5):1226–35.
32. Everts P, Onishi K, Jayaram P, et al. Platelet-rich plasma: new performance understandings and therapeutic considerations in 2020. Int J Mol Sci 2020;(20):21.
33. Scully D, Matsakas A. Current insights into the potential misuse of platelet-based applications for doping in sports. Int J Sports Med 2019;40(07):427–33.
34. Andrade BM, Baldanza MR, Ribeiro KC, et al. Bone marrow mesenchymal cells improve muscle function in a skeletal muscle re-injury model. PLoS One 2015; 10(6):e0127561.
35. Tsuji W, Rubin JP, Marra KG. Adipose-derived stem cells: implications in tissue regeneration. World J Stem Cells 2014;6(3):312–21.
36. Mizuno H, Zuk PA, Zhu M, et al. Myogenic differentiation by human processed lipoaspirate cells. Plast Reconstr Surg 2002;109(1):199–209 [discussion: 10-1].
37. Yu D, Cai Z, Li D, et al. Myogenic differentiation of stem cells for skeletal muscle regeneration. Stem Cells Int 2021;2021:8884283.
38. Pinheiro CH, de Queiroz JC, Guimarães-Ferreira L, et al. Local injections of adipose-derived mesenchymal stem cells modulate inflammation and increase angiogenesis ameliorating the dystrophic phenotype in dystrophin-deficient skeletal muscle. Stem Cell Rev Rep 2012;8(2):363–74.
39. Lee EM, Kim AY, Lee EJ, et al. Therapeutic effects of mouse adipose-derived stem cells and losartan in the skeletal muscle of injured mdx mice. Cell Transplant 2015;24(5):939–53.
40. Wexler SA, Donaldson C, Denning-Kendall P, et al. Adult bone marrow is a rich source of human mesenchymal 'stem' cells but umbilical cord and mobilized adult blood are not. Br J Haematol 2003;121(2):368–74.
41. Amati E, Sella S, Perbellini O, et al. Generation of mesenchymal stromal cells from cord blood: evaluation of in vitro quality parameters prior to clinical use. Stem Cell Res Ther 2017;8(1):14.
42. Mishra S, Sevak JK, Das A, et al. Umbilical cord tissue is a robust source for mesenchymal stem cells with enhanced myogenic differentiation potential compared to cord blood. Sci Rep 2020;10(1):1–12.
43. Taghizadeh R, Cetrulo K, Cetrulo C. Wharton's Jelly stem cells: future clinical applications. Placenta 2011;32:S311–5.
44. Conconi MT, Burra P, Di Liddo R, et al. CD105(+) cells from Wharton's jelly show in vitro and in vivo myogenic differentiative potential. Int J Mol Med 2006;18(6): 1089–96.
45. Su W-H, Wang C-J, Fu H-C, et al. Human umbilical cord mesenchymal stem cells extricate bupivacaine-impaired skeletal muscle function via mitigating neutrophil-mediated acute inflammation and protecting against fibrosis. Int J Mol Sci 2019; 20(17):4312.
46. Barlow S, Brooke G, Chatterjee K, et al. Comparison of human placenta- and bone marrow-derived multipotent mesenchymal stem cells. Stem Cells Dev 2008;17(6):1095–107.
47. Magatti M, Vertua E, Cargnoni A, et al. The immunomodulatory properties of amniotic cells: the two sides of the coin. Cell Transpl 2018;27(1):31–44.

48. Winkler T, Perka C, von Roth P, et al. Immunomodulatory placental-expanded, mesenchymal stromal cells improve muscle function following hip arthroplasty. J Cachexia Sarcopenia Muscle 2018;9(5):880–97.
49. Cruciani M, Franchini M, Mengoli C, et al. Platelet-rich plasma for sports-related muscle, tendon and ligament injuries: an umbrella review. Blood Transfus 2019; 17(6):465–78.
50. Mautner K, Malanga GA, Smith J, et al. A call for a standard classification system for future biologic research: the rationale for new PRP nomenclature. PM&R 2015; 7(4):S53–9.
51. Miroshnychenko O, Chang W-t, Dragoo JL. The use of platelet-rich and platelet-poor plasma to enhance differentiation of skeletal myoblasts: implications for the use of autologous blood products for muscle regeneration. Am J Sports Med 2017;45(4):945–53.
52. Chahla J, Cinque ME, Piuzzi NS, et al. A call for standardization in platelet-rich plasma preparation protocols and composition reporting: a systematic review of the clinical orthopaedic literature. J Bone Joint Surg Am 2017;99(20):1769–79.
53. Le AD, Enweze L, DeBaun MR, et al. Platelet-rich plasma. Clin Sports Med 2019; 38(1):17–44.
54. Rossi L, Murray I, Chu C, et al. Classification systems for platelet-rich plasma. Bone Joint J 2019;101(8):891–6.
55. Denapoli PMA, Stilhano RS, Ingham SJM, et al. Platelet-rich plasma in a murine model: leukocytes, growth factors, Flt-1, and muscle healing. Am J Sports Med 2016;44(8):1962–71.
56. Martins RP, Hartmann DD, de Moraes JP, et al. Platelet-rich plasma reduces the oxidative damage determined by a skeletal muscle contusion in rats. Platelets 2016;27(8):784–90.
57. Terada S, Ota S, Kobayashi M, et al. Use of an antifibrotic agent improves the effect of platelet-rich plasma on muscle healing after injury. J Bone Joint Surg Am 2013;95(11):980–8.
58. Bubnov R, Yevseenko V, Semeniv I. Ultrasound guided injections of platelets rich plasma for muscle injury in professional athletes. Comparative study. Med Ultrason 2013;15(2):101–5.
59. Hamilton B, Tol JL, Almusa E, et al. Platelet-rich plasma does not enhance return to play in hamstring injuries: a randomised controlled trial. Br J Sports Med 2015; 49(14):943–50.
60. Martinez-Zapata MJ, Orozco L, Balius R, et al. Efficacy of autologous platelet-rich plasma for the treatment of muscle rupture with haematoma: a multicentre, randomised, double-blind, placebo-controlled clinical trial. Blood Transfus 2016; 14(2):245–54.
61. Hamid MSA, Mohamed Ali MR, Yusof A, et al. Platelet-rich plasma injections for the treatment of hamstring injuries: a randomized controlled trial. Am J Sports Med 2014;42(10):2410–8.
62. Reurink G, Goudswaard GJ, Moen MH, et al. Rationale, secondary outcome scores and 1-year follow-up of a randomised trial of platelet-rich plasma injections in acute hamstring muscle injury: the Dutch Hamstring Injection Therapy study. Br J Sports Med 2015;49(18):1206–12.
63. Reurink G, Goudswaard GJ, Moen MH, et al. Myotoxicity of injections for acute muscle injuries: a systematic review. Sports Med 2014;44(7):943–56.
64. Bezuglov E, Maffulli N, Tokareva A, et al. Platelet-rich plasma in hamstring muscle injuries in professional soccer players: a pilot study. Muscles Ligaments Tendons J 2019;9(1):112–8.

65. Guillodo Y, Madouas G, Simon T, et al. Platelet-rich plasma (PRP) treatment of sports-related severe acute hamstring injuries. Muscles Ligaments Tendons J 2015;5(4):284–8.
66. Rettig AC, Meyer S, Bhadra AK. Platelet-rich plasma in addition to rehabilitation for acute hamstring injuries in NFL players: clinical effects and time to return to play. Orthop J Sports Med 2013;1(1). 2325967113494354.
67. Zanon G, Combi F, Combi A, et al. Platelet-rich plasma in the treatment of acute hamstring injuries in professional football players. Joints 2016;4(1):17–23.
68. Güleçyüz MF, Macha K, Pietschmann MF, et al. Allogenic myocytes and mesenchymal stem cells partially improve fatty rotator cuff degeneration in a rat model. Stem Cell Rev Rep 2018;14(6):847–59.
69. Takase F, Inui A, Mifune Y, et al. Effect of platelet-rich plasma on degeneration change of rotator cuff muscles: in vitro and in vivo evaluations. J Orthop Res 2017;35(8):1806–15.
70. Hotfiel T, Seil R, Bily W, et al. Nonoperative treatment of muscle injuries-recommendations from the GOTS expert meeting. J Exp Orthop 2018;5(1):1–11.
71. Sciorati C, Rigamonti E, Manfredi AA, et al. Cell death, clearance and immunity in the skeletal muscle. Cell Death Differ 2016;23(6):927–37.
72. Peetrons P. Ultrasound of muscles. Eur Radiol 2002;12(1):35–43.
73. Trunz LM, Landy JE, Dodson CC, et al. Effectiveness of hematoma aspiration and platelet-rich plasma muscle injections for the treatment of hamstring strains in athletes. Med Sci Sports Exerc 2022;54(1):12–7.
74. Ling X, Ma X, Kuang X, et al. Lidocaine inhibits myoblast cell migration and myogenic differentiation through activation of the notch pathway. Drug Des Devel Ther 2021;15:927–36.
75. Bedi A, Trinh TQ, Olszewski AM, et al. Nonbiologic injections in sports medicine. JBJS Rev 2020;8(2):e0052.
76. Ljungqvist A, Schwellnus MP, Bachl N, et al. International Olympic Committee consensus statement: molecular basis of connective tissue and muscle injuries in sport. Clin Sports Med 2008;27(1):231–9, x-xi.
77. Engebretsen L, Steffen K, Alsousou J, et al. IOC consensus paper on the use of platelet-rich plasma in sports medicine. Br J Sports Med 2010;44(15):1072–81.
78. Cole BJ, Gilat R, DiFiori J, et al. The 2020 NBA orthobiologics consensus statement. Orthop J Sports Med 2021;9(5). 23259671211002296.
79. Finnoff JT, Awan TM, Borg-Stein J, et al. American Medical Society for sports medicine position statement: principles for the responsible use of regenerative medicine in sports medicine. Clin J Sport Med 2021;31(6):530–41.
80. Rodeo SA, Bedi A. 2019-2020 NFL and NFL physician society orthobiologics consensus statement. Sports Health 2020;12(1):58–60.

Special Populations in Orthobiologics

Athletic, Elderly, and Pediatrics Populations

Arthur Jason De Luigi, DO, MHSA[a,*], Stephanie Tow, MD[b], Ryan Flowers, DO[c], Andrew H. Gordon, MD, PhD[d]

KEYWORDS

• Orthobiologics • Regenerative medicine • Elite athletes • Elderly • Pediatrics

KEY POINTS

- Orthobiologics have gained popularity in the treatment of elite athletes in hopes to accelerate recovery and return to play.
- Orthobiologics are being used with the elderly in hopes to regenerate degenerative cartilage and tendons.
- There is still some resistance to the use of orthobiologics in the pediatric population due to fear of unknown adverse effects and efficacy.

INTRODUCTION/HISTORY/DEFINITIONS/BACKGROUND

Although the term "Regenerative Medicine" was first coined in 1992[1] and platelet-rich plasma (PRP) was first reported to help with bone repair,[2] the use of orthobiologics for the treatment of musculoskeletal conditions was in limited use and did not gain in popularity until 2009. Just before the kickoff for Super Bowl XLIII, one of the sports reporters shared a surprising report of Hines Ward's recovery from a grade 2 medial collateral ligament sprain revealing he had undergone a PRP injection enabling him to play 2 weeks after his injury instead of missing 4 to 6 week to recovery.[3–5] The acronym, PRP, was all over the mainstream media because many wanted to know what it was and could it help other musculoskeletal injuries. There were already publications on PRP in the sports medicine literature at the time including publications by Dr Mishra on PRP for chronic tendinopathy in 2006 and a few reviews on PRP just before that Super Bowl.[6–8] However, the term orthobiologics was already being

[a] Department of PM&R, Sports Medicine, Mayo Clinic Arizona, 13400 East Shea Boulevard, Scottsdale, AZ 85259, USA; [b] University of Texas Southwestern, Scottish Rite for Children Orthopedic and Sports Medicine Center, 5323 Harry Hines Boulevard, Dallas, TX 75390, USA; [c] University of Texas Southwestern, 5323 Harry Hines Boulevard, Dallas, TX 75390, USA; [d] US Physiatry, 1850 Town Center Parkway, Reston, VA 20190, USA

* Corresponding author.

E-mail address: ajdeluigi@gmail.com

Phys Med Rehabil Clin N Am 34 (2023) 199–237

https://doi.org/10.1016/j.pmr.2022.08.013

used in bone healing literature[9,10] as early as 2005 but did not first appear in sports medicine literature until 2008.[7] The spark ignited a flame of hope for patients suffering a wide variety of conditions. The social popularity of PRP grew faster than the studies could be performed, and this coupled with opportunities of a new treatment opened the door for financial gain by a wide array of practitioners because insurances withheld coverage for these treatments.

As the news grew of more athletes getting this treatment for a wide variety of conditions, the general population sought care for these conditions as well as many others that had not yet been studied. The growth, however, was not limited to the sports injuries as persons with chronic musculoskeletal pain were hopeful this treatment would help them. There was also renewed hope that these treatments can heal and reverse both acute injuries as well as chronic degenerative conditions such as osteoarthritis. The growth of PRP began to spread across the spectrum of the pediatric to the elderly population. Our goal is to share the current research in these populations for various conditions and highlight some areas in which there is still a paucity of literature.

DISCUSSION

The authors will review the literature of the special populations of athletes, pediatric, and the elderly, highlighting conditions with more robust literature as well as some that are frequently treated despite a paucity of supportive data.

Athletic Population

Anyone who exercises or participates in recreational sports can be defined as an athlete. The However, the scope of the section will be limited to studies that targeted elite, high-level athletes span all age groups and levels of competition ranging from high school, collegiate, international, and professional. Major professional leagues (National Basketball Association [NBA], National Football League [NFL]) have come out with position statements regarding orthobiologics, and there have been studies assessing their utilization in professional, collegiate, and Olympic sports.[11–14] Because the world of sports is broad and diverse, the use of orthobiologics in the athletic population could theoretically include many musculoskeletal conditions. The focus of this section will be on those conditions that are commonly treated and have been studied.

Ulnar Collateral Ligament of the Elbow-Tommy John Injury

An injury to the ulnar collateral ligament (UCL) used to be career ending, before Tommy John, who successfully returned as a Major League Baseball (MLB) pitcher after reconstruction by Frank Jobe.[15] However, despite the "relative success" of the surgery, this injury can still be career threatening and altering because there is a prolonged course of postoperative rehabilitation. A review of 178 MLB pitchers demonstrated that the average return to at least 1 game was 20.5 $\pm$ 9.72 months and the length of their career postoperatively was only another 3.9 $\pm$ 2.84 seasons.[16] Although frequently and popularly quoted by surgeons that 80% of MLB Pitchers return to the majors, they frequently omit the second half of the statement, which is "for at least one game." The retrospective case review of 147 MLB pitchers who underwent Tommy John reveals that although 80% pitch at least 1 game, only 67% become established (10+ games). Of this 67%, another 57% of these pitchers return to the disabled list (DL) because of throwing injuries to the same arm. Unfortunately, the statistical metrics of success in a pitcher also decline after Tommy John surgery both compared with the uninjured counterparts but most importantly compared with those who opted for a nonsurgical management of the UCL injury. The postoperative pitchers' performance declined across several metrics after surgery compared with preinjury levels, such as earned run average, batting average against, walks plus hits per inning pitched, percentage of pitches thrown in the strike zone, innings pitched, percentage fastballs thrown, and average fastball velocity ($P < .05$ for all).[17] There is not any sport that considers 33% of the players who can come back for less than 10 games or 57% to returning to the DL a "success." Additionally, in a sport that emphasizes everything on statistical measurement metrics, a decline in every pitching metric is not "successful." Therefore, those who care for elite athletes began to look for alternative options such as orthobiologics.

The scientific evaluation on the use of PRP for UCL injuries originated in the practice built by Dr Jobe. Podesta and colleagues published a study in 2013 on 34 overhead throwing athletes following a single PRP resulting in 88% return to play within 12 weeks with statistically significant improvements in pain and function[18] (**Table 1**). The findings of this study demonstrated a reduction of a typically 2-year recovery period to allow for return in 3 months. The study provided a potential alternative to surgery and began being used in clinical settings. As such, it led to numerous retrospective reviews and cohorts as well as other prospective studies totaling 1121 overhead athletes and 3 hockey players[19–26] (see **Table 1**). Dines and colleagues completed a retrospective review on 44 baseball players (6 pro, 14 college, 24 high school), who had partial UCL tear by MRI and subsequently underwent PRP injection. The number of injections varied with 16 having a single injection, 6 having 2, and 22 undergoing 3 PRP injections. They used a Modified Conway Scale (73% excellent/good outcome), return to throwing (5 weeks), and return to competition (RTC; 12 weeks) without any complications.[19] The following study by Deal and colleagues was designed as a prospective cohort of 25 throwing athletes with grade 2 UCL tears who underwent treatment with a varus-loading brace, activity restriction, physical therapy, and as series of 2 PRP injection 2 weeks apart with a follow MR arthrogram 2 weeks after the second injection. The results revealed 96% of the athletes had stability of the UCL with reconstitution of the ligament in all patients allowing all patients to return to the same or higher level of competition at 6 weeks after injury, which is significantly sooner that the historical surgical management.[20] There was a smaller prospective case series of 3 professional hockey players with grade 2 or 3 tears who were treated with brace, graduated physical therapy, 2 leukocyte poor (LP)-PRP at 2 days postinjury and 1 week later. All 3 players returned to professional hockey at a mean of 36 days after the injury.[21] A large retrospective cohort was completed using 977 MLB or Minor League Baseball (MiLB) players diagnosed with UCL tear during a 5-year period. The author compared all treatments with 433 surgical and 544 nonsurgical patients with 133 having one or more PRP injections followed by rehab versus rehab alone in the remaining 411 players. The study looked at return to throwing, last throwing date, date of first throw after PRP, first throw after rehab, return to play at any level, failed nonop care, UCL surgery, reinjury rate for all treatments, and players released or retired. Unfortunately, there was too much heterogeneity in the data to make conclusive recommendations.[22] A separate retrospective review of professional baseball players included 3 studies with a high success of return to play (RTP; 66%–100%) after PRP for grade 1 injuries and 66% to 94% in grade 2 or 3 injuries.[23] A different retrospective review included 8 articles in high level (elite HS, college, MiLB, MLB) baseball players and concluded that PRP is promising in the RTP after UCL injury but more robust studies are needed.[24] A third review included 3 case series (25 grade 2, 44 baseball-any grade, 34 grade 1 or 2) totaling 103 overhead throwing athletes with varying numbers of injections, volumes of PRP, and postinjection rehabilitation

Table 1
Platelet-rich plasma injections for elite athletes

Reference	Study Type	Population	Injury Type	System	Methods	Outcome Measures	Results	Conclusion
Podesta L, et al,[18] AJSM 2013	Prospective cohort	Overhand-throwing athletes	UCL elbow	Magellan arteriocyte PRP (leukocyte rich)	34 athletes (28 men, 6 women) symptomatic grade 1 or 2 partial UCL by examination and MRI who failed 2 mo nonoperative tx w/NSAIDs and >6 wk. Single USG PRP. 12 wk of graduated exercises	Baseline KJOC and DASH, US measurement of h-u joint space w/wo 10 lbs valgus stress at 30° elbow flexion. KJOC/DASH q4weeks and after RTP	30 of 34 athletes (88%) returned to play without complaints at average of 12 wk (range 10–15). Statistically significant improvement of KJOC, significant improvement of DASH	PRP is an effective treatment for partial UCL. Success rate similar to UCL reconstruction, avoids substantial time away (12 mo) for rehabilitation. PRP patients return sooner
Dines JS, et al,[19] AJO 2016	Retrospective review	Baseball players	UCL elbow	Varied	44 baseball players (6 professionals, 14 college, 24 HS) treated with PRP for partial UCL diagnosed by examination and MRI. 16 had 1 injection, 6 had 2 injections, and 22 had 3 injections. Started on interval throwing program once asymptomatic	Modified Conway Scale, Return to Throw, Return to Competition	32 (73%) had excellent or good outcome. Return to throwing average time was 5 wk, return to competition 12 wk (range 5–24 wk), no injection-related complications	PRP for UCL insufficiency produced outcomes much better that earlier reported outcomes for conservative treatments. Particularly beneficial for young athletes and athletes who are unable or unwilling to undergo extended rehab after surgical UCL reconstruction
Deal JB, et al,[20] OJSM 2017	Prospective cohort	Throwing athletes	UCL elbow	Harvest (leukocyte rich)	25 throwing athletes (23 baseball, 2 softball). Symptomatic UCL instability with MR arthrography demonstrating grade 2 UCL tears. Tx w/varus-loading elbow brace,	MRI findings, exam, symptoms, Return to Play	23 (96%) of grade 2 demonstrated stability of UCL with reconstitution of ligament in all patients and return to play at same or higher level of competition. All	Treatment of Grade 2 UCL injuries with 2 PRP-LR injections with bracing and PT proves to be safe and effective in reconstituting tears on MRI with a high return to play rate significantly sooner

					activity restriction, PT, 2 PRP injections 2 wk apart. MR arthrogram repeated 2 wk after the second injection		released to play at 6 wk	that surgical management
McCrum CL, et al,[21] OJSM 2018	Case series	Professional hockey players	UCL elbow	Arthrex Autologous conditioned plasma (ACP) leukocyte poor	3 hockey players with grade 2 or 3 tear had a trial of brace, PT, PRP, and progressive RTP. Immediate bracing and removal from competition. 2 ACP injections at 2 d postinjury and 1 wk later. Graduated PT	Physical examination, MRI, Return to Play	All 3 players returned to professional hockey at a mean of 36 days after injury with 2 injections of ACP, bracing, and graduated PT	Two injections of leukocyte-reduced PRP was successful in the return to play of 3 professional hockey players to the same level of play
Chauhan A, et al,[22] AJSM 2019	Retrospective cohort	MLB and MiLB players	UCL elbow	Varied	977 MLB/MiLB players diagnosed with physical examination and MRI between 2011 and 2015, 433 elected surgery, 544 (56%) opted for nonoperative tx; 133 had 1 or more PRP before rehab vs 411 had just rehab	Return to throwing, last throwing date, first throw after PRP, first throw after nonop tx, return to play at any level, failed nonop, UCL surgery, reinjury, released, retired	Heterogenous data with varying grades, PRP preparations, injection protocols, required time to withhold throwing post-PRP, rehabilitations protocols	Inconclusive due to significant heterogeneity regarding numerous aspects of the comparison groups
Cascia N, et al,[23] J Sports Rehab 2019	Retrospective review	Professional baseball players	UCL elbow	Varied	3 retrospective reviews met inclusion criteria, of which 2 reported RTP rates following nonop rehab whereas 1 reported	Successful RTP	High success with RTP rates up to 100% (66%–100%) after PRP nonoperative tx of Grade 1 UCL injuries in professional	High RTP rates following nonoperative tx of partial UCL injuries in professional baseball players

(*continued on next page*)

Table 1
(continued)

					RTP rates after injection after failed conservative rehab only		baseball players and 66%–94% in Grade 2 and above	
Carr JB, et al,[24] Arthroscopy 2020	Review	Baseball players	UCL elbow	Not reported	Review of 8 articles related to all treatments related to UCL injuries in high level (elite HS, college, MiLB, MLB) baseball players	Return to Play	No results reported	PRP has shown effectiveness in treatment of partial UCL in multiple studies, however, more robust clinical data in needed
Conant BJ, et al,[25] J Sports Rehab 2020	Retrospective review	Overhand-throwing athletes	UCL elbow	Varied	3 case series (25 grade 2, 44 baseball-any grade, 34 grade 1 or 2) met inclusion criteria, of which there was heterogeneity of number of injections, amount of PRP injection, and postinjection rehab protocols	Return to competition rates, recovery time	PRP injections led to higher return-to-competition rates and shorter recovery times compared with rehab only; PRP demonstrates comparable return to competition rate compared with surgery	PRP is an effective treatment for partial UCL with faster return to competition and shorter recovery times than rehab alone and comparable rates to surgery
Baker Mills F, et al,[26] OJSM 2021	Retrospective cohort	Elite high school, collegiate, and professional throwing athletes	UCL elbow	Emycte PurePRP (leukocyte rich)	50 patients (50 male, 2 female; 50 baseball, 2 javelin) Grades I–IV UCL injuries, one PRP-LR injection; No NSAIDs × 6 wk, light ROM/ isometric exercise for 2 wk, Active Wrist ROM week 3,	RTP, 2-y follow-up after PRP injection, 4 groups (A-grade 1/2 w/o surgery, B-grade 3/4 w/o surgery, C-grade 1/2 repeat injection, surgery, or retire, D-grade 3/4 repeat injection, retired, or surgery)	26 patients (52%) of any Grade returned to baseline level of play or better at 2-y follow up after single PRP-LR injection and standard rehab protocol. 24 (48%) had to have at least	Success with single PRP for grades 1–2 UCL tears, great promise for single injection for grade 3, dismal response in grade 4 with 7 of the 8 patients requiring surgery or retired

					gradual buildup of strength exercises w/o valgus forces at elbow from weeks 4–7, UE plyometrics week 8, light tossing week 9, full throwing symptom free and cleared by surgeon		one more PRP, retired, or surgery. 60% of grades 1–3 returned to baseline with one PRP-LR and rehab; 7 of 8 grade 4 did not respond to single PRP	
Bubnov R, et al,[41] Med Ultrason 2013	RCT	Professional athletes	Hamstring	Not reported	30 consecutive professional athletes had a single 5-mL USG PRP injection for extremity injuries (18 hamstrings) with conservative management vs conservative management alone	VAS, physical assessment, global functional assessment	Day 1: 28% pain relief on VAS in PRP group compared with 10% in no injection group; Day 7: significant improvement of physical assessment in PRP group, Day 14: significantly superior response in physical assessment in PRP group; Day 28: 93% reduction in pain by VAS in PRP vs 80% in conservative alone group and significant improvement of function at 28 days in PRP group comparatively	PRP as part of conservative management is superior to conservative management alone for hamstrings in pain relief, physical assessment, and global functional assessment
Rettig AC, et al,[42] OJSM 2013	Retrospective case control study	NFL players	Hamstring	Biomet GPS III	Retrospective chart review of a single NFL team found 10 players with	Return to Play	No significant difference in RTP of treatment group (20 days) and	Significant flaws in the report of results and lack of reporting of the

(*continued on next page*)

Table 1
(*continued*)

					hamstring tear. *Divided into Tx* (PRP + rehab) and control group (rehab Only) with PRP within 24–48 h of injury		control group (17 days), although the control started with 5 the results only report data on 4 patients without any mention at all what happened to the fifth player and why the data were not included, also there was imbalance of skill position players (3 of 5 in tx, only 1 of 4 in control) because there is a significant difference in requirements of the position to help with RTP in QB/DB vs OL/DL	fifth player in control group may have artificially lowered the days of RTP; however, the conclusion was no difference between groups based on this exclusion
Wetzel RJ, et al,[43] Ortho 2013	Retrospective case series	Competitive (collegiate and high-level) athletes	Hamstring	Biomet GPS III	17 hamstring injuries, 5 successfully responded to conservative treatment 6–12 wk PT + scheduled NSAIDs, 12 failed and had one 6-mL PRP injection, followed by PT	Pre-VAS and Post-VAS, Nirschl Phase Rating Scale, and Return to Sport	Players treated with PRP reported reduction of post-tx VAS and Nirschl Phase Rating, whereas the PT + NSAIDs did not have the same reduction, all players returned to play to their desired activity level	PRP provided reduction in VAS and Nirschl Phase Rating, traditional treatment did not

Hamid MS, et al,[44] AJSM 2014	RCT	High level athletes	Hamstring	Biomet GPS III	28 players randomized to PRP + rehab vs rehab only; PRP group had a single injection	Return to play	PRP + rehab returned to play at a mean time of 26.7 games, whereas the rehab only group returned to play in 42.5 days	Athletes with hamstring injuries returned (statistically and clinically) significantly earlier than the control group
Zanon G, et al,[45] Joints 2016	Prospective cohort	Professional football (soccer) players	Hamstring	Not reported	57 football (soccer) players on a team were followed during a 31-mo periods for any muscles injury; of which 18 players sustained hamstring injury with 25 hamstrings, only grade 2 injuries were included; first PRP injected 48–72 h after the injury, grade 2A (2 injections with second 7 d later), 2B/C (3 injections at 7-d intervals); MRIs at days 14, 21, 28, Classification-specific rehab protocols	Healed (Return to Play), SPA in days	All hamstring mean SPA 36.7 d, mean SPA BF 31.7 d for 2a, 61.3 for 2b, and 49.3 for 2c; mean SPA SM was 15.5 for 2a, 69 for 2c, there were not any 2b SM injuries	PRP was successful in helping recovery of hamstring injury and RTP; however, there was not a control to provide info related to improved time to recovery
Rossi LA, et al,[46] Knee Surg Sports Traumatol Arthrosc 2016	RCT	Competitive (college and professional) athletes	Hamstring	Not reported	75 Athletes with hamstring injury by MRI were randomized into intervention (single	Return to play, VAS at rest, VAS during resistive motion	RTP for intervention was 21 days compared with 25 days for control,	PRP group had a faster RTP and a significant difference of pain reduction

(*continued on next page*)

Table 1
(*continued*)

					PRP + rehab) or control (rehab only)		greater reduction of VAS in PRP group	compared with rehab alone
Bradley JP, et al,.[47] OJSM 2020	Cohort	NFL players	Hamstring	ACP leukocyte poor	108 NFL players from single team had hamstring injury by MRI, 69 had grade 2 of which 30 had LP-PRP + rehab and 39 underwent rehab only	Return to play (time missed)	PRP group returned in mean time of 22.5 d, 18.2 practices, 1.3 games compared with control group which missed 25.7 d, 22.8 practices, and 2.9 games. 1 recurrent injury in each group, but the 1 s/p PRP returned earlier than recommended due to playoff game	PRP reduces the time for RTP and amount of practices and games missed compared with rehab alone
A Hamid MS, et al,[48] BMJ Open 2020	Double-blind placebo-controlled randomized control trial	High performance national level athletes	Hamstring	Biomet	68 athletes with MRI confirmed grade 2 hamstring injuries were randomized into a PRP vs control group. PRP group received one LR-PRP injection followed by rehab. Control group was rehab only	Primary outcome: RTP Secondary outcomes: Pain intensity and Brief Pain Inventory-Short Form, injury recurrence	Final results have not been published	Pending
Lee KY, et al,[39] AJSM 2019	Case series	Collegiate athletes	Hamstring	Arthrex Angel	15 cases of PT or hamstring pathology at a single university	Return to play	All 8 athletes treated with PRP had faster recovery time and RTP	PRP helps to lessen recovery time and allows the athletes

					treated with PRP of which 8 were hamstring injuries treated with PRP			to return to play sooner
Trunz LM, et al,[50] MSSE 2021	Retrospective case series	High level athletes	Hamstring	Biomet GPS III	55 athletes with MRI confirmed grade 2 hamstring injuries. 28 treated conservatively, 27 had hematoma aspiration and PRP injection	Return to play, recurrence rate	The average RTP was 23.5 d in the PRP group and 32.4 d in the conservative (no PRP) group; Recurrence rate was 28.65 in the conservative group and <4% in the PRP group	PRP significantly shortened the RTP time and as well as a markedly lower recurrence rate
Seow D, et al,[41] AJSM 2021	Systematic review and meta-analysis	High level athletes	Hamstring	Varied	2 authors systematically reviewed 10 publications following PRISMA protocol	Varied	A total of 10 studies with 207 hamstring injuries in the PRP group and 149 in the control group; PRP group has a return to play that was a mean difference of 5.67 d earlier than the control group with a lower risk of reinjury rate	PRP significantly shortened the RTP time and lowered the recurrence rate
Vetrano M et al,[44] AJSM 2013	RCT	Elite athletes	Patellar tendon	Not reported	46 patients who had previous failed at least 12 wk of conservative management were randomized into a PRP (two 2-mL injections 1 wk apart) group vs Extracorporeal Shock Wave Therapy-ESWT (3 treatments	VISA-P questionnaire, VAS after 5 single leg squats, Blazina scale to assess response to treatment, prevention of surgery	Both groups have improvement with greater improvement with PRP at both 6 and 12 mo; PRP has had a Blazina scale rating of good or excellent in 91.3% of patients compared with 60.8% in the ESWT group. No patients in either group	Both PRP and ESWT are effective in improving symptoms of PT and surgery prevention with significantly greater improvements in PRP at 6 and 12 mo as well as patient satisfaction

(*continued on next page*)

Table 1
(*continued*)

					separated by 48–72 h) groups followed by the same rehab protocol		proceeded to surgery	
Charousset C, et al,[45] AJSM 2014.	Case series	Professional athletes	Patellar tendon	Arthrex ACP	28 professional athletes with chronic refractory PT received 3 consecutive LP-PRP injections 1 wk apart	VAS, VISA-P, Lysholm, Return to Practice, MRI at 1 and 3 mo to assess tendon healing	21 of 28 returned to play within 3 mo; VISA-P, VAS, and Lysholm scores had statistically significant improvement at a 2-y follow-up; Tendon returned to normal structural integrity in 16 patients	PRP provides long-term improvement in pain and function at 2 y
Lee KY, et al,[39] AJSM 2019	Case series	Collegiate athletes	Patellar tendon	Arthrex Angel	15 patients had either PT or hamstring pathology at a single university treated with PRP of which 7 patients (9 knees with 2 bilateral) were PT injuries treated with PRP	Return to play	All 7 athletes treated with PRP returned to play, although one PRP occurred at the time of surgery, and 2 had recurrence of symptoms after RTP which later proceeded to surgery	PRP helps to lessen recovery time and allows the athletes to return to play
Andriolo L, et al,[46] AJSM 2019	Systematic review and meta-analysis	Elite athletes	Patellar tendon	Varied	70 studies involving 2530 patients comparing PRP (1 or 2 injection) with eccentric exercise and ESWT	Varied	Multiple injections of PRP had the best long term (>6 mo) results followed by single injection of PRP, then ESWT and eccentric exercises; although eccentric	PRP had the best long-term results in treating PT with multiple injections having the best results

							exercises had the best short term (< 6 mo) results	
Blanke F, et al,[47] M, L & T Journal 2015	Case series	High level athletes	Meniscus	Arthrex ACP	10 athletes with Grade 2 meniscal lesions on MRI received 3 fluoroscopic-guided injections of PRP at 7 day intervals without any physical therapy after	Numeral rating scale (	60% had significant improvement of pain relief and 40% had healing on MRI at 6 mo; only 20% had worsening of Meniscus on MRI but these patients did not have any improvement in pain as well	PRP was shown to be effective in decreasing pain, healing the meniscus, and preventing surgery in the majority of patients; however, some players did not respond
Samra DJ, et al,[49] BMJ Open Sport Exerc Med 2015	Cohort controlled pilot	Professional Rugby Union players	Syndesmotic ankle	Manual centrifuge	10 Rugby Union players with MRI confirmed AITFL syndesmotic injuries underwent a single PRP followed by a rehab program and were compared with a historical group	Return to play, VAS, Dorsiflexion ROM (weight bearing lunge), Balance-Star Excursion Balance Test, Ankle Power (Vert Jump), Ankle Power (VJ), Fear of Injury: Fear Avoidance Beliefs Questionnaire, Illinois Agility Test and Triple Hop test	PRP group had a mean difference of an earlier RTP of 20.7 d compared with the historical group	PRP significantly shortened the RTP for athletes with syndesmotic ankle sprains
Laver L, et al,[50] Knee Surg Sports Traum Arthrosc 2015	RCT	Elite athletes	High ankle	Not reported	16 elite athletes with MRI confirmed torn AITFL were randomized into a treatment (PRP + rehab) or control group (rehab only); The treatment group had 2 US-guided PRP 7 d	Return to play	The mean RTP time for the PRP group was 40.8 d compared with 59.6 d in the rehab group with 6 out of 8 PRP patients returning to play under 6 wk	PRP group had a markedly significant improvement of RTP of nearly 3 weeks compared to rehab alone

(*continued on next page*)

Table 1
(continued)

					apart into the syndesmosis at the level of the tear followed by the same rehab protocol as the rehab only group			
Tiwari M, and Bhargava R,[54] J Clin Orth & Trauma 2013	RCT	Athletes and nonathletes	Plantar fasciitis	PRP FAST System (BIO)	60 patients randomized into PRP and steroid (40 mg methyl prednisolone) groups	VAS (0, 1, 3, and 6 mo)	Both groups had a statistically significant reduction of VAS at 1 mo but greater reduction in PRP group, at 3 mo the VAS increased and remained at 6 mo in steroid group, whereas there was a significant reduction in the PRP group at both 3 and 6 mo	PRP is superior to steroids in pain reduction at 1, 3, and 6 mo. Steroids only provided a reduction of pain at the 1 mo interval then increased at 3 mo
Mahindra P et al,[55] Orthopedics 2016	Double-blind placebo-controlled RCT	Athletes and nonathletes	Plantar fasciitis	Not reported	75 patients randomized into 3 groups: PRP, corticosteroid, and placebo groups followed at 3 wk and 3 mo	VAS, AOFAS	Both groups had improvement to placebo at 3 wk, 3 mo with PRP group have a significantly greater improvement in both outcomes at these intervals	PRP is significantly more effective than corticosteroid and placebo in reducing pain and improving function for plantar fasciitis
Gogna P, et al,[56] The Foot 2016	Randomized comparative study	Sportspersons	Plantar Fasciitis	GPS (cell factor tech)	40 patients with 6 mo or more of failed conservative treatment were	VAS, AOFAS, PF thickness by US	PRP group had a greater reduction in Pain and AOFAS compared with	A single PRP injection into the PF provides greater pain relief and functional

					randomized into a PRP (single injection with 2-wk rest from sports) and ESWT (2 treatments/wk for 3 wk)		ESWT group and had relative equal reduction of PF thickness	improvement at both 3 and 6 mo compared with a 3-wk series of 6 ESWT treatments
Kalia RB, et al,[57] Indian J Orth 2021	Prospective case series	Athletes and nonathletes	Plantar fasciitis	Manual centrifuge	30 patients underwent a single PRP injection and followed for 12 wk	VAS, AOFAS, Foot and Ankle Disability Index (FADI), and PF thickness at 0, 6 and 12 wk	PRP provided statistically significant reduction of Pain (VAS), functional improvement (AOFAS, FADI) and reduction of PF thickness	A single PRP injection provides statistically significant relief of pain, improved function, and reduced PF thickness at 6 wk and continues to improve at 12 wk

Abbreviations: AITFL, Anterior Inferior Talofibular Ligament; DB, Defensive Back; DL, Defensive Line; KJOC, Kerlan Jobe Orthopedic Clinic; OL, Offensive Line; QB, Quarterback; USG, Ultrasound Guided.

protocols. The review concluded that the PRP injections led to higher RTC rates with shorter recovery times compared with rehab alone and comparable RTC compared with surgery.[25] The most recent study published on elite (High School [HS], College, MiLB, MLB) throwing athletes was a retrospective cohort with grade I–IV UCL injuries who had one LR-PRP. Following the injection, they were not allowed any Non-Steroidal Anti-Inflammatory Drug (NSAIDs) for 6 weeks, started active wrist range of motion (ROM) at week 3 with graduated strength exercises with valgus forces from weeks 4 to 7, upper extremity plyometrics at week 8, light tossing at week 9, and return to full throwing once cleared by the surgeon. They followed the players for 2 years with 52% at baseline or higher level of competition after one injection, 48% either had a repeat injection, retired, or had surgery. Evaluating the response by grade, 60% of the players with grades 1 to 3 injuries responded to a single PRP, whereas 7 of 8 players with grade 4 injuries responded poorly and needed a repeat injection, had surgery, or retired.[26]

Overall, the data and results are promising for RTC following PRP for grades 1 or 2 UCL injuries. Additional prospective studies are encouraged regarding the number of injections and the use of LR-PRP versus LP-PRP (**Table 2**).

Hamstring

Hamstring injuries are a common soft tissue injury in athletes and have been reported to make up 15% of injuries in Australian Rules Football,[27] 12% of British professional soccer,[28] and 2.2 injuries per 1000 athlete exposures second only to knee sprains.[29,30] As the incidence and time lost can be high, the providers caring for these athletes continue to investigate treatment options to accelerate their recovery as well as prevention of reinjury leading to an opportunity to trial and studied the potential benefits of using orthobiologics. There is a relatively robust amount of research on the use of orthobiologics for hamstring injuries in the athlete population compared with most other conditions.

An RCT on 30 consecutive professional athletes who were randomized into a single PRP with conservative management versus conservative management alone revealed some immediate effect on Day 1 (28% relief vs 10%), superior physical assessment in the PRP group on days 7 and 14, 93% relief compared with 80% as well as significant improvement of function by day 28.[31] There was a retrospective case control study on NFL players that the researcher divided into a treatment group (PRP + rehab) and a control group (rehab only); however, there were flaws with the reporting because the results only reported on 4 of the 5 players in the control group and 3 of the 5 players in the treatment group played skills positions, whereas only 1 of 4 in the control group was a skills player because there are vastly different requirements to perform at an NFL level at a speed versus strength position following a hamstring injury. Despite these flaws, the recovery time was comparable.[32] Another retrospective case series of 17 collegiate athletes were reviewed with all athletes starting with 6 to 12 weeks of patellar tendinopathy (PT) and NSAIDs. Of the 17 athletes, only 5 were able to return to play after PT alone with the remaining 12 receiving one LR-PRP injection and additional PT with all 17 athletes returning to their desired level of competition. Despite PRP only being introduced to only those who failed 12 weeks of therapy, the athletes had PRP had greater reduction of visual analog scale (VAS) and a better Nirschl Phase Rating.[33] Another RCT of 28 high-level athletes with hamstring injuries was randomized into a single LR-PRP with rehab versus rehab alone with the PRP group return to play at 26.7 days compared with 42.5 days for the rehab only group.[34] A prospective cohort of 57 professional football (soccer) players from a single team were followed for 31 months with 18 players sustaining hamstring injuries and 25 total

Table 2
Platelet-Rich Plasma Injections for Elderly Patients

Reference	Study Type	Population	Injury Type	Preparation	Methods	Outcome Measures	Results	Conclusion
Osteoarthritis								
Costa, et al,[62] AJSM 2022	Systematic review and meta-analysis	Various	Knee osteoarthritis	Varied	5 authors systematically reviewed 40 studies comparing PRP with hyaluronic acid, corticosteroid, and saline	Varied	40 studies with 3035 participants were included. PRP was as effective and/or more effective than other therapies when treating pain, improving function and knee stiffness	Studies suggest PRP may be more effective or at least as effective as other methods of nonsurgical treatment but limitations/methodological flaws considerable in current literature
Lin, et al,[63] Arthroscopy 2019	Randomized, double-blind, triple-parallel placebo-controlled trial	Mean age 61–62 y	Knee osteoarthritis	RegenKit-THT (Leukocyte-poor PRP)	87 osteoarthritic knees (57 patients) were randomized to 1 of 3 groups receiving 3 weekly injections of either leukocyte-poor PRP, hyaluronic acid, or saline	Western Ontario and McMaster Universities Osteoarthritis Index (WOMAC), International Knee Documentation Committee (IKDC) subjective score	All 3 groups had statistically significant improvements in WOMAC, IKDC after 1 mo. Only the PRP group had sustained improvement in the scores after 12 mo	Intra-articular leukocyte-poor PRP injections may provide clinically significant functional improvement of at least 1 y in patients with mild-to-moderate knee osteoarthritis

(*continued on next page*)

Table 2
(*continued*)

Anz et al,[64] AJSM 2022	Randomized controlled trial	Age range 18–80 y	Knee osteoarthritis	EmCyte Pure PRP (Monocyte/ leukocyte-rich, neutrophil-poor)	90 participants between 18 and 80 y of age with symptomatic knee osteoarthritis were randomized into 2 study groups: PRP and bone marrow aspirate concentrate (BMAC)	WOMAC, IKDC subjective score	Both groups had significantly improved IKDC and WOMAC scores from baseline to 24 mo after injection. Improvements plateaued at 3 mo, with no difference between PRP and BMAC at any time point	For treatment of knee osteoarthritis, PRP, and BMAC performed similarly over a 24-mo period, with neither being superior to the other
Bennell, et al,[65] JAMA 2021	Randomized controlled trial	Age range 50 y and older	Knee osteoarthritis		288 adults aged 50 y or older (mean age 62 y) with symptomatic medial knee osteoarthritis were injected with either leukocyte-poor PRP or saline placebo at weekly intervals for 3 wk	12-mo change in overall average knee pain scores and percentage change in medial tibial cartilage volume as assessed by MRI	After 12 mo, treatment with PRP or placebo resulted in a mean change of knee pain scores of -2.1 vs -1.8 points, respectively, and mean change in medial tibial cartilage volume was -1.4% vs -1.2%, respectively	Patients with symptomatic mild-to-moderate radiographic knee osteoarthritis did not have a significant difference in symptoms or joint structure after 12 mo, whether injected with PRP or placebo

Dorio, et al,[66] BMC Musculoskeletal Disord. 2021	Double-blind, placebo-controlled randomized controlled trial	Mean age 65 y	Knee osteoarthritis	Standard collection of blood with vacuum centrifuge tubes, subsequent centrifugation	62 patients with mean age of 65 y were divided into 3 groups: PRP, platelet poor plasma (PPP), and placebo. Two ultrasound-guided knee injections were performed within a 2-wk interval	VAS for overall pain at week 24, with intermediate assessments at weeks 12 and 24. Secondary outcomes were KOOS, OMERACT-OARSI, and TUGT	There were no differences among the 3 groups at weeks 6 and 12. Similarly, there were no differences between groups regarding secondary outcomes. The PRP group showed higher frequency of adverse events, mostly mild transitory increase in pain	PRP and PPP were not superior to placebo for pain and function improvement during 24 wk
Rossi, et al,[67] JBJS Reviews. 2020	Review	Various	Glenohumeral osteoarthritis	Various				Evidence for use of orthobiologics in GH arthritis is scarce, with most available options demonstrating only partial to short-term relief of symptoms
Kirschner et al,[67] Clin J Sport Med 2022	Double-blind, RCT	Mean age 68–69 y	Glenohumeral osteoarthritis	Harvest-TerumoBCT SmartPReP Clear PRP System	70 patients with chronic GH osteoarthritis were randomized to receive single injection of hyaluronic acid or leukocyte poor PRP	Shoulder and Pain Disability Index (SPADI), American Shoulder and Elbow Surgeons Score (ASES), current/average numeral rating scale (NRS) pain scores, satisfaction, side effects evaluated at 5 follow-up time points over 12 mo	No significant differences between HA and LP-PRP regarding SPADI, ASES, and current/average NRS pain scores up to 12 mo postinjection ($P>.05$. However, improvements within each group were statistically significant beginning 1–2 mo after injection, regardless of OA severity	No differences in pain, functional outcomes after single injection of HA or LP-PRP; however, significant improvements in pain and function were observed in both treatment groups

(*continued on next page*)

Table 2
(continued)

Abbas et al,[61] JBJS 2022	Network meta-analysis	Various	Knee osteoarthritis	Various	23 studies: 20 RCTs and 3 prospective comparative studies with a total of 2260 patients and mean follow-up period of 9.9 mo	WOMAC, IKDC subjective score, VAS score for patient outcomes. Treatment modalities ranked with the SUCRA probabilities. Risk of bias assessed with the relevant Cochrane tools	No significance differences in all outcome measures and local adverse reactions between LR-PRP and LP-PRP. SUCRA rankings revealed that, for all outcome measures, LP-PRP was preferred to LR-PRP across follow-up periods	Leukocyte concentration of PRP was not significant in patient-reported outcome measures for knee OA. LP-PRP is preferred to LR-PRP according to SUCRA rankings but may not be important for clinical practice/ outcomes
Tendinopathy								
Oudelaar etal,[71] Am J Sports Med 2021	Double-blinded, RCT	Mean age 49 y	Rotator cuff (calcific) tendinitis	PRP	80 patients included with symptomatic rotator cuff calcific tendinitis received either PRP or corticosteroids after needle aspiration of calcific deposits (NACD)	Numeric rating scale for pain (NRS); the Constant-Murley score; the Disabilities of the Arm, Shoulder and Hand questionnaire (DASH); the Oxford Shoulder Score (OSS); and the EuroQol 5-dimension scale (EQ-5D). Additionally, resorption of calcific deposits and the integrity of rotator cuff tendons were assessed by using standard radiographs and ultrasound examination, respectively	Both groups showed improvement of clinical scores at 2-y follow-up. NACD+PRP was overall found to be noninferior to NACD + corticosteroids. Six complications, of which 5 were frozen shoulders, occurred in the NACD + PRP group compared with 1 complication in the NACD + corticosteroids group	NACD+PRP resulted in worse clinical scores at the 6-wk follow-up but better clinical scores at the 6-mo follow-up compared with NACD + corticosteroids. At the 1-y and 2-y follow-ups, the results were comparable between groups. PRP potentially reduces need for additional treatments over long-term but was associated with more complications

Robinson et al,[70] Journal of Back and Musculoskeletal Rehab. 2021.	Systematic review	Various	Rotator cuff tendinitis	Various	Systematic review using PRISMA guidelines. 20 articles met inclusion criteria for rotator cuff pathology, none for glenohumeral osteoarthritis. 16 studies were RCTs and 4 were cohort studies	Outcomes assessed included VAS, Constant Shoulder Score (CSS), Western Ontario Rotator Cuff index (WORC), and SPADI, ASES	Efficacy results were mixed for rotator cuff tendinitis. No studies met inclusion criteria for glenohumeral osteoarthritis	Orthobiologics including PRP offer a relatively safe management option with inconclusive evidence for or against its use for rotator cuff tendinitis. Standardized preparation reporting and consistent use of functional outcome measures are needed in future studies
A Hamid, et al,[38] PLoS One. 2021	Systematic review and meta-analysis	Various	Rotator cuff tendinopathy	Various	Eight RCTs were reviewed after systematic literature review according to PRISMA guidelines, and assessed for methologic quality using Cochrane Collaboration tool	VAS, numerical rating pain scale, CSS, American Shoulder and Elbow Score (ASES), Disability of the Arm, Shoulder and Hand (DASH), shoulder range of movement (ROM)	No difference in short-term (3 wk) pain symptom control between PRP and control interventions. PRP injection (s) performed significantly better for medium (6 mo) and long-term (12 mo) pain symptom control	PRP injection was safe and effective for long-term pain control and shoulder function in patients with rotator cuff tendinopathy

(*continued on next page*)

Table 2
(continued)

Kirschner et al,[67] PM R 2021	Randomized controlled trial	Various	Various chronic tendinopathy	Harvest SmartPrep Platelet Concentration System	40 participants with chronic tendinosis (rotator cuff, wrist extensor, wrist flexor, hip abductor, proximal hamstring, patellar, or Achilles) confirmed via ultrasound were randomly assigned to PNT only group vs PNT +LR-PRP	Primary outcome was current numerical rating scale pain at 6 wk. Secondary outcomes were average pain, function, general well-being, and sleep quality at 6, 52, and 104 wk	No significant differences among groups over time for any of the outcomes. Significantly lower current and average pain after PNT compared with PNT + LR-PRP at 6 wk only	While pain scores were initially lower for PNT only vs PNT + LR-PRP groups, there was no long-term between-group differences in outcomes at 52 and 104 wk

hamstrings were injured. Only grade 2 injuries were included in the PRP group, and the injection regimen varied on the grade (2A, 2B, 2C). The grade 2A injuries received a single PRP within 48 to 72 hours of the injury, whereas grades 2 B/2C received 3 injections at 7-day intervals. The athletes were followed with serial MRIs at days 14, 21, and 28, and the outcome measures were healed (return to play) and sports participation absence (SPA) in the number of days. The mean SPA for all hamstrings was 36.7 days, and then was further broken down into biceps femoris (BF) or semimembranosus (2C) and grades 2A, 2B, or 2C. The SPA BF were 31.7 (2A), 61.3 (2B), and 49.3 days (BC) compared with SPA SM, which were 15.5 (2A) and 69 days (2C) without any athletes having a 2B SM injury.[35] Another RCT included 75 collegiate and professional athletes with hamstring injury by MRI and were randomized into a single PRP with rehab versus rehab only. They measured RTP, VAS at rest, and VAS with resistive motion with the PRP group having an RTP at 21 days versus 25 days with a significant difference in VAS reduction in the PRP group.[36] One of the largest cohorts was completed in a study of 108 NFL players on a single team who had hamstring injuries by MRI with 69 grade 2 injuries. The athletes with grade 2 injuries either had a single LP-PRP (30 players) followed by rehab or had rehab only (39 players). The only outcome was RTP (time missed) and the PRP group returned in 22.5 days, 18.2 practices, and 1.3 games, whereas the rehab only group missed 25.7 days, 22.8 practices, and 2.9 games.[37] A double-blind, placebo-controlled RCT has been completed using 68 national performance elite level athletes with grade 2 hamstring injuries. They were randomized into a PRP (one LR-PRP + rehab) or control (rehab alone) groups with the primary outcome being RTP and secondary outcomes of Pain Intensity, Brief Pain Inventory-Short Form, and injury recurrence, however, the final results of the study have not been published.[38] A case series of 15 collegiate athletes was completed at single university for either hamstring or patellar tendon injury with 8 of the 15 having hamstring injuries with 8 athletes receiving a single PRP and had a faster recovery and RTP.[39] Another retrospective case series reviewed 55 athletes who had sustained a grade 2 hamstring injury with 27 having hematoma aspiration followed by PRP and 28 athletes being treated conservatively. The athletes in the PRP group had an RTP at 23.5 days compared with 32.4 days in the conservative group. Additionally, only 1 of the 27 athletes (3.7%) in the PRP group had a reoccurrence of hamstring injury compared with 28.7% in the conservative group.[40] The most recent study was a systematic review, which included 10 studies with 207 hamstring injuries in the PRP group and 149 in a control group. The PRP group returned to play 5.67 days earlier with a lower risk of reinjury.[41]

Overall, there is strong evidence that PRP is effective in the treatment of hamstring injuries with a faster recovery, less time lost, and lower recurrence rates.

Patellar Tendon

PT typical responds to conservative management and therapeutic exercises; however, recalcitrant cases can be challenging and may require injections or surgery.[42,43] There is an increased risk of tendon rupture with corticosteroid injection, which has led to physicians finding safer and potentially more effective options.[43] Orthobiologics have been compared with some of these other options and has been a promising treatment alternative.

The literature search revealed an RCT, 2 case series, and a systematic review regarding the use of orthobiologics in athletes. The RCT randomized 46 patients, who previously failed conservative management, into a PRP group (2 injections 1 week apart) and an extracorporeal shock wave treatment (ESWT) group (3 treatments 48–72 hours apart). Both groups had improvement of 6 and 12 months with

PRP having greater improvement in VAS after 5 single-leg squats and the Victorian Institute of Sports Assessment-Patella (VISA-P) questionnaire. The PRP group also had a Blazina Ratings Score of 91.3% of good–excellent compared with 60.8% in the ESWT group. There were not many patients in either group who proceeded to surgery, which was another outcome measure.[44] The first case series was performed on 28 professional athletes with chronic refractory PT who received a series of 3 LP-PRP 1 week apart followed by therapy with 21 of 28 athletes returning to play within 3 months. There was statistically significant improvement of the VISA-P, VAS, and Lysholm scores, which continued out to the end of a 2-year follow-up.[45] The other case series included college athletes with hamstring or PT. Focusing on data for the PT patients, there were 7 patients (9 knees-2 bilateral) who received a single LR-PRP injection with all 7 returning to play; however, 2 patients later had surgery.[39] The systematic review included 70 studies with 2530 patients (athletes and nonathletes) revealing that PRP had the best long-term (>6 months) outcomes particularly the studies with multiple injections, followed by ESWT, and eccentric exercises, although eccentric exercises were best in the short term (<6 months).[46]

The results of these studies are promising but there was heterogeneity in the type of PRP (LR vs LP) and the number injections. The review highlighted that PRP is beneficial for the treatment of PT but also a multimodal approach may provide the best short-term and long-term benefits.

Meniscus

There has been significant clinical interest in the use of orthobiologics for the meniscus, the research for the use in elite athletes is still sparse. In the review of the literature, we were only able to identify a single case series that included 10 athletes with grade 2 meniscal injuries who underwent a series of 3 fluoroscopic-guided PRP injections at 7-day intervals followed by a course of physical therapy. Although the meniscus cannot be visualized with fluoroscopy, the treatment significantly reduced pain in 60% and 40% healed on MRI at 6 months. Only 2 patients had neither improvement of pain nor any healing on MRI.[47] These findings are encouraging and warrant further research. The authors would recommend a study using ultrasound guidance as well as a control group in future studies.

Syndesmosis (High Ankle)

Although high ankle sprains only account for about 10% of all ankle sprains, the impact on sports participation and time for recovery is significant.[48] Most high ankle sprains respond to conservative management with more severe cases requiring surgery. The recovery time ranges from 6 to 8 weeks to several months. This has led to clinicians and investigators to evaluate orthobiologics as possible treatment to help reduce recovery time and return to play because literature have revealed 2 studies (RCT and cohort controlled) with relatively small sample sizes. The first was a pilot study on 10 professional rugby players who had a single PRP followed by rehabilitation and compared with the historical group of 11 players with rehab alone. The primary outcome measure was return to play but also included VAS, dorsiflexion ROM with a weight-bearing lunge, Star Excursion Balance Test, Ankle Power with a vertical jump, Illinois Agility Test, Triple Hop Test, and the Fear Avoidance Beliefs Questionnaire. There was improvement in all of these metrics but the most impactful was the PRP group was able to return to play 20.7 days sooner than the historical group who had rehab alone.[49] The RCT included 16 elite athletes who were randomized into a rehab only control group versus a PRP and rehab group with RTP because its only outcome measure. The PRP group underwent 2 ultrasound-guided injections

7 days apart and then both groups completed the same rehab protocol. The mean RTP time for the PRP group was 40.8 days compared with 59.6 days in the rehab group with 6 out of 8 PRP patients returning to play under 6 weeks demonstrating that use of PRP provided markedly significant improvement of RTP of nearly 3 weeks compared with rehab alone.[50]

These initial studies are of small sample size but both have demonstrated the same outcome with the RTP 3 weeks sooner (20.7 and 18.8 days faster). Additional studies with a larger enrollment and time follow-up for potential recurrent injuries are encouraged.

Plantar Fasciitis

Plantar fasciitis typically responds to conservative management without the need for intervention; however, there is a growing subset of patients with recalcitrant symptoms. As corticosteroids increase the risk of plantar fascia rupture, there have been other agents, such as botulinum toxin, studied with positive outcomes with pain and function.[51–53] These treatments have been promising and effective but have been limited by cost and insurance coverage. Given the nature of the pathophysiology of plantar fasciitis, it has led to clinicians and investigators to evaluate orthobiologics for this condition.

In the review of the literature, studies related to the use of orthobiologics of plantar fasciitis include 2 RCTs and a prospective cohort. An RCT, of 60 athletes/nonathletes, was randomized into a steroid or PRP group and was followed by VAS pretreatment and at 1-month, 3-month, and 6-month revealing pain relief in both groups with a statistically significant reduction in pain in the PRP group compared with the steroid group.[54] Another randomized controlled trial (RCT) comparing PRP versus steroids also had a placebo-controlled group and revealed both PRP and steroids provided significant reduction of VAS and improvement of function with the American Orthopedic Foot and Ankle Score (AOFAS) with greater improvements in the PRP group compared with corticosteroid.[55] An RCT, of 60 sportspersons, was randomized into a PRP group versus ESWT group revealing a greater reduction in VAS and the AOFAS with the PRP group compared with ESWT.[56] Finally, there was a prospective cohort who had PRP with improvement at 12 weeks in VAS, AOFAS, Foot and Ankle Disability Index, and reduction of plantar fascia thickness.[57]

Although the number of studies and total number of patients has been limited, the results of these level 1 studies have demonstrated thus far that PRP is superior to corticosteroid, ESWT, and placebo for the treatment of plantar fasciitis that is not responding to conservative management. Although these short-term results are promising, additional studies with more patients and longer follow-up time are still encouraged to determine long-term effectiveness.

Elderly Patients

Increases in life expectancy will simultaneously increase the number of elderly people living with chronic musculoskeletal conditions that need to be treated. These conditions are potentially amenable to orthobiologic therapies.[58] The growth factors arising from platelet activation in PRP, and other biologics, are particularly valuable to elderly patients with waning biologic response to healing.

The most common musculoskeletal complaints in the elderly include osteoarthritis and tendinopathies including knee, hip, and shoulder pain from osteoarthritis, and shoulder, hip, knee, and ankle pain from tendinopathy.[58] Degenerative disc disease of the spine and spinal stenosis are also very prevalent in the elderly. More severe cases of osteoarthritis and tendinopathy may not be amenable to orthobiologic treatment, and sometimes mandate referral to a surgeon for joint replacement and/or primary surgical repair.

Different regenerative treatment strategies in the elderly can include injection of viscosupplements with hyaluronic acid to assist in ameliorating degenerative joint disease, mechanical tenotomy or tendon fenestration to provoke a healing response in diseased tendons, prolotherapy with chemical irritants such as hyperosmolar dextrose, and autologic biologics such as PRP and stem cell therapies from bone marrow aspirate and micronized adipose tissue with each have their own use in the elderly, aging adult.[58]

Osteoarthritis

The most common joints affected by osteoarthritis include the shoulder, hip, and knee.[59] In the 55 and older population, 80% have radiographic evidence of osteoarthritis with 30% of those with radiographic present with significant pain and/or disability.[58]

Knee osteoarthritis is the most widely studied arthritic process using orthobiologics. However, there is still debate regarding the evidence of efficacy of PRP and other orthobiologics (ie, bone marrow concentrate aspirate) in knee osteoarthritis and other arthritic processes. A meta-analysis of 6 RCTs including 1055 patients have previously concluded that LP-PRP has superior outcome measures because they did significantly better in Western Ontario and McMaster Universities Osteoarthritis Index compared with hyaluronic acid and placebo, however, no difference was observed when comparing LR-PRP to these other treatments.[60] LP-PRP had the highest-ranking treatment based on the surface under the cumulative ranking (SUCRA) probabilities.[60] However, a different meta-analysis demonstrated no significant differences in patient reported outcomes when treating knee osteoarthritis with LR-PRP versus LP-PRP but also concluded that SUCRA rankings in their meta-analysis revealed for all outcome measures, LP-PRP is preferred to LR-PRP across all follow-up periods.[61] A larger systematic review examined 40 studies including 3035 patients comparing PRP with hyaluronic acid, steroid, and saline in treating knee osteoarthritis.[62] Although the authors thought that the studies included has some limitations, flaws, and potential risk of bias, their conclusion was that PRP demonstrate that PRP is superior to and as effective as other nonsurgical treatments for knee osteoarthritis in terms of pain, function, and adverse events.[62] There are also significant challenges and flaws with meta-analysis and systematic reviews when comparing such studies, including type of PRP preparation used, volume of PRP injected, and time course over which treatment outcomes were measured.[62]

However, despite these 2 reviews, which made a conclusion that is contradictory to their data, there are numerous other randomized clinical trials that demonstrated PRP to be superior to several alternative treatment options for knee osteoarthritis, including bone marrow–derived stem cells, placebo, platelet poor plasma, and hyaluronic acid.[63–66]

The distribution of primary glenohumeral (GH) osteoarthritis related to age reveals that 90% of the cases occur in patients in the 65 years and older age group, whereas younger patients with GH osteoarthritis develop it from secondary causes such as previous dislocation/trauma or obesity. It is characterized by articular cartilage damage.[59] An RCT of 70 patients with GH osteoarthritis were randomized into a single LP-PRP or a single viscosupplement injection with both groups some improved pain and functional outcomes; however, there were no differences between the results of the 2 groups.[67]

Overall, the summary of the studies shows that LP-PRP and LR-PRP have both improvement of pain and functional outcomes. In knee OA, LP-PRP was superior to LR-PRP as well as other injections and conservative treatments; however, the singular study on LP-PRP in the GH OA showed that there was no difference in the overall improvements achieved with hyaluronic acid injections.

Tendinopathy

The most common source of shoulder pain in all age groups is rotator cuff tendinopathy. This is largely originating from overuse over time in combination with suboptimal postural control and the prevalence of rotator cuff tears increases dramatically after 50 years of age.[58] In these regards, orthobiologics such as PRP also hold promise. The philosophic use of orthobiologics to help initiate an inflammatory healing cascade was proven to promote human tenocyte proliferation and migration in a concentration-dependent manner.[68] A systematic review and meta-analysis of 8 randomized controlled trials demonstrated that PRP was significantly better for medium-term and long-term pain control as opposed to control interventions.[69] In another systematic review/meta-analysis, PRP was deemed to be a safe management option in rotator cuff tendinopathy; however, the authors thought it was inconclusive due to the significant variance in the aspect of these studies.[70] Unfortunately, this review too had methodological flaws because it included 4 blind, palpation injections where the researchers had no idea if the PRP was delivered to the proper location and included another which did not offer therapeutic exercise after the procedure. Despite these flaws and limitations in these studies, PRP was still found to be superior in most of the included studies. Therefore, the results of the data demonstrate PRP was superior to exercise, steroids, and dry needling in most of these studies, despite the "inconclusive" conclusion.

Regarding studies treating calcific rotator cuff tendinosis with barbotage and needle aspiration, use of PRP versus corticosteroid seemed to yield comparable outcomes after 1 and 2 years; however, the PRP-treated group was found to yield a higher incidence of frozen shoulder as a complication.[71]

Another study that examined various types of chronic tendinopathy (rotator cuff, wrist extensor, wrist flexor, hip abductor, proximal hamstring, patellar, Achilles) treated with percutaneous needle tenotomy (PNT) randomized patients into groups that received PRP or not. Patients who received PNT only without PRP had lower pain scores initially, and no long-term between-group differences in pain and function were observed at 52 and 104 weeks.[72] Studies examining gluteal tendinopathy, which is also more common in the elderly, have not yielded sufficient evidence to support the use of PRP.[58]

DISCUSSION

The use of orthobiologics in geriatric and elderly patients has been studied more rigorously than in pediatric/adolescent populations. However, the results of these studies in elderly patients are promising but additional longer term studies with larger cohorts are still warranted.

Pediatric Patients

There is an increasing incidence of nonsurgical and overuse injuries among pediatric athletes.[73] Musculoskeletal conditions accounted for 10.9% of parent-reported health conditions among the 0 to 17-year-old population in the United States in 2012, with an estimated cost of US$213 billion in 2011.[73] As the prevalence of injuries increase in the pediatric population, parents and physicians are seeking alternative options to surgery and steroids, including increased interest in the benefits and risks of orthobiologic treatments.[74] However, because the global orthobiologics market is growing, the need for safety oversight and quality RCTs among young athletes has never been greater.[74] With different anatomic and physiologic considerations related to growth and regeneration in children and adolescents, research findings from adult orthobiologics studies may not be necessarily applicable to the pediatric population. Currently there is a paucity of research on the application of orthobiologics in pediatric sports medicine, but the clinical applications are advancing despite the trailing data.

The clinical use of orthobiologics in the pediatric population has been predominantly in orthopedic surgery as osteoconductive autograft substitutes and, to a lesser extent, osteogenic autologous bone marrow aspirate to treat unicameral bone cysts,[75] as well as in benign bone lesions, congenital pseudoarthrosis of the tibia, and spine surgery.[74] Use in pediatric sports medicine is limited by a combination of factors. To date, there are not any large RCTs for this population from which to draw meaningful conclusions on efficacy and safety. Although several studies exist on the use of PRP and mesenchymal stem cells in adults and equine populations, extrapolating results to the unique physiology of children remains problematic.[73] Furthermore, data on the use of PRP in adolescent athletes is limited to a few small case studies and RCTs with suboptimal methodology.

Ligaments

Ligamentous injuries are increasing in pediatric sports.[74] Increased participation in athletics, year-round engagement, and a greater focus on sports specialization are all thought to contribute to this observation. Among the major ligamentous injuries sustained include the ACL, medial patellofemoral ligament (MPFL), and the UCL.[74]

ACL injuries vary in type and severity among athletes, with tibial spine avulsion fractures and partial or full-thickness tears commonly seen in the pediatric population. The role for orthobiologics in this setting largely pertains to reconstruction or augmentation of the repair. Data from the Multicenter Orthopedic Outcomes Network (MOON) Knee Group revealed that younger patients, aged 10 to 19 years, who underwent ACL reconstruction with an allograft had a 4-fold increased risk of graft rupture.[76] In a separate adult cohort study by the MOON group,[77] augmentation with PRP at the end of allograft ACL reconstruction had only short-term benefits: Participants had decreased effusion at 10 days—a difference that disappeared by 8 weeks, with no significant differences in postoperative measures related to symptoms such as pain and mechanical symptoms, functional levels in activities of daily living, function in sport/recreation, quality of life, or number of additional operative procedures at 2 years between the PRP and control groups.[77] Although PRP is the most extensively studied augmentative orthobiologic agent for ACL injuries, these results have shown short-term benefits and cannot provide definitive conclusions on its use in pediatric patients.

Data are scarce on any treatments of MPFL and UCL injuries in the pediatric population, despite an increasing prevalence.[74] Several adult studies have examined the role of PRP in partial UCL tears with promising clinical outcomes. There is one case report in the literature of a 14-year-old male pitcher with medial elbow pain and a low-grade partial UCL tear, confirmed by ultrasound and MRI.[78] A single ultrasound-guided PRP injection was performed followed by a 12-week rehabilitation protocol. At 16 weeks after injection, ultrasound evaluation demonstrated nearly complete healing without laxity on physical or sonographic examination and return to play without pain or limitations in function. A retrospective mixed cohort study conducted in 2016 by Dines, and colleagues[19] reviewed 44 high-level throwing baseball athletes who had been treated with either 1, 2, or 3 PRP injections for a partial UCL tear, followed by 2 weeks of rest, 1 month of progressive stretching and strengthening, and then an interval throwing program once asymptomatic. Overall, the mean time for returning to throw was 5 weeks and the mean time for RTC was 12 weeks for all study participants; however, the age-specific results for the Modified Conway Scale, return to throw, or the RTC timing were not reported.[79] High-quality RCTs focused on youth athletes with strong methodology are needed to accurately assess the effects of PRP augmentation compared with rehabilitation alone.

Tendons

Tendon injuries are common in children and adolescents but there remains minimal evidence available for the use of orthobiologics in this population. Albano and colleagues reported gradual resolution of pain with incremental return to a competitive level of play over 6 months following PRP, bone marrow aspirate, and autologous fat grafting in a 17-year-old male basketball player with insertional patellar tendinosis with large complex interstitial tears.[80] In a separate case study, Scollon-Brieve and colleagues treated a partial-thickness patellar tendon tear in an 18-year-old lacrosse player with an ultrasound-guided PRP injection after multiple nonoperative treatment failures and pain for 1 year.[81] At 1 month, he was pain-free with 90% clinical improvement based on a functional analog scale, and by 2 months, he returned to play without pain or limitation in sports performance. Despite evidence in apparent support of orthobiologics for tendon injuries, there remains a significant need for quality RCTs with consistent methodological strength that include pediatric populations.

Cartilage

Injury to cartilage in children and adolescents is potentially problematic. The frequency of knee chondral injuries in adolescents is high, often after acute trauma.[82,83] Due to the lack of cartilage calcification in the immature structure, forces are transmitted through the subchondral bone in developing pediatric patients.[74] In addition, other symptomatic lesions may include repetitive microtrauma, osteochondritis dissecans (OCD), and chondromalacia patellae.[74] Generally, asymptomatic, stable lesions are addressed nonoperatively due to a more favorable healing prognosis, whereas symptomatic or unstable chondral lesions should be treated to avoid long-term sequelae, including chronic pain, poor function, and premature osteoarthritis.[74]

Despite limited evidence, multiple treatment approaches have been developed with relative support in surgical management including microfracture (proposed to release pluripotent stem cells from within subchondral bone), osteochondral autograft, osteochondral allografts, and autologous chondrocyte implantation (ACI), which implants chondrocytes harvested from the patient's articular cartilage to form hyaline-like cartilage that resembles the cartilage of the native joint.[74,84]

Although comparative evidence and long-term efficacy are lacking with these surgical procedures, similarly, there are also limited initial data in the pediatric population to support further investigation of orthobiologics for cartilage repair. Knutson and colleagues studied the use of the microfracture technique in comparison to ACI in a pediatric RCT, evaluating clinical outcomes at 5 years.[85] The microfracture group had significant improvement in their subjective physical health from baseline to 5 years, as measured by the Short Form-36 (SF-36)[86] physical component score, whereas the ACI group had no significant improvement in the SF-36 physical component score.[85] Otherwise, the results suggest equivalence between microfracture and ACI at 5 years when looking at clinical outcomes of failure rates of surgery, development of early osteoarthritis, or subjective measurements of impact on daily quality of life measured by the Lysholm Knee Scoring Scale[87] and the Tegner form.[85,88] Although microfracture leads to the development of fibrocartilage rather than hyaline, and theoretically may not possess the same long-term characteristics, Knutsen, and colleagues did not find a correlation between the histology quality and the aforementioned clinical outcomes.[88] In a different study, microfracture effectiveness was only supported by subjective reports of function and healing measured on MRI when performed at the femoral condyle (compared with the trochlea, tibia, and patella) in patients aged younger than 35 years with smaller lesions.[89] Questions remain about the application on larger lesions, durability, and possible damage to subchondral bone.

There are currently only case series and retrospective studies demonstrating that ACI provides beneficial outcomes in adolescent patients.[74] Among these are an adolescent retrospective review concluding that patients postoperatively after ACI had significant improvement in symptoms such as pain and function compared with preoperative levels, as measured by multiple validated clinical inventory scores included in the studies reviewed.[84] A level IV case series with a control group assessed 20 adolescent athletes underwent ACI and were followed at a mean of 47 months post-ACI. The results showed 96% were able to return to high-impact sports, 96% reported good or excellent results with significant improvement in symptoms and function postoperatively as measured by the Tegner activity[85] and Lysholm scores,[87] and 60% reported returned to sports at or above preinjury level.[90] There is another retrospective case review of 23 patients who previously had ACI augmented with cultured bone marrow stem cells. The findings suggested that ACI is associated with significant improvements in symptoms and function as measured by the International Knee Documentation Committee (IKDC),[91] Lysholm-Gillquist,[87] and Tegner-Lysholm[85,87] scores during the first 12 to 24 months postoperatively for patellar OCD in patients 12 to 21 years of age.[92] Unfortunately, there are not any RCTs or studies with a control group, and the evidence is limited only to case reports, case series, and retrospective reviews. However, based on the preliminary findings with these studies, there is a hypothesis that PRP may offer stimulatory effects to accelerate healing for cartilage lesion but similar to these surgical techniques, there is currently limited evidence.[74]

FUTURE DIRECTIONS: SUGGESTED AREAS OF FOCUS

Based on studies in the adult population demonstrating potential efficacy and common injuries among young athletes, there are anatomic sites proposed by Best and colleagues[73] that warrant particular attention for further research regarding the use of orthobiologics in the pediatric population. A list of upper and lower extremity regions with a current summary of evidence is attached in **Table 3**.

Risks and Adverse Effects

Owing to the paucity of research for the use of orthobiologics in pediatric sports medicine, the incidence of adverse effects from such agents is unknown. In general, some pediatric health-care professionals may be concerned of potential adverse effects such as the ability of cells to migrate from placement sites and differentiate into inappropriate cell types or excessive multiplication and tumor growth; however, these concerns are theoretic and not evidence based. There is one case report in which Latalski and colleagues[93] document an allergic reaction in a 14-year-old patient following the administration of PRP formulation into a distal tibia simple bone cyst, resulting in a cutaneous rash in association with pharyngitis, tonsillar enlargement, mucopurulent

Table 3
Best et al. Summary of Recommendations in Pediatric Applications

Region	Support	Needs More Evidence	No Evidence
ACL		• Limited data supports PRP for faster graft maturation, but the long-term clinical significance of this remains unclear (Figueroa et al, 2015) • Majority of studies reviewed by Figueroa et al. (2015) do not show statistically significant clinical outcomes • Inconsistent variables, including volume/concentration of PRP, injection location, surgical techniques, and rehabilitation protocols, make it difficult to compare studies quantitatively (Figueroa et al, 2015) • RCTs with larger sample size and sound methodology are needed	
Meniscal Repair		Table 3. Best et al. Summary of Recommendations in Pediatric Applications (Data from Best TM, Caplan A, Coleman M, et al. Not Missing the Future: A Call to Action for Investigating the Role of Regenerative Medicine Therapies in Pediatric/Adolescent Sports Injuries. Curr Sports Med Rep. 2017;16(3):202-210. doi:10.1249/JSR.0000000000000357)	

(*continued on next page*)

Table 3 (*continued*)

Articular Cartilage	• Level 2 evidence of improved symptoms and function as measured by Tegner (Tegner et al, 1985), IKDC (Higgins et al, 2007) and Knee Injury and Osteoarthritis Outcome (KOOS) (Ross and Lohmander, 2003) scores following stem cell therapy versus microfracture (Gobbi and Whyte, 2016) • Microfracture with adipose-derived stem cells provided radiologic and KOOS (Ross and Lohmander, 2003) pain and symptom sub-score improvement compared with microfracture alone (Koh et al, 2016)		
OCD of the Knee			• No evidence to guide use of PRP or stem cell therapy (Best et al, 2017)
Partial UCL Rupture	• Evidence suggests PRP may be useful for healing, but more rigorous RCTs needed (Dines et al, 2016, Gordon and De Luigi, 2018) • Treatments with mesenchymal stem cells (MSC), with or without PRP, warrants further investigation		
OCD of the Capitellum			• No current evidence available for use of orthobiologics (Best et al, 2017)
Internal impingement (Subacromial/SLAP repair/ Rotator Cuff)			• MSC treatment may have a role, but no evidence to date (Best et al, 2017)
Distal Clavicle		• MSC treatment may have a role in reducing surgical need, but further research is needed (Best et al, 2017)	

(*Data from* Best TM, Caplan A, Coleman M, et al. Not Missing the Future: A Call to Action for Investigating the Role of Regenerative Medicine Therapies in Pediatric/Adolescent Sports Injuries. Curr Sports Med Rep. 2017;16(3):202-210. doi:10.1249/JSR.0000000000000357)

Table 4
Vail, Colorado 2016 Meeting Action Items: A discussion on regenerative medicine and its role in youth sports injuries

Action 1	Exercise caution in treating youth as research continues
Action 2	Improve regulatory oversight
Action 3	Expand governmental and other funding of research
Action 4	Create a system of registries
Action 5	Develop a multiyear policy and build support for it
Action 6	Build a multidisciplinary consortium
Action 7	Develop and pursue a clear collective impact agenda

discharge in the posterior pharynx, and swelling of the eyelids. PRP was separated according to the manufacturer's manual, with the addition of calcium citrate as an anticoagulant agent. Skin prick and intradermal testing for PRP was negative but intradermal testing for calcium citrate was positive. Although this is clearly not a direct adverse effect of the PRP, the case highlights the importance of awareness of potential side effects of adjunct agents.

SUMMARY

The use of orthobiologics in the athlete population has accelerated the overall usage in the general population. While seeking opportunities to have an athlete heal and return to play and with the potential of preventing reinjury, orthobiologics have gained some favor and support in this arena. The studies have been led by many leaders in the professional sports world by physicians at major academic institutions. Although there has not been complete evidence or universal acceptance, major sports organizations have released consensus statements in support of the use of orthobiologics.[11–14]

The elderly population has embraced the use of orthobiologics as an alternative treatment partly due to a desire to delay surgery but also when comorbidities may prevent surgical option. The number of studies on this population has steadily increased with favorable results. Although there is clear and definitive success for all, there has been enough evidence to support the use as part of the spectrum of care for arthropathies and tendinopathies in the elderly population.

The efficacy and safety of orthobiologics in pediatric sports medicine remain unknown. The theory underlying its use to promote primary repair of ligaments and tendons, augment cartilage regeneration, decrease the time to return to sport, and reduce reinjury rates is promising; however, the ability to extrapolate pediatric-specific data from mixed adult and pediatric studies is limited, and quality RCTs in the pediatric population are currently scarce. Multiple factors need to be addressed, and despite the media attention and presumed benefits, there are currently limited data to elucidate efficacy and safety. It will require a collective effort to further evaluate the emerging field of regenerative medicine and its application in pediatric sports medicine (**Table 4**).

CLINICS CARE POINTS

Athletes

- Platelet-rich plasma (PRP) has been shown to be effective in treating grade 1 and 2 UCL and hamstring injuries with faster recovery and return to play; more studies are needed to demonstrate the most effective protocol and PRP type (LR vs leukocyte poor [LP]).

- Although there is only a small volume of studies regarding the usage of PRP for patellar tendinopathy, meniscal injury, high ankle sprains, and plantar fasciitis; the preliminary results are favorable. Additional studies are still warranted to demonstrate efficacy in this population.

Elderly

- PRP has been shown to be effective in the use of osteoarthritis and tendinopathy in the elderly population.
- Most studies support LP-PRP over LR-PRP for osteoarthritis but there is less clear guidance for tendinopathy.
- The results of these studies in elderly patients are promising but additional longer term studies with larger cohorts are still warranted.

Pediatrics

- We should exercise caution when attempting to extrapolate findings from adult studies to apply in the pediatric population because characteristics of anatomy and physiology are unique to this subpopulation.
- There is need for formulation of robust methodology in study designs, with larger sample sizes, matched controls, and standardized administration and rehabilitation protocols.
- Special populations, including youth adaptive athletes, may benefit greatly from orthobiologic innovations but standardized research is needed in this area.

DISCLOSURE

The authors have nothing to disclose.

ACKNOWLEDGMENT

.

REFERENCES

1. Kaiser L. The Future of Multihospital Systems." *Top Health Care Finance.* Summer 1992;18(4):32–45.
2. Marx RE, Carlson ER, Eichstaedt RM, et al. Platelet-rich plasma – Growth factor enhancement for bone grafts. Oral Surg Oral Med Oral Pathol Oral Radiol Endod 1998;85:638–46.
3. Florio M. Hines Ward's Blood Treatment." Pro football Talk. NBC sports. Available at: https://profootballtalk.nbcsports.com/2009/02/03/hines-wards-blood-treatment/. Accessed on March 16, 2022.
4. Dines J, Positano R. Plasma helps Hines ward Be super. New York Daily News 2009.
5. Schwarz A. A Promising Treatment for Athletes, In Blood. New York Times 2009.
6. Mishra A, Pavelko T. Treatment of chronic elbow tendinosis with buffered platelet-rich plasma. Am J Sports Med 2006;34(11):1774–8.
7. Sampson S, Gerhardt M, Mandelbaum B. Platelet rich plasma injection grafts for musculoskeletal injuries: a review. Curr Rev Musculoskelet Med 2008;1(3–4): 165–74.
8. Mishra A, Woodall J, Vieira A. Treatment of Tendon and Muscle Using Platelet-Rich Plasma. Clin Sports Med 2009;28(1):113–25.
9. Schoelles K, Snyder D, Kaczmarek J, et al. "The role of bone growth stimulating Devices and orthobiologics in healing Nonunion fractures." Technology assessment report. Rockville (MD): Agency for Healthcare Research and Quality (US); 2005.

10. Toolan BC. Current Concepts Review: Orthobiologics. Foot Ankle Int 2006;27(7): 561–6.
11. Cole BJ, Gilat R, DiFiori J, et al. The 2020 NBA Orthobiologics Consensus Statement. Ortho J Sports Med 2021;9(5). https://doi.org/10.1177/23259671211002296. 23259671211002296.
12. Rodeo SA, Bedi A. The 2019-2020 NFL and NFL Physician Society Orthobiologcis Consensus Statement. Sports Health 2020;12(1):58–60.
13. Murray IR, Makaram NS, Rodeo SA, et al. Biologics in Professional and Olympic Sport: A Scoping Review. Bone Joint J 2021;103-B(7):1189–96.
14. Kantrowitz DE, Padaki AS, Ahmad CS, et al. Defining Platelet-Rich Plasma Usage by Team Physician in Elite Athletes. Ortho J Sports Med 2018;6(4). https://doi.org/10.1177/2325967118767077. 2325967118767077.
15. Available at: https://www.mlb.com/news/tommy-john-surgery-pioneer-frank-jobes-hall-of-fame-life/c-54371126. Accessed July 8 2022.
16. Erickson BJ, Gupta AK, Harris JD, et al. Rate of Return to Pitching and Performance After Tommy John Surgery in Major League Baseball Pitchers. Am J Sports Med 2014;42(3):536–43.
17. Makni EC, Lee RW, Morrow ZS, et al. Performance, Return to Competition, and Reinjury After Tommy John Surgery in Major League Baseball Pitchers: A Review of 147 Cases. Am J Sports Med 2014;42(6):1323–32.
18. Podesta L, Crow SA, Volkmer D, et al. Treatment of partial ulnar collateral ligament tears in the elbow with platelet-rich plasma. Am J Sports Med 2013;41(7): 1689–94.
19. Dines JS, Williams PN, ElAttrache N, et al. Platelet-Rich Plasma Can Be Used to Successfully Treat Ulnar Collateral Ligament Insufficiency in High-Level Throwers. Am J Orthop 2016;45(5):296–300.
20. Deal JB, Smith E, Heard W, et al. Platelet-Rich Plasma for Primary Treatment of Partial Ulnar Collateral Ligament Tears: MRI correlation with results. Ortho J Sports Med 2017;5(11). 2325967117738238.
21. McCrum C.L., Costello J., Onishi K., et al., Return to Play After PRP and Rehabilitation of 3 Elite Hockey Players with Ulnar Collateral Ligament Injuries of the Elbow, Orthop J Sports Med, 6 (8), 2018, 2325967118790760, doi:10.1177/2325967118790760.
22. Chauhan A, McQueen P, Chalmers PN, et al. Nonoperative Treatment of elbow ulnar collateral ligament injuries with and without platelet-rich plasma in professional baseball players: a comparative and matched cohort analysis. Am J Sports Med 2019;47(13):3107–19.
23. Cascia N, Uhl TL, Hettrich CM. Return to Play Following Nonoperative Treatment of Partial Ulnar Collateral Ligament Injuries in Professional Baseball Players: A Critically Appraised Topic. J Sports Rehab 2019;28(6):660–4.
24. Carr JB, Camp CL, Dines JS. Elbow Ulnar Collateral Ligament Injuries: Indications, Management, and Outcomes. Arthroscopy 2020;36(5):1221–2.
25. Conant BJ, German NA, David SL. The Use of Platelet-Rich Plasma for Conservative Treatment of Partial Ulnar Collateral Ligament Tears in Overhead Athletes: A Critically Appraised Topic. J Sports Rehab 2020;29:509–14.
26. Baker Mills F, Misra AK, Goyeneche N, et al. Return to Play After Platelet-Rich Plasma Injection for Elbow UCL Injury. Orthop J Sports Med 2021;9(3). https://doi.org/10.1177/2325967121991135. 2325967121991135.
27. Orchard J, Seward H. Epidemiology of injuries in the Australian Football League, seasons 1997–2000. Br J Sports Med 2002;36(1):39–44.

28. Hawkins RD, Hulse MA, Wilkinson C, et al. The association football medical research programme: an audit of injuries in professional football. Br J Sports Med 2001;35(1):43–7.
29. Feeley BT, Kennelly S, Barnes RP, et al. Epidemiology of National Football League training camp injuries from 1998 to 2007. Am J Sports Med 2008;36(8):1597–603.
30. Chu S, Rho M. Hamstring Injuries in the Athlete: Diagnosis, Treatment, and Return to Play. Curr Sports Med Rep 2016;15(3):184–90.
31. Bubnov R, Yevseenko V, Semeniv I. Ultrasound Guided Injections of Platelet Rich Plasma for Muscle Injury in Professional Athletes. Comparative Study. Med Ultrason 2013;15(2):101–5.
32. Rettig A.C., Meyer S. and Bhadra A.K., Platelet-Rich in Addition to Rehabilitation for Acute Hamstring Injuries in NFL Players. Clinical Effects and Time to Return to Play, Ortho J Sports Med, 1 (1), 2013, 2325967113494354, doi:10.1177/2325967113494354.
33. Wetzel RJ, Patel RM, Terry MA. Platelet-Rich Plasma as an Effective Treatment for Proximal Hamstring Injuries. Orthop 2013;36(1):e64–70.
34. Hamid MS, Ali MRM, Yusof A, et al. Platelet-Rich Plasma Injections for the Treatment of Hamstring Injuries: A Randomized Controlled Trial. Am J Sports Med 2014;42(10):2410–8.
35. Zanon G, Combi F, Combi A, et al. Platelet-Rich Plasma in the Treatment of Acute Hamstring Injuries in Professional Football Players. Joints 2016;4(1):17–23.
36. Rossi LA, Romoli ARM, Altieri BAB, et al. Does Platelet-Rich Plasma Decrease Time to Return to Sports in Acute Muscle Tear. Knee Surg Sports Traumatol Arthrosc 2017;25:3319–25.
37. Bradley JP, Lawyer TJ, Ruef S, et al. Platelet-Rich Plasma Shortens Return to Play in National Football League Players with Acute Hamstring Injuries. Orthop J Sports Med 2020;8(4). 2325967120911731.
38. Hamid A, Ali MRM, Yusof A, et al. Platelet-Rich Plasma (PRP): An Adjuvant to Hasten Hamstring Muscle Recovery. A Randomized Controlled Trial Protocol (ISCRTN66528592). BMC Musculoskel Disord 2012;13:138.
39. Lee KY, Baker HP, Hanaoka CM, et al. Treatment of Patellar and Hamstring Tendinopathy with Platelet-Rich Plasma in Varsity Collegiate Athletes: A Case Series. J Orthop 2020;18:91–4.
40. Trunz LM, Landy JE, Dodson CC, et al. Effectiveness of Hematoma Aspiration and Platelet-Rich Plasma Muscle Injections for the Treatment of Hamstring Strains in Athletes. MSSE 2022;54(1):12–7.
41. Seow D, Shimozono Y, Yusof TNBT, et al. Platelet-Rich Plasma Injection for the Treatment of Hamstring Injuries. A Systematic Review and Meta-Analysis with Best-Worst Case Analysis. Am J Sports Med 2021;49(2):529–37.
42. Rodriguez-Merchin EC. The Treatment of Patellar Tendinopathy. J Orthop Traumatol. 2013;14(2):77–81.
43. Schwartz A, Watson JN, Hutchinson MR. Patellar Tendinopathy. Sports Health 2015;7(5):415–20.
44. Vetrano M, Castorina A, Vulpiani MC, et al. Platelet-rich plasma versus focused shock waves in the treatment of jumper's knee in athletes. Am J Sports Med 2013;24:89–803.
45. Charousset C, Zaoui A, Bellaiche L, et al. Are Multiple Platelet-Rich Plasma Injections Useful for Treatment of Chronic Patellar Tendinopathy in Athletes? A Prospective Study. Am J Sports Med 2014;42(4):906–11.

46. Andriolo L, Altamura SA, Reale D, et al. Nonsurgical Treatments of Patellar Tendinopathy: Multiple Injections of Platelet-Rich Plasma Are a Suitable Option. A Systematic Review and Meta-Analysis. Am J Sports Med 2019;47(4):1001–18.
47. Blanke F, Vavken P, Haenle M, et al. Percutaneous injections of Platelet rich plasma for treatment of intrasubstance meniscal lesions. Musc Lig Tend J 2015;5(3):162–6.
48. Dubin JC, Comeau D, McClelland RI, et al. Lateral and syndesmotic ankle sprain injuries: a narrative literature review. J Chiropractic Med 2011;10:204–19.
49. Samra JC, Sman AD, Rae K, et al. Effectiveness of a single platelet-rich plasma injection to promote recovery in rugby players with ankle syndesmosis injury. BMJ Open Sport Exerc Med 2015;0:e000033. https://doi.org/10.1136/bmjsem-2015-000033.
50. Laver L, Carmont MR, McConkey MR, et al. Plasma rich in growth factors (PRGF) as a treatment for high ankle sprain in elite athletes: a randomized control trial. Knee Surg Sports Traum Arthrosc 2015;23:3383–92.
51. Babcock MS, Foster L, Pasquina P, et al. Treatment of pain attributed to plantar fasciitis with botulinum toxin a: a short-term, randomized, placebo-controlled, double-blind study. Am J Phys Med Rehabil 2005;84(9):649–54.
52. Peterlein CD, Funk JF, Holscher A, et al. Is botulinum toxin A effective for the treatment of plantar fasciitis? Clin J Pain 2012;28(6):527–33.
53. Ahmad J, Ahmad SH, Jones K. Treatment of Plantar Fasciitis With Botulinum Toxin. Foot Ankle Int 2017;38(1):1–7.
54. Tiwari M, Bhargava R. Platelet Rich Plasma Therapy: A Comparative Effective Therapy with Promising Results in Plantar Fasciitis. J Clin Orthop Traum 2013; 4:31–5.
55. Mahindra P, Yamin M, Selhi HS, et al. Chronic Plantar Fasciitis: Effect of Platelet-Rich Plasma, Corticosteroid, and Placebo. Orthopedics 2016;39:e285–9.
56. Gogna P, Gaba S, Mukhopadhyay R, et al. Plantar Fasciitis: A Randomized Comparative Study of Platelet Rich Plasma and Low Dose Radiation in Sportspersons. Foot 2016;28:16–9.
57. Kalia RB, Singh V, Chowdhury N, et al. Role of Platelet Rich Plasma in Chronic Plantar Fasciitis: A Prospective Study. Ind J Orthop 2021;55(S1):S142–8.
58. Ciancia JC, Jayaram P. Musculoskeletal Injuries and Regenerative Medicine in the Elderly Patient. Phys Med Rehabil Clin N Am 2017;28(4):777–94.
59. Rossi LA, Piuzzi NS, Shapiro SA. Glenohumeral Osteoarthritis: The Role for Orthobiologic Therapies. JBJS Rev 2020;8(2):e0075.
60. Riboh JC, Saltzman BM, Yanke AB, et al. Effect of Leukocyte Concentration on the Efficacy of Platelet-Rich Plasma in the Treatment of Knee Osteoarthritis. Am J Sports Med 2016;4(3):792–800.
61. Abbas A, Du JT, Dhotar H. The Effect of Leukocyte Concentration on Platelet-Rich Plasma Injections for Knee Osteoarthritis: A Network Meta-Analysis. JBJS 2022; 104(6):559–70.
62. Costa LAV, Lenza M, Irrgang JJ, et al. How Does Platelet-Rich Plasma Compare Clinically to Other Therapies in the Treatment of Knee Osteoarthritis? A Systematic Review and Meta-analysis. Am J Sports Med 2022 (Online ahead of print).
63. Lin KY, Yang CC, Hsu CJ, et al. Intra-articular Injection of Platelet-Rich Plasma Is Superior to Hyaluronic Acid or Saline Solution in the Treatment of Mild to Moderate Knee Osteoarthritis: A Randomized, Double-Blind, Triple-Parallel, Placebo-Controlled Clinical Trial. Arthroscopy 2019;35(1):106–17.

64. Anz AW, Plummer HA, Cohen A, et al. Bone Marrow Aspirate Concentrate is Equivalent to Platelet-Rich Plasma for the Treatment of Knee Osteoarthritis at 2 Years: A Prospective Randomized Trial. Am J Sport Med 2022;50(3):618–29.
65. Bennell KL, Paterson KL, Metcalf BR, et al. Effect of Intra-articular Platelet Rich Plasma vs. Placebo Injection on Pain and Medial Tibial Cartilage Volume in Patients with Knee Osteoarthritis. JAMA 2021;326(20):2021–30.
66. Dorio M, Pereira RMR, Luz AGB, et al. Efficacy of platelet-rich plasma and plasma for symptomatic treatment of knee osteoarthritis: a double-blinded placebo-controlled randomized clinical trial. BMC Musculoskelet Disord 2021;22(1):822.
67. Kirschner JS, Cheng J, Creighton A, et al. Efficacy of Ultrasound-Guided Glenohumeral Joint Injections of Leukocyte-Poor Platelet-Rich Plasma Versus Hyaluronic Acid in the Treatment of Glenohumeral Osteoarthritis: A Randomized, Double-Blind Controlled Trial. Clin J Sports Med 2022 (Online ahead of print).
68. Berger DR, Centeno CJ, Steinmetz NJ. Platelet lysates from aged donors promote human tenocyte proliferation and migration in a concentration-dependent manner. Bone Joint Res 2019;8(1):32–40.
69. Hamid A, Sazlina SG. Platelet-rich plasma for rotator cuff tendinopathy: A systematic review and meta-analysis. PLoS One 2021;16(5):e0251111.
70. Robinson DM, Eng C, Makovitch S, et al. Non-operative orthobiologic use for rotator cuff disorders and glenohumeral osteoarthritis: A systematic review. J Back Musculoskelet Rehabil 2021;34:17–32.
71. Oudelaar BW, Huis In't Veld R, Ooms EM, et al. Efficacy of Adjuvant Application of Platelet-Rich Plasma After Needle Aspiration of Calcific Deposits for the Treatment of Rotator Cuff Calcific Tendinitis: A Double-Blinded, Randomized Controlled Trial with 2-Year Follow-up. Am J Sports Med 2021;49(4):873–82.
72. Kirschner JS, Cheng J, Hurwitz BS, et al. Ultrasound-guided percutaneous needle tenotomy (PNT) alone versus PNT plus platelet-rich plasma injection for the treatment of chronic tendinosis: A randomized controlled trial. PM R. 2021; 13(12):1340–9.
73. Best TM, Caplan A, Coleman M, et al. Not Missing the Future: A Call to Action for Investigating the Role of Regenerative Medicine Therapies in Pediatric/Adolescent Sports Injuries. Curr Sports Med Rep 2017;16(3):202–10.
74. Bray CC, Walker CM, Spence DD. Orthobiologics in pediatric sports medicine. Orthop Clin North America 2017;48(3):333–42.
75. Murphy RF, Mooney JF. Orthobiologics in pediatric orthopedics. Orthop Clin North America 2017;48(3):323–31.
76. Fabricant PD, Jones KJ, Delos D, et al. Reconstruction of the anterior cruciate ligament in the skeletally immature athlete: a review of current concepts. J Bone Joint Surg Am 2013;95(5):e28.
77. Magnussen RA, Flanigan DC, Pedroza AD, et al. Platelet rich plasma use in allograft ACL reconstructions: Two-year clinical results of a moon cohort study. Knee 2013;20(4):277–80.
78. Gordon AH, De Luigi AJ. Adolescent pitcher recovery from partial ulnar collateral ligament tear after platelet-rich plasma. Curr Sports Med Rep 2018;17(12):407–9.
79. Dines JS, Williams PN, ElAttrache N, et al. Platelet-Rich Plasma Can Be Used to Successfully Treat Elbow Ulnar Collateral Ligament Insufficiency in High-Level Throwers. Am J Orthop (Belle Mead Nj) 2016;45(5):296–300.
80. Albano JJ, Alexander RW. Autologous fat grafting as a mesenchymal stem cell source and living Bioscaffold in a patellar tendon tear. Clin J Sport Med 2011; 21(4):359–61.

81. Scollon-Grieve KL, Malanga GA. Platelet-rich plasma injection for partial patellar tendon tear in a high school athlete: A case presentation. PM&R. 2011;3(4): 391–5.
82. Macmull S, Parratt M, Bentley G, et al. Autologous chondrocyte implantation in the adolescent knee. Am J Sports Med 2011;39(8):1723–30.
83. Oepenn RS, Connolly SA, Bencardino JT, et al. Acute injury of the articular cartilage and subchondral bone: a common but unrecognized lesion in the immature knee. AJR Am J Roentgenol 2004;182:111–7.
84. DiBartola AC, Wright BM, Magnussen RA, et al. Clinical outcomes after autologous chondrocyte implantation in adolescent's knees: a systematic review. Arthroscopy 2016;32(9):1905–16.
85. Tegner Y, Lysholm J. Rating systems in the evaluation of knee ligament injuries. Clin Orthop Relat Res 1985;198:43–9.
86. Ware JE Jr, Sherbourne CD. The MOS 36-item short-form health survey (SF-96) I. Conceptual framework and item selection. Med Care 1992;30:473–83.
87. Lysholm J, Gillquist J. Evaluation of knee ligament surgery results with specialemphasis, 1982 emphasis on use of a scoring scale. Am J Sports Med 1982;10: 150–4.
88. Knutsen G, Drogset JO, Engebretsen L, et al. A randomized trial comparing autologous chondrocyte implantation with microfracture. Findings at five years. J Bone Joint Surg Am 2007;89(10):2105–12.
89. Kreuz PC, Steinwachs MR, Erggelet C, et al. Results after microfracture of full-thickness chondral defects in different compartments in the knee. Osteoarthritis and Cartilage 2006;14:1119–25.
90. Mithöfer K, Minas T, Peterson L, et al. Functional outcome of knee articular cartilage repair in adolescent athletes. Am J Sports Med 2005;33(8):1147–53.
91. Higgins LD, Taylor MK, Park D, et al. Reliability and validity of the International Knee Documentation Committee (IKDC) Subjective Knee Form. Joint Bone Spine 2007;74(6):594–9.
92. Teo BJ, Buhary K, Tai BC, et al. Cell-based therapy improves function in adolescents and young adults with patellar osteochondritis dissecans. Clin Orthop Relat Res 2013;471(4):1152–8.
93. Latalski M, Walczyk A, Fatyga M, et al. Allergic reaction to platelet-rich plasma (PRP). Medicine 2019;98(10). https://doi.org/10.1097/md.0000000000014702.

Clinical Rationale and Rehabilitation Guidelines for Post Biologic Therapy

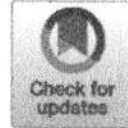

Eric S. Honbo, PT, DPT, OCSDN[a], Raymond Mattfeld, PT, OCS, ATC[b], Michael Khadavi, MD, RSMK[c], Luga Podesta, MD[d,*]

KEYWORDS

• Orthobiologics • Tissue healing • Tissue loading • Rehabilitation

INTRODUCTION

Orthobiologic therapies such as platelet-rich plasma (PRP) have been increasingly studied as a treatment for several musculoskeletal and orthopedic injuries Involving tendons, ligaments, muscles, the intervertebral disk, and synovial joints. In the United States, PRP was first used in 1987 to control wound healing after cardiac surgery.[1] Over the last decade, there has been a significant increase in the utilization of orthobiologic therapies and cell-based therapies by orthopedic, musculoskeletal, and sports medicine physicians. Despite promising clinical results and the widespread use of PRP to treat musculoskeletal and orthopedic injuries, its use remains controversial due to the heterogeneity in study designs, lack of reporting standardization, and evidence of publication bias.[2,3]

ORTHOBIOLOGIC FORMULATIONS

PRP is the supinate fraction processed from autologous peripheral whole blood that has a platelet concentration above the normal baseline.

There are substantial differences in the content of platelet concentrations produced by the various automated and manual PRP recovery systems. PRP is produced by either single spin or double spin density gradient centrifugation producing platelet concentrations ranging from 1.7 to 12× baseline. There are substantial differences in the content of platelet concentrations produced by the various automated and

[a] Advanced Physical Therapy & Sports Medicine- Spine & Sport PT, USC Department of Biokinesiology & Physical Therapy, Consultant- Chinese Olympic Committee/Team, 101 Hodencamp Road Suite #102, Thousand Oaks, CA 91360, USA; [b] Sports Rehab Consultants & Bright Bay Physical Therapy, 160 Orinoco Drive, Brightwaters, NY 11718, USA; [c] Kansas City Orthopedic Alliance, Leawood, Kansas, USA; [d] Regenerative Sports Medicine, Bluetail Medical Group Naples, Podesta Orthopedic & Sports Medicine Institute, Florida Everblades, 1875 Veterans Park Drive, Suite 2201, Naples, FL 34109, USA
* Corresponding author.
E-mail address: lugamd13@gmail.com

Phys Med Rehabil Clin N Am 34 (2023) 239–263
https://doi.org/10.1016/j.pmr.2022.08.014
1047-9651/23/

manual PRP recovery systems. The most common methods of PRP production use of either a plasma-based system or a buffy coat system, which produce either a leukocyte-poor PRP (LP-PRP) or a leukocyte-rich PRP (LR-PRP), respectively. Regardless of the system used, all systems must release growth factors from platelets. However, they all differ in platelet, white blood cells, red blood cells, and plasma concentrations.

Today, there has been a significant amount of literature published on the effects of PRP. We currently know that PRP has an analgesic effect by diminishing inflammation, it can augment the proliferation of tenocytes, osteoblasts, and myocytes and can augment the secretion of hyaluronic acid by synovial joints, and when used in combination with hyaluronic acid creating a synergistic effect. Finally, PRP through its paracrine effect can augments stem cell migration.

TISSUE HEALING

The healing process is defined as a complex and dynamic biologic progression that results in the restoration of anatomic structure and function. Tissue healing is a process characterized by a predictable cascade of biological tissue responses triggered by the injury itself. Physiologic healing progresses through four overlapping stages: stage 1, Hemostasis, stage 2, the acute inflammatory phase; stage 3, the proliferative or repair phase; and stage 4, the remodeling phase (**Fig. 1**).

Hemostasis, stage 1, is the first and shortest phase of the healing cascade occurring within seconds to minutes, and this is the process of forming a blood clot to stop bleeding. Platelets are vital to hemostasis, also functioning as the physiologic trigger to activate acute inflammation and program tissue repair.[4]

The *inflammatory phase*, stage 2, begins immediately following the injury and continues for 48 to 72 h. Platelets are stimulated to provide hemostasis by forming a clot. Platelets in the clot then degranulate and secrete several growth factors, hemostatic factors, and cytokines from alpha granules that are necessary for the early stages of the clotting cascade. Histamine and serotonin are released from the dense granules and function to increase capillary permeability, activate macrophages, and allow inflammatory cells greater access to the injury site[5,6] The inflammatory phase can last up to 72 h and is characterized by localized pain, swelling, erythema, and increased local tissue temperature.

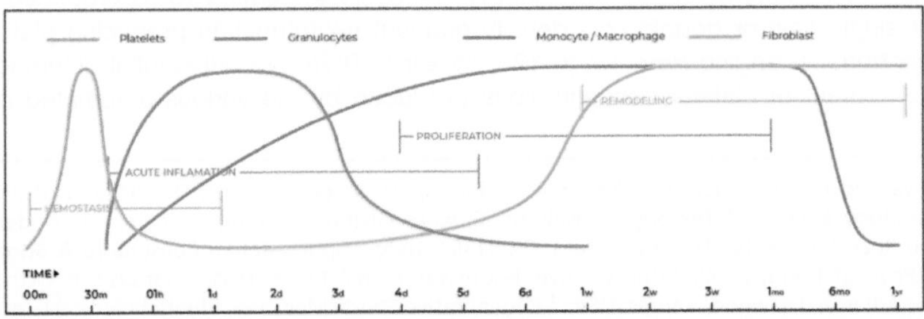

Fig. 1. Healing Cascade. The four stages of the healing cascade consisting of four partially overlapping stages- hemostasis, acute inflammation, proliferation, and remodeling. The particular cell type activity within each phase is crucial for the progression and successful execution of the healing cascade leading to tissue repair. (*Adapted from* Parrish WR, Roides B. Physiology of Blood Components in Wound Healing: an Appreciation of Cellular Co-Operativity in Platelet Rich Plasma Action. J Exec Sports Orthop.4(2):1–14. DOI:10.15226/2374-6904/4/2/00156.)

The *proliferative phase* (stage 3) begins with the activation of fibroblasts by growth factors and inflammatory mediators released during the acute inflammatory phase.[7] The proliferative phase is defined by cell proliferation, neovascularization, and matrix synthesis in addition to other metabolic processes that aid and remodeling and organization of the healing tissue.[8] During the ensuing 48 h to 6 weeks, anatomic structures begin to be restored, whereas tissue generation occurs. Fibroblasts begin to synthesize scar tissue and capillary neoformation begins to reestablish nutrients to the injured tissue. Stage 3 ends with the beginning of wound contracture.

The *remodeling phase,* stage 4, is the longest phase of the healing cascade, beginning several weeks after the initial injury and may last months to over a year depending on the severity of the initial injury.[7] Fibroblasts are responsible for remodeling, replacing the type 3 collagen matrix with the stronger type 1 collagen matrix. Fibroblasts either die through apoptosis or differentiate into myofibroblasts that align to the direction of force within the tissue. Failure to properly transition from the proliferation phase may lead to excessive or hypertrophic scarring.[7]

As with orthobiologic therapy such as PRP, there is great variability in reporting post-orthobiologic rehabilitation in return to activities. Several articles have proposed a standardized rehabilitation program following treatment with PRP.[9–11]

Townshend and colleagues,[2] performed a systematic review of post-procedure protocols following PRP injections for tendinopathy. They discovered significant variability in reporting periods of relative rest, weight-bearing restrictions, rehabilitation exercises, full return to play, and the use of nonsteroidal anti-inflammatory drug (NSAID) medications pre- and post-treatment.

THERAPY GUIDELINES FOR REHABILITATION

Prehabilitation or prehab is a concept that is not foreign to physical therapy. Prehabilitation was first mentioned in the literature in 1946.[12] The authors reported how a period of training for warfare, physical therapy, and strength training for the whole body, improved the physical and mental well-being of army recruits during the Second World War. Recently, prehabilitation has been mentioned in various orthopedic conditions and settings—ACL injury, joint replacements, regenerative cartilage surgery, and running.[13–18]

The intent of prehabilitation is to prepare a patient for optimal recovery from some type of procedure. The focus of this time period is on the restoration of osteokinematic and arthrokinematic mobility, soft-tissue extensibility, muscle flexibility, strength, balance, and proprioception. It also gives the clinician an opportunity to focus on improvement on other areas of the body that the patient would benefit from.

Emphasis is given to determine the reason for the injury-what, how, and why. In the case of ligament injuries, before biologic treatment, dynamic imaging/ultrasound is performed to establish baseline measurements of ligament morphology and joint stability. Baseline metrics include stressed and non-stressed ligament tensioning in comparison to the contralateral joint. These measurements are repeated at key time periods post-injection per Podesta and colleagues.[20] These metrics are then used to confirm tissue healing and joint stability for the purpose of rehabilitation progression.

A key component to prehabilitation with respect to biologics is patient education regarding the overall phases, time frames, and expectations for recovery from biologic treatment[19] (**Box 1**).

Rehabilitation progression following PRP injection is based on several individual factors—the combinations of time since injection, physiologic healing mechanism,

Box 1
Pre–Post Injection Treatment Instructions

Before PRP Treatment:

1. Stop all nonsteroidal anti-inflammatory medications NSAIDs 2 to 3 weeks before the procedure.
2. Prehab-gain general understanding of the healing process, time frames, use of heat to facilitate vascularization and local metabolism, and set patients up for best outcome.
3. Use of functional outcome tools such as the Kerlan–Jobe Orthopedic Score (KJOCS), Shoulder Pain and Disability Index (SPADI), Lower Extremity Functional Scale, Patellofemoral Index (SCOR), etc., are commonly used to establish the patient's baseline subjective functional status.
4. Establish baseline with imaging (dynamic MSK ultrasound, fluoroscopy, MRI)

Post-PRP Treatment:

1. Apply a thermal heat agent for 15 min four times per day when awake for 2 weeks.
2. Acetaminophen for pain as needed.
3. Increased pain and inflammation are expected in the treated tissue after the procedure.
4. Range-of-motion exercises as tolerated after the procedure.
5. Continue to use any braces, splints or crutches as recommended by your physician after the treatment.
6. Dynamic MSK ultrasound at 6 to 7 weeks to determine tissue continuity, integrity, and joint stability to safely progress later phase rehabilitation and higher-level functional activities.

patient's health and age, severity of injury, tissue integrity, response to physical therapy treatment dosage, as well as adherence to appropriate home programs. Characteristics of optimal loading include controlled and directed force to the selective tissue; early loading through functional ranges; an appropriate blend of compressive, tensile, and shear loading; variability in magnitude, direction, duration, and intensity; includes neural overload; needs to be dynamic and reflect demands of that tissue; and is functionally appropriate. Optimal loading is tissue and adaptation specific. It improves the mechanical properties of tissue and creates better fiber alignment and less disorganized matrix formation. The goal of rehabilitation following PRP injections is to progressively and therapeutically place appropriate amounts of physical stress and optimally load through and along the injured tissue to help facilitate healing.[20]

Loading is tissue-specific (**Table 1**). For instance, ligament, muscle, and tendon soft-tissues require linear loading due to fiber alignment. However, articular cartilage requires controlled and progressive compressive loading due to osteochondral matrix physiology. It responds optimally to progressive compression or shear, which creates a 'pumping effect' that provides joint cell nutrition, molecule transport, and joint lubrication. Successful functional outcomes for cartilage repair necessitate the correct quantity of loading. For example,:

- *Insufficient loading*: leads to adverse effects, delays healing, thinning and softening articular cartilage, decreases matrix content, chondrocytes, and yields less lubrication (immobilization)
- *Moderate loading*: *essential for cartilage health* and aides repair (low impact, bike, and swim)
- *Excessive loading*: detrimental to cartilage (high impact, Plyometrics)

General guidelines, expectations, and treatment interventions following orthobiologic injections are based on loading and tissue healing cascade and repair principles. A clinical framework that includes criteria-based progressions, goals within the healing phases, and clinical rationales for progression following orthobiologic injections are suggested in **Table 2**.[20]

Table 1
Tissue-specific loading and healing timeline

Tissue:	Healing Capacity Vascularity	Force to Facilitate Healing	Tissue Healing Time	Loading Protection
Muscle	Good, abundant	*Contractile Loading* Isometric- > Concentric- > Eccentric muscle	6–8 wk	ROM parameters, SubMax Isometrics- > Max Isometrics- > Concentrics- > Eccentrics- > Ballistic progressions
Tendon	Fair, less	*Contractile Loading* Isometric- > Concentric- > Eccentric	8–12 wk	ROM parameters, SubMax Isometrics- > Max Isometrics- > Concentrics- > Eccentrics- > Ballistic progressions
Ligament	Less, Diminished	*Tension* Controlled fiber Tension in line of stress	7–14 wk	Bracing with protected ROM parameters
Cartilage Labrum Intervertebral Disc	Limited/absent	*Cyclical Compression, Decompression & Shear* Imbibing pumping effect; controlled	6–12 wk	Bracing, Unloading, progressing weight bearing, Aquatics, Stationary Bike, weight bearing loading and controlled torsional stress
Subchondral Bone/Bone		Controlled Weight Bearing	6–12 wk	Weight Bearing Status, Unloading

Controlled physical stress to the tissue (muscle, tendon, ligament, and bone) is imparted throughout the rehabilitation duration to facilitate repair and may include tension, torsion, compression, and shear.[20] The stress or loading is imparted via manual therapy techniques, dosed medical exercise therapy progressions, as well as functional strengthening and return to play phase exercises. There is limited evidence in the literature defining specific protocols following PRP injection and limited documentation regarding tissue healing time frames following PRP injection.[10,11,21,22] There is no absolute progression or transition between phases and there can be variability between patients pending each individual case.

The goal following orthobiologic injection is to promote adequate tissue healing such that the tissue is able to once again maximally withstand the physiologic stresses and forces placed upon it with daily functional demands or sporting activities.[20] Collagen fibers run in parallel alignment that affords the tissue to withstand tensile forces and unilateral stress placed upon it.[23] The following information is based on the authors' clinical experience treating patients who have undergone orthobiologic injections with PRP and bone marrow-derived progenitor cells to ligament, tendon, muscle, intra-articular joints, and subchondral bone since 2006.

Phase I–II (Hemostasis/Inflammatory)

Time: 0 to 7 days.

Goals:

- Allow the PRP to absorb the injected tissue.
- Avoid cross-link disruption.
- Facilitate integrity of cross-link formation.

Phase One consists of early mobilization, gentle self-stretching, and protected or unloaded weight-bearing functional activities to prevent the deleterious effects of immobilization and to promote tissue healing.[20] Owing to the elevated inflammatory response, the patient commonly feels an increase in pain for the next 1 to 3 days following the injection. Following PRP injection the majority of the growth factors are released within the first hour of injection but continued release occurs up until about 7 days following injection.[24,25] Thus, the home program for the first 7 days following PRP injection is aimed at avoiding disruption of this physiologic mechanism and includes: rest, gentle active motion, submaximal isometric holds in all pain-free planes and ranges to help fiber alignment, pain medications such as over-the-counter analgesics avoiding NSAIDs, to control symptoms. Use of a heating agent at home following biologics injection is recommended. Thermotherapy increases tissue temperature, blood flow, and metabolism (providing a closer physiologic environment). Increased blood flow facilitates tissue healing by supplying protein, nutrients, and oxygen at the site of injury. A 1°C increase in tissue temperature is associated with a 10% to 15% increase in local tissue metabolism.[25] This increase in metabolism aids the healing process by increasing both catabolic and anabolic reactions needed to degrade and remove metabolic by-products of tissue damage and provides the milieu for tissue repair.[26]

Phase II (Inflammatory/Early Proliferation Phase)

Time: 8 to 21 days.

Goals:

- Avoid disruption of collagen cross-link bridging and formation.
- Initiate early motion.

Table 2
Criteria-based progressions and clinical rationale for rehab phases

Rehabilitation Phase	Criteria to Progress to this Phase	Anticipated Impairments and Functional Limitations	Intervention	Goal	Rationale
Phase I-II Hemostasis/ Inflammatory Phase Post Injection (0–7 d)	• Post Injection with no signs of infection	• Day 1–2: painful in the tissue/joint • Day 3–6: Diminishing pain and improving significantly • Day 7: Minimal pain, improved quality of ROM	*Restrictions:* ***Avoid all varus, valgus, A-P & rotational loads & ligament stressing, or and any loaded contractile activities or exercises*** ***Maintain any limited weight bearing precautions*** • Tissue/joint specific protected bracing & weight bearing • No exercise except for rehab program • UE injections - no lifting > body wt. • Tylenol for pain • Heat pack for 15 min, 4x/day for 1–2 wk. • Avoid ice over treatment site • Shower ok 24 h after procedure	• Protect tissue • Allow biologic to absorb • Daily activity as tolerated within provided brace • Avoid excess loading or stress to treated area • Improve tissue vascularity and joint synovialization via gentle movement of extremity to improve • Avoid tissue overload or exercise unless approved by doctor	• Minimizes stress on injection site • Cross link initiation and homeostasis occurring as biologic activating to preparing for cross bridging

(*continued on next page*)

Table 2
(continued)

Rehabilitation Phase	Criteria to Progress to this Phase	Anticipated Impairments and Functional Limitations	Intervention	Goal	Rationale
			• No submersion in water, bath, pool, hot tub or ocean for 1 wk. *PT Progression: (Home Based)* • Progress PROM to AROM, to point of initial resistance, within brace restraints, and only within physician ROM restraints • Gentle sub maximum Isometrics (lower to mid-range sub maximal holds) twice a daily		
Phase II Inflammatory/Early Proliferation Phase (8–21 d)	• No signs of infection *2-4-wk delay/slower progression with ligament injections due to decreased vascularization	• Pain • Limited ROM ○ pain with light UCL stress tests and ADL's ○ Limited UE strength	*Restrictions:* ***Avoid all varus, valgus, A-P & rotational loads & ligament stressing, or and any loaded contractile activities or exercises*** ***Maintain any limited weight*	• Facilitate collagen deposition • Avoid homeostasis • Avoid disruption of collagen crosslink • Maintain any restricted weight bearing status • Continue Phase 1 Rehabilitation recommendations	• Minimizes stress on injection site • Allow the PRP to absorb at the location • Prepare for cross bridging • Tissue is not yet ready for excessive weight bearing, compression, shearing, tensile, and contractile loads

		*bearing precautions*** • Tissue/joint specific protected bracing & weight bearing • No exercise except for rehab program • No concentric contractions or exercises to affected tissue except for unloaded ADLs and/ or ambulation • For UE procedures, no lifting more than a dinner plate. *PT Progression: (Home Based)* • Gradually progress AROM to point of initial resistance ◦ Obtain > 90% full ROM by end of week 2 ◦ AAROM to point of resistance or pain • Continue Phase 1 exercises, (gentle submax. isometrics) • Gradually progress to full weight bearing with protective brace if applicable	• Consult physician regarding cross-training and return to exercise options • Improve tissue vascularity and joint synovialization by initiating upper body exercise if you had lower body procedure or LB exercise for UB

(*continued on next page*)

Table 2
(continued)

Rehabilitation Phase	Criteria to Progress to this Phase	Anticipated Impairments and Functional Limitations	Intervention	Goal	Rationale
			• Continue Heat pack as in Phase I		
Phase III Proliferative Phase (3–6 wk)	• Full pain-free ROM • Able to tolerate full weight bearing (dependent on treated tissue)	• Limited UE/LE strength and cardiovascular endurance • Limited tissue tolerance to weight bearing, compression, shearing, tensile, and contractile loads or functional activities • Pain (diminishing) • Limited tolerance with heavier lifting, pushing, pulling functional activities	*Restrictions:* ***Avoid all valgus loads or ligament stressing activities/ exercises x 7 wk*** ***Avoid all compressive torsional loads for articular cartilage tissue x 5–6 wk*** • Continue use of assisted devices as instructed by physician procedures • No over stressing of tissue through exercise or impact activity • Initiate high repetition low load therapeutic concentric exercises for muscle/tendon • Initiate unloaded cyclical high volume compression-	• Protect tissue • Facilitate collagen deposition • Avoid disruption of collagen cross-link and facilitate parallel fiber alignment • Minimize deconditioning • Communication among physician, physical therapist & patient is essential during this key transitional phase	• Pain threshold significantly reduced • Collagen synthesis occurring, aligning in the longitudinal axis Nominal tables that are really just one-column lists are best represented as boxes, so Table 1 and 4 has been converted to Box 1 and 2, and subsequent tables have been renumbered sequentially. Please verify. • Cross bridging occurring and matrix integrity improving • Tissue beginning to withstand tensile forces and loads • Use modalities to facilitation collagen

	decompression exercises for cartilage/ joint • Improve tissue vascularity and joint synovialization by initiating upper body cardiovascular exercise if you had lower body procedure or LB exercise for UB • No exercises except for supervised rehab program • (3–6 wk) *PT Progression Overview:* • Pain should not increase > 2 points on 10-point VAS • Modalities for collagen synthesis & pain control: • Moist heat, nonthermal ultrasound, cold laser, Russian stim, ES, Shock Wave Therapy (ESWT) Manual Therapy Techniques • Gentle Soft-tissue Mobilization along	formation & remodeling • Soft-tissue mobilization techniques have mechanical, physiologic, histologic, and neurologic effects on the tissue which facilitate the healing mechanism and fiber alignment • Progress toward light ligamentous loading by end of phase III • Tissue tensile strength should be strong enough to initiate stress loading exercises • BFR enables strengthening using a light load and a relatively low volume of work • Cardiovascular training to improve endurance & tissue repair

(*continued on next page*)

Table 2
(continued)

Rehabilitation Phase	Criteria to Progress to this Phase	Anticipated Impairments and Functional Limitations	Intervention	Goal	Rationale
			the line of tissue fibers • Joint Mobilizations to maintain arthrokinematics Therapeutic Exercises: • AROM to point of initial resistance sub maximum to max isometrics • Emphasize proper postural alignment, distal joint position Adjust exercise progression based on severity of injury • Gradual progression of early to mid-phase weight bearing activities (aquatics, unloaded treadmill, elliptical) • Initiate low resistance, high repetition, concentric, open chain exercise		

			• Initiate Blood Flow Restriction (BFR) exercises • Initiation and progression of eccentric exercises as concentric strength increases Neuromuscular Re-education: • PNF and rhythmic stabilization exercises • Proprioceptive training • Use of taping techniques as indicated for facilitation/inhibition		
Phase IV Remodeling Phase (6–15 wk)	Overlap of timelines is based on the patient's condition and severity of injury • Pain-free ligament provocation tests • Improving to no pain with resisted contractile tests	• Limited UE/LE strength • Limited ligament & tendon tensile strength during early phase IV • Diminished but improving weightbearing or joint compressive exercise loading tolerance • Limited joint proprioception • Altered timing and mechanics with sports	*Diagnostic imaging:* • Diagnostic Ultrasound (~6–8 wk) to determine extent of healing and exercise progression and return to activity or sports status *PT Progression: (Physical Therapy)* *Modalities*: • Continue as needed *Manual Therapy;* • Continue Deep transverse friction mobilization/massage	• Restore normal tissue integrity & fiber alignment • Maximize tissue vascularity and joint synovialization • Increase tissue tensile strength • Improve joint proprioception • Improve force production, tissue elasticity and ability to withstand tensile stretching	• Increased tissue integrity & strength of repaired tissue • Improved ability to produce force, withstand tensile stretching, absorb shock, and increased tissue elasticity • Reassess Functional Index Score and dynamic imaging to correlate with objective exam findings to determine soft-tissue and

(*continued on next page*)

Table 2
(*continued*)

Rehabilitation Phase	Criteria to Progress to this Phase	Anticipated Impairments and Functional Limitations	Intervention	Goal	Rationale
	• Pain-free joint stability with stress testing • Show tissue integrity & joint stability with dynamic imaging • Subjective Functional Index Tool indicates patient is ready to progress through Phase IV to return to play status • Functional Testing performed to determine return to activity	specific & functional activities	to increase tissue vascularization and break up tissue adhesions *Therapeutic Exercise:* • Progress exercise and functional mobility integrating UE/LE CKC exercises as appropriate • Progress eccentric exercise • Progressive plyometric loading from <body weight to full body weight-bilateral to single • Progress to ballistic, explosive training • Sport specific training ○ ≸ 50% effort up to week 8 ○ ≸ Below 75% effort up to week 10 ○ ≸ Below 90% effort up to week 12	*Critical Decision-Making Period-determine if tissue has sufficiently healed via dynamic imaging or if a second injection and/or surgical intervention is warranted* • Prepare for return to activity, sports	subchondral bone healing, joint stability and pace of current exercise progression can continue, or if a second injection and/or surgical intervention is warranted

- Initiate Interval Sport Programs (Throwing, running, on field drills) pending results of Diagnostic US
- Return to sports 10–15 wk depending on the sport/activity

Neuromuscular Reeducation:

- Light concentric resistance pulley or tubing patterns with controlled speed emphasis
- Light Resistance PNF exercises performed manually using distal hand placements and initiating joint specific motions and adding pulleys or tubing/bands
- Progress proprioception exercises to unstable surfaces

Week 6–7 Critical Decision-Making Period

**Dynamic imaging (MSK ultrasound) is used to confirm ligament healing,

(continued on next page)

Table 2
(*continued*)

Rehabilitation Phase	Criteria to Progress to this Phase	Anticipated Impairments and Functional Limitations	Intervention	Goal	Rationale
			joint stability, and load progression. • Initiate ligament and joint loading when healing and joint stability are determined, exercise progression is initiated. • Initiate eccentric tendon loading If sufficient healing and stability has not occurred at 6–7 wk, a second injection vs surgical stabilization may be warranted *Week 8–10*: Progress to fast twitch and dynamic exercises • Increase speed, resistance, and functional strengthening • Add kinetic chain functional and sport specific loading progressions		

**Pending repeated US imaging findings progress to return to play phase 4

Week 10–12:

Reassess Objective Exam results, Functional Testing, and Subjective Functional Tool Scores to determine return to higher level activity and/or sport-specific play

- Begin interval Return to Sport program. Start interval throwing, batting, tennis serves, volleyball hitting programs pending repeat US imaging findings,

Weeks 12–16:

Progress from 75-90+ % in controlled setting. Gradual return to sport at 12–15 wk

- Initiate high repetition no resistance loading exercises.
- Obtain 90% full range of motion.

Phase Two consists of continued gentle active motion and increased activity at home. The patient should obtain 90% of full ROM by the end of week 2.[20] Light soft-tissue mobilizations should commence toward the end of week 3 to the injected tissue and surrounding fascia at this time. However, to avoid disruption of collagen cross-link bridging and formation, deeper soft-tissue techniques (transverse friction, etc.) are not implemented until the sixth week following injection.[20] Gentle early motion of the local joints facilitates the physiologic tissue healing response following PRP injection that proceeds through the inflammatory, reparative, and remodeling phases. Furthermore, early motion and self-stretching prevents joint adhesions, increases muscle contraction, muscle fiber size, and tension, as well as increases resting levels of glycogen and protein synthesis. Mechanical stimulation (ie,: motion and controlled external loading) is a prerequisite for platelet effect in the early post-injection phase. Platelets influence the early stages of tissue repair, and this allows mechanical stimulation to further drive the reparative phase healing.[27]

Submaximal-maximal effort isometrics performed three times per day are also initiated in attempts to create light tension in the direction of the tendon fibers. However, any tensioning forces to injected ligament tissue are avoided at this time (valgus elbow stress to ulnar collateral ligament [UCL]) and until 7 weeks post-injection. Intermittent rest and care with resuming work and normal daily functional activities are also encouraged at home to help control post-injection symptoms and early inflammatory elevation.

Progressive full arc motion in the first two phases prevents ligament atrophy and increases ligament linear tissue stress and stiffness-particularly at a bone-ligament junction. Ligament stressing exercises or functional activities as well as excessive muscle or tendon tension is avoided during this phase. There may be a 2- to 4-week delay with ligament healing due to decreased tissue vascularization **Table 3**.[20] Exercises that exert tension on the UCL (Valgus stress) are not begun until later phase 3.

Early motion restoration aids connective tissue lubrication between collagen cross-links, increases collagen mass, decreases abnormal collagen cross-links, and prevents adhesion development. Following PRP injections, articular cartilage responds to early motion, intermittent compression, and decompression loading with improved metabolic activity and increased health of the cartilage matrix. Muscle, tendon, ligament, and bone tissue all respond favorably to motion. Restoring full range of motion during the first 10 to 14 days following PRP injection is advocated.[20]

Modalities used in the first two phases of PRP rehabilitation can include ultrasound, laser, and electrical stimulation. The use of modalities during this phase is aimed to further stimulate tissue healing and increase local perfusion and oxygen delivery to the site. Nonthermal ultrasound is commonly used to facilitate tissue repair and regeneration in damaged tissue. There is research that supports the use of therapeutic ultrasound to increase boney and muscle tissue regeneration.[28–30] However, most

Table 3
Tissue vascularization

Tissue Vascularization			
Ligament	Tendon	Bone	Muscle
Less			More

studies that support the use of nonthermal ultrasound and laser to aid tissue healing are based on animal studies. It is still unclear if using a pulsed nonthermal ultrasound is more effective than a low-intensity continuous protocol in terms of proliferation and tissue healing. The use of laser treatment in patients with lateral epicondylosis was found to lower subjective overall pain levels with reports of 90% to 100% relief in more than 45% of the patients who were treated with laser.[31] In addition, studies have found the use of low-energy laser improves tensile strength and stiffness in repairing medial collateral ligament in rats at 3 and 6 weeks after injury.[32] When rehabilitating after tendon PRP, to help increase endorphin release and minimize tissue response to loading and manual mobilizations, the authors have found positive results using Russian electrical stimulation with the following parameters: 2500 Hz frequency, 50 pps, 10/10 s duty cycle, 2 s ramp time for 10 to 12 min.

Progressive loading with shoulder, elbow, and wrist exercises during phases 2 to 4 is a critical component of the post-PRP injection treatment plan. The first two phases include use of concentric low-load higher repetition exercise dosage—three sets of 20 to 25 repetitions is recommended. Once the patient reaches three sets of 25 repetitions the weight is increased by 1 pound and progresses from there. Proper postural alignment, proximal and distal joint positioning, and control throughout the range, etc. are emphasized. This submaximal intensity using higher repetition progression improves tissue vascularization, helps align collagen cross-links, promotes tissue healing, and enables the tissue to start adapting to controlled amounts of stress.[20] Endurance training versus strengthening has been used in the early phases with success following PRP injections. Submaximal loading exercises reduce homeostasis and tissue breakdown and symptom exacerbation during the first 2 to 4 weeks. Studies have shown that resistance exercise is more effective in inducing acute muscle anabolism than high-load low volume or work matched resistance exercise modes (isometrics).[33]

Phase III (Proliferative/Reparative Phase)

Time: 3 to 6 weeks.

Goals:

- Adjust exercise progression based on type of tissue and severity of injury
- Use of modalities to aide tissue proliferation (recommend pulsed US, laser, electrical stimulation, extracorporeal shockwave therapy [ESWT], blood flow restriction [BFR] therapy)
- Begin high repetition loading and concentric
- Begin functional activities
- *Avoid Ligament stress for 7 weeks with activities of daily living and exercise*
- **Progress to Eccentrics week 4 to 6**

Pain levels have typically lessened by the third week. Collagen synthesis is occurring and aligning in the longitudinal axis. At this point, the tissue is beginning to withstand tensile forces and loads. However, it is important to adjust exercise progression based on the type of tissue and the severity of injury (ligament healing and proliferation take longer).[20] BFR has been shown to increase loading and training capacity for those who are not ready or may not tolerate heavier training loads and is often initiated in week 3 following orthobiologic injection. Specifically, BFR has been shown to produce increased muscle mass, strength, as well as cross-sectional patellar and Achilles tendon stiffness at comparable levels to conventional high-load resistance training.[34] The ability to provide the skeletal muscle with a sufficient exercise stimulus using a light load and a relatively low volume of work is helpful for muscle, tendon, ligament, and joint that is important in the earlier post-injection phase of healing.[35]

Soft-tissue mobilizations and progressive loading via resisted exercise are key components of the post-injection reparative and remodeling phases[20]. The primary pathologic mechanism that leads to tendinopathy includes chronic microscopic tearing in hypovascular tendon tissue. These repetitive tears heal by scar formation versus the normal tendon-healing pathways of vascularization and inflammation mechanisms.[36] Thus, during the reparative and remodeling phase of muscle and tendon tissue, the use of soft-tissue mobilizations techniques (ASTYM, deep transverse friction mobilization, Active Release, Graston Technique) in conjunction with appropriate exercise progressions is an important component of the healing process to help minimize this scar formation and promote anatomic tissue fiber healing in line of stress.[20] These techniques, however, should be used with caution to avoid tissue alignment disruption and once in the remodeling phase after 6 to 8 weeks post-injection.

Deep transverse tissue mobilization (DTFM) and friction massage had been implored with positive results. As described by Cyriax, DTFM is an aggressive form of soft-tissue mobilization in which localized pressure or distractive manipulation of tissues is directed tangentially across the longitudinally oriented collagen component of the injured tissue. To promote normal resolution of the collagen tissue, the tissue to be treated should be in a moderate stretch position (not painful).[37] Deep Transverse Friction mobilizations and other soft-tissue manipulation techniques have mechanical, physiologic, histologic, and neurologic effects on the tissue which facilitate the healing mechanism of PRP injections (**Box 2**). Reaction to DTFM may include rapid desensitization, latent post-treatment soreness, and moderate tissue bruising covering the area of tissue contact is acceptable.[38]

The use of extracorporeal shockwave therapy is effective in reducing pain and improving function.[39–41] The proposed mechanisms of ESWT involve inducing suppression of inflammatory reactions and oxidative stress and eliciting neovascularization in degenerative tissues.[42] The use of ESWT combined with PRP injection are beneficial on pain reduction and recovery of physical activity of patients with insertional Achilles tendinopathy and can relieve the pain synergistically for KOA.[43,44]

Eccentric loading is initiated early in the reparative and remodeling phases at approximately weeks 5 to 6 for muscle belly and 6 to 8 for tendon pending individual patient status. Owing to its positive effect on improving tissue integrity, strength, and improved function, eccentric loading is the other important component of the post-PRP injection rehabilitation.[20] Eccentric contractions function to decelerate a limb, provide shock absorption, and generate forces 14% to 50% greater than a maximal concentric contraction does.[45] This increased force generation improves musculotendinous integrity by inducing muscle hypertrophy and increased tensile strength or by lengthening the musculotendinous unit.[46]

Unlike concentric phase 1 to 2 exercises, eccentric loading has been shown to aid in stable angiogenesis in early tendon injury.[47] Daily eccentric loading was found to not have any detrimental effect on tendon vascularity or microcirculation.[47] A systematic review of tendinopathy found that eccentric exercises had the most clinical efficacy in regenerating function.[48] Other studies have found that eccentric exercise progressions are an effective treatment for chronic tendinosis.[49,50] Eccentric tendon loading exercise progressions are thus implemented into the post-injection rehabilitation by week 4 to 5 pending individual patient response.[20]

There is no clear consensus on the best non-operative treatment for muscle injuries beyond immediate rest and anti-inflammatory medications or modalities.[29] In chronic tendinosis injuries, rest has been found to be a less effective treatment efficacy.[48,51] In turn, eccentric exercise and loading have been shown in many studies to be beneficial in treating patients with tendinosis.[46,47] The optimal dosage and frequency of

Box 2
Effects of deep transverse tissue mobilization

Mechanical
- Distortion and elongation of collagen fibers
- Increased interstitial mobility

Physiologic
- Localized hyperemia
- Stimulate white blood cell invasion and healing production
- Destruction of substance P

Histologic
- Prevents scar formation and haphazard collagen orientation
- Stimulate collagen orientation along lines of stress via "Piezzo-electric effect"

Neurologic
- Initial nociceptor stimulation
- Mechanoreceptor stimulation
- Pain inhibition via "Central Biasing Mechanism"

eccentric loading for treating chronic tendinosis have not yet been established.[52] However, the literature indicates that to optimize treatment PRP injection should be combined with the mechanical stimulus of the tissue in order to promote optimal post-injection tissue healing and repair.[20]

Phase IV (Remodeling Phase)

Time: 6 to 12 weeks.
Goals:

- Eccentric loading, plyometric training return to sport/activity (pending individual sport and post-injection status variable from patient to patient)
- Continue tissue remodeling facilitation with deep transverse friction and soft-tissue mobilizations
- *Diagnostic ultrasound (~ 6 to 7 weeks) may be repeated to determine the extent of healing
- Resume full functional or sporting activity for 10 to 12 weeks pending progress with the post-injection program

The injected tissue commonly shows increased tensile strength during the remodeling phase.[20] Tissue remodeling facilitation is continued in phase four with the use of deep transverse friction and soft-tissue mobilizations. Depending on the response to the eccentric strengthening progression, the patient progresses to speed and coordination drills, plyometrics, ballistics, and more explosive sport-specific phase 4 exercises.

At this point, connective tissue has improved tensile strength as its fiber orientation is better aligned and suited to withstand more demanding tensile stress.[53] The functional strengthening, plyometrics, ballistics, neuromuscular power, and coordination exercises are performed at more intense levels to enable the patient to meet the demands of his or her sport or job activity. Typically, selective tissue tension tests (ligament stress tests, resisted muscle-tendon tests in a lengthened position, weight-bearing, and compression tests for bone) are non-provocative. Use of follow-up functional tools to ascertain patient readiness to resume higher level exercises, and return to sport or work is recommended. Studies regarding the efficacy of using scores on

Table 4
Estimated average tissue healing response time

Tissue Recovery Time			
>4–8 wk.	>6–8 wk.	>10–12 wk.	>11–15 wk.
Joints	Muscle belly	Ligaments[a]	Tendons

[a] Ligament healing may be delayed 2 to 4 wk; avoid varus/valgus.

subjective functional tools or questionnaires to help determine when a patient is ready to safely resume a particular activity or sport given a certain subjective score have not yet been published.

There are no clearly defined or objective means of determining when an athlete is able to safely return to play or when a patient is able to return to a functional activity (job duty). A grading system has been used to describe tendinopathy.[54] However, the use of a detailed clinical examination together with the repeat ultrasound imaging findings, as well as the patient's subjective assertions and functional index score as to whether the patient is ready to resume certain activities or sports are all used to assist the physician, therapist, and athletic trainer in determining when the patient is ready to resume the desired activity. Interval running programs, on-field agility progressions, and interval throwing programs are initiated in phase 4. Although there are several notable documented cases in which an athlete has returned to play at an earlier time period following PRP injection, most patients have been able to resume full functional or sporting activity by 10 to 12 weeks (**Table 4**).[20]

SUMMARY

The use of orthobiologic modalities such as PRP in orthopedics and sports medicine to deliver high concentrations of naturally occurring biologically active growth factors and proteins to the site of injury is very promising and continues to evolve. Early protection and tissue-specific progressive loading are critical components to successful outcomes following orthobiologic intervention. Each tissue heals and responds differently. Ligament, tendon, muscle, and articular cartilage each have unique healing properties that require tissue-specific loading. The authors have found using a criteria-based loading and exercise progression guided by dynamic imaging when appropriate to further advance the goal-oriented rehabilitation program. Each patient and injured tissue are unique and require specificintervention and rehabilitation.

DISCLOSURE

L. Podesta, MD, Editor, Biologic Orthopedic Journal E. Honbo, PT, DPT, OCS, Cert. DN, The Authors have nothing to disclose. R. Mattfeld, PT, DPT, OCS, ATC, The Authors have nothing to disclose.

REFERENCES

1. Ferrari M, Zia S, Valbonesi M, et al. A new technique for hemodilution, preparation of autologous platelet-rich plasma and interoperative blood salvage in cardiac surgery. Int J Artif Org 1987;10:47–50.
2. Townsend C, Von Rickenbach KJ, Bailowitz Z, et al. Post-procedure protocols following platelet rich plasma injections for tendinopathy: a systematic review. PMR 2020;(12):904–15.

3. Moraes VY, Lenza M, Tamaoki M, et al. Platelet-rich therapies for musculoskeletal soft-tissue injuries. Cochrane Data-base Syst Rev 2014;40:CD010071.
4. Broughton G 2nd, Janis JE, Attinger CE. The basic science of wound healing. Plast Reconstr Surg 2006;117(7 Suppl):12S–34S.
5. Foster T, Puskas B, Mandelbaum B, et al. Platelet-rich plasma-from basic science to clinical applications. Am J Sports Med 2009;37(11):2258–72.
6. Bennett NT, Schultz GS. Growth factors and wound healing: biochemical properties of growth factors and their receptors. Am J Surg 1993;165(6):728–37.
7. Parrish WR, Roides B. Physiology of Blood Components in Wound Healing: an Appreciation of Cellular Co-Operativity in Platelet Rich Plasma Action. J Exec Sports Orthop 2017;4(2):1–14. https://doi.org/10.15226/2374-6904/4/2/00156.
8. Dean R, DePhilliPhysiology of Blood Components in Wound Healing: an Appreciation of Cellular Co-Operativity in Platelet Rich Plasma Action. J Exec Sports Orthop.4(2):1-14. po N, LaPrade R. Ligament Lesions: Cell Therapy. In G. Filardo et al. (eds), Orthobiologics, Chap 20, 245-255, https://doi.org.org/*10.1007/978-3-084744-9_20.*
9. Finnoff J, Fowler S, Lai J, et al. Treatment of chronic tendinopathy with ultrasound-guided needle tenotomy and platelet-rich plasma injection. PM R 2011;3:900–11.
10. van Ark M, van den Akker-Scheek I, Meijer L, et al. An exercise-based physical therapy program for patients with patellar tendinopathy after platelet-rich plasma injection. Phys Ther Sport 2013;14:124–30.
11. Kaux J-F, Forthomme B, Namurois M-H, et al. Description of a standardized rehabilitation program based on sub-maximal eccentric following a platelet-rich plasma infiltration for jumper's knee. Muscles Ligaments Tendons J 2014;4:85–9.
12. Prehabilitation. rehabilitation, and revocation in the army. Br Med J 1946;1:192–7.
13. Shaarani S, O'Hare C, Quinn A, et al. Effect of Prehabilitation on the Outcome of Anterior Cruciate Ligament Reconstruction. Am J Sports Med 2013;41(9): 2117–27.
14. Carter H, Littlewood C, Webster K, et al. The Effectiveness of Preoperative Rehabilitation Programmes on Postoperative Outcomes Following Anterior Cruciate Ligament (ACL) Reconstruction: A Systematic Review. BMC Musculoskelet Disord 2020;21(647):1–13.
15. Potts G, Reid D, Larmer P. The Effectiveness of Preoperative Exercise Programmes on Quadriceps Strength Before and Following Anterior Cruciate Ligament (ACL) Reconstruction: A Systematic Review. Phys Ther Sports 2022;54: 16–28.
16. Linton L, Valentin S. Running Coaches and Running Group Leaders' Engagement with, and Beliefs and Perceived Barriers to Prehabilitation and Injury Prevention Strategies for Runners. Phys Ther Sports 2020;46:54–62.
17. Villers J, Burch J, Scheller M, et al. Physical therapy Prehabilitation on a Reverse Total Shoulder Replacement Candidate: A Case Study. J Phys Ther Sci 2020;32: 197–205.
18. Hirschmüller A, Schoch W, Baur H, et al. Rehabilitation Before Regenerative Cartilage Knee Surgery: A New Prehabilitation Guideline Based on the Best Available Evidence. Arch Orthop Trauma Surg 2019;139:217–30.
19. Honbo E, Podesta L. Clinical Applications of Platelet Rich Plasma Therapy. In: Maxey L, Magnusson J, editors. Rehabilitation for the Postsurgical Orthopaedic patient. 3rd ed. Mosby; 2012. p. 171–92.
20. Podesta L, Crow S, Volkner D, et al. Treatment of Elbow Partial Ulnar Collateral Ligament Tears with Platelet Rich Plasma. Am J Sports Med 2013;41(7):1689–94.

21. Bagwell M, Wilk K, Colberg R, et al. The Use of Serial Platelet Rich Plasma Injections with Early Rehabilitation to Expedite Grade III Medial Collateral Ligament Injury in a Professional Athlete: A Case Report. IJSPT 2018;13(3):520–5.
22. Mautner K, Malanga G. Optimization of Ingredients, Procedures, and Rehabilitation for Platelet-Rich Plasma Injections for Chronic Tendinopathy. Pain Manage 2011;1(6):523–32.
23. Donatelli R, Owens-Burkhart A. Effects of immobilization on the extensibility of periarticular connective tissue. J Orthop Sports Phys Ther 1981;3:67–72.
24. Hammond JW, Hinton RY, Curl LA, et al. Use of autologous platelet-rich plasma to treat muscle strain injuries. Am J Sports Med 2009;37:1135–11342.
25. Cameron MH. Thermal agents: physical principles, cold and superficial heat. In: Physical agents in rehabilitation: from research to Practice. Philadelphia: Saunders; 1999. p. 149–75.
26. Nadler S, Weingand K, Kruse R. The Physiologic Basis and Clinical Applications of Cryotherapy and Thermotherapy for the Pain Practitioner. Pain Physician 2004;395–9.
27. Virchenko O, Aspenberg P. How can one platelet injection after tendon injury lead to a stronger tendon after 4 weeks? Interplay between early regeneration and mechanical stimulation. Acta Orthop 2006;77(5):806–12.
28. Byl NN, Mckenzie AL, West JM, et al. Pulsed microamerage stimulation: A controlled study of healing of surgically induced wounds in Yucatan pigs. Phys Ther Arch Phys Med Rehab 1994;74:201–13 [discussion: 213-218].
29. Chan YS, Li Y, Foster W, et al. The use of suramin, an antifibrotic agent, to improve muscle recovery after strain injury. Am J Sports Med 2005;33:43–51.
30. Gum S, Reddy G, Stehno-Bittel L, Enwemeka C. Combined ultrasound, electrical stimulation, and laser promote collagen synthesis with moderate changes in tendon biomechanics. Am J Phys Med Rehab 1997;76:288–96.
31. Zlato S, Tatjana T. Comparison Between Low Level Laser Therapy, Transcutaneous Electro-Neural Stimulation, Visible Incoherent Polarized Light, and Placebo in the Treatment of Lateral Epicondylitis: A Pilot Clinical Study on 120 Patients. Lasers Surg Med 2002;Supplement:14.
32. Fung DT, Ng GY, Leung MC, et al. Therapeutic low energy laser improves the mechanical strength of repairing medial collateral ligament. Lasers Surg Med 2002; 31:91–6.
33. Burd NA, West DWD, Staples AW, et al. Low-Load High Volume Resistance Exercise Stimulates Muscle Protein Synthesis More Than High-Load Low Volume Resistance Exercise in Young Men. PLoS ONE 2010;5(8):e12033. https://doi.org/10.1371/journal.pone.0012033.
34. Song JS, Spitz RW, Yamada Y, et al. Loenneke JP Exercise-induced hypoalgesia and pain reduction following blood flow restriction: a brief review. Phys Ther Sport 2021;(50):89–96.
35. Centner C, Jerger S, Lauber B, et al. Low-Load Blood Flow Restriction and High-Load Resistance Training Induce Comparable Changes in Patellar Tendon Properties. Med Sci Sports Exerc 2022;54(4):582–9.
36. Courville XF, Coe MP, Hecht PJ. Current concepts review: noninsertional Achilles Tendinopathy. Foot Ankle Int 2009;30(11):1132–42.
37. Cyriax JH. Textbook of orthopaedic medicine: volume 2 Treatment by Manipulation, Massage, and injection. 10th edition. London: Bailliere Tindall; 1980.
38. Mattingly GE, Mackarey PJ. Optimal methods for shoulder tendon palpation: a cadaver study. Phys Ther 1996;76(2):166–74.

39. Li W, Pan Y, Yang Q, et al. Extracorporeal Shockwave Therapy for The Treatment of Knee Osteoarthritis: A Retrospective Study. Medicine 2018;97(27):1–4.
40. Vulpani M, Trischitta D, Trovato P, et al. Extracorporeal Shockwave Therapy (ESWT) in Achilles Tendinopathy: A Long-term Follow-up Observational Study. J Sports Med Phys Fitness 2009;49(2):171–6.
41. Aldajah S, Alashram A, Annino G, et al. Analgesic Effect of Extracorporeal Shock-Wave Therapy in Individuals with Lateral Epicondylitis: A Randomized Controlled Trial. J Funct Morphol Kinesiol 2022;7(29):1–8.
42. Chang C, Chen L, Chou Y, et al. The Effectiveness of Platelet-Rich Plasma and Radial Extracorporeal Shock Wave Compared with Platelet-Rich Plasma in the Treatment of Moderate Carpal Tunnel Syndrome. Pain Med 2020;21(8):1668–75.
43. Erroi D, Sigona M, Suarez T, et al. Conservative treatment for Insertional Achilles Tendinopathy: platelet-rich plasma and focused shock waves. A Retrospective Study Muscles, Ligaments Tendons J 2017;7(1):98–106.
44. Wenzhen S, Yongjie L, Guowei W, et al. Prospective clinical study on extracorporeal shock wave therapy combined with platelet-rich plasma injection for knee osteoarthritis. Chin J Reparative Reconstr Surg Dec. 2019;33(12):1527–8.
45. Dean E. Physiology and therapeutic implication of negative work. Phys Ther 1988;68:233–7.
46. Alfredson H, Tendon Pietila, Jonsson P, et al. Heavy-load eccentric calf muscle training for the treatment of chronic Achilles Tendinosis. Am J Sports Med 1998;26:360–6.
47. Nakamura K, Kitaoka K, Tomita K. Effect of eccentric exercise on the healing process of injured patellar tendon in rats. J Orthop Sci 2008;13:371–8.
48. Magnussen RA, Dunn WR, Thompson AB. Nonoperative treatment of midportion Achilles tendinopathy: a systematic review. Clin J Sport Med 2009;19:54–64.
49. Purdam CR, Jonsson P, Alfredson H, et al. A pilot study of the eccentric decline squat in the management of painful chronic patellar tendinopathy. Br J Sports Med 2004;38:395–7.
50. Young MA, Cook JL, Purdam CR, et al. Eccentric decline squat protocol offers superior results at 12 months compared with traditional eccentric protocol for patellar tendinopathy in volleyball players. Br J Sports Med 2005;39:102–5.
51. Rompe JD, Nafe B, Furia JP, et al. Eccentric loading versus eccentric loading plus shock-wave treatment for midportion Achilles tendinopathy: a randomized controlled trial. Am J Sports Med 2009 Mar;37(3):463–70.
52. Andres BM, Murrell GA. Molecular and clinical developments in tendinopathy: editorial comment. Clin Orthop Rel Res 2008;466:1519–20.
53. Kellet J. Acute soft-tissue injuries- A review of the literature. Med Sci Sports Exerc 1986;18:489–500.
54. Blazina ME, Kerlan RK, Jobe FW, et al. Orthop Clin North Am 1973;4:665–78.

Orthobiologic Techniques for Surgical Augmentation

Kenneth M. Lin, MD, Christopher S. Frey, MD, Ran Atzmon, MD, Kinsley Pierre, BS, Monica S. Vel, BS, Seth L. Sherman, MD*

KEYWORDS

• Orthobiologics • Cell-based augmentation • PRP • LR-PRP • Tissue healing

KEY POINTS

- Biologic augmentation may carry a benefit in altering the biologic potential of repaired tissue in surgical treatments of cartilage, meniscus, and intra-articular tendons because intra-articular milieu is generally less favorable for tissue healing.
- The three types of biologic augmentation include: cell-based augmentation for tendon and ligament repair, cartilage restoration, and bony nondelayed or delayed union, factor-based augmentation which intra-operatively utilizes the use of growth factors such as PRP and fibrin clots, and biomechanical augmentation where various forms of tissue scaffolds are used for tendon and ligament repair.
- The use of orthobiologics in surgical settings shows promise for reducing treatment failure rates and improving patient outcomes, however, research to improve basic science and clinical understanding of injury, healing, and limitations of native tissue biology will guide targets and treatment algorithms for biologic therapy.

INTRODUCTION

General awareness and clinical utilization of orthobiologic therapy has increased sharply in the recent years, both as stand-alone treatment of various conditions, and also in the setting of surgical augmentation. Orthobiologics can be broadly defined as "biological materials and substrates that promote bone, ligament, muscle, and tendon healing."[1] Conceptually, there are 3 major strategies by which orthobiologics are thought to augment tissue repair or native biologic potential: factor-based, cell-based, and biomechanical augmentation. The purpose of this review is to synthesize the recent literature on orthobiologic techniques for surgical augmentation, with focus on several key areas including meniscus repair, osteochondral grafting, and rotator cuff repair.

Sports Medicine Service, Department of Orthopedic Surgery, Stanford University, 430 Broadway, MC 6342, Redwood City, CA 94063, USA
* Corresponding author. 450 Broadway, MC 6342, Redwood City, CA 94063.
E-mail address: shermans@stanford.edu

Phys Med Rehabil Clin N Am 34 (2023) 265–274
https://doi.org/10.1016/j.pmr.2022.08.015
1047-9651/23/Published by Elsevier Inc.

PRINCIPLES OF TISSUE HEALING AND RATIONALE FOR AUGMENTATION

Although certain tissues such as bone and skin have the potential to truly regenerate with regrowth of native tissue, it is known that cartilage, and tendon and ligament insertional tissue do not have the capacity to regenerate in the postnatal human.[2] Rather, healing occurs through fibrovascular scar formation, and the native tissue architecture and function are not completely restored.[3] Furthermore, the biological milieu of any particular tissue affects its healing potential. For instance, midsubstance ruptures of extra-articular ligaments such as the medial collateral ligament of the knee are known to heal with native ligament tissue; however, midsubstance ruptures of the anterior cruciate ligament (ACL), an intra-articular ligament, do not typically heal.[2] It is known that the intra-articular milieu is generally less favorable for tissue healing. Thus, in surgical treatment of cartilage, meniscus, and intra-articular tendons and ligaments, it follows that biological augmentation may carry potential benefit in altering the biologic potential of the repaired tissue, or the local biological milieu.

Research interest in the use of biologics to improve healing in various orthopedic conditions is sharply increasing.[4] The improving basic science and clinical understanding of injury, healing, and limitations of native tissue biology in the setting of regeneration will guide targets and treatment algorithms for biologic therapy. There remain many fundamental unanswered questions, as indications, delivery method, mechanism of action, and patient-specific differences in harvest yield for autologous agents are still to be determined.

CELL-BASED AUGMENTATION

Autologous cell-based therapies have gained popularity in several disciplines of orthopedic surgery including tendon and ligament repair, cartilage restoration, and bony nondelayed or delayed union. There are several methods of obtaining autologous progenitor cells, most commonly from bone marrow and from peripheral adipose tissue.[5] Hematopoietic or adipose tissue is obtained and processed to isolate mononuclear cells to concentrate progenitor cells. For bone marrow aspirate concentrate (BMAC), the classically described harvest site is the iliac crest, although bone marrow is also easily obtained from the distal femur, proximal tibia, proximal humerus, or other long bones.[2] BMAC has been shown to improve bony healing in the setting of fractures and nonunions.[6] (**Fig. 1**). Although there is theoretical benefit in the setting of tendon and ligament healing, the current data is primarily preclinical in the setting of animal studies,[7] with a rabbit model showing increased bone formation at the rotator cuff footprint during repair,[8] and a separate rabbit model showing increased fibrocartilage formation at the bone–tunnel interface in an ACL reconstruction model.[9] Mechanistically, there is variability and poor standardization among preparation protocols and systems,[2] so the exact formulation of each harvest is thus unpredictable. It is thought that the true concentration of cells based on formal criteria is low, with a 0.001% to 0.01% yield; however, numerous growth factors are present, such as platelet-derived growth factor (PDGF), transforming growth factor (TGF)-B, and bone morphogenetic protein (BMP)-2 and BMP-7.[7]

A recent target of interest for cell-based augmentation is osteochondral allograft transplantation (OCA). This is indicated for symptomatic focal chondral or osteochondral lesions in a nonarthritic knee that have failed nonoperative treatment. Although there are numerous options, including microfracture, particulated cartilage, matrix-induced autologous chondrocyte implantation, osteochondral autograft transfer, or OCA, the indications for each individual procedure are beyond the scope of this review. OCA has the advantages of allowing more rapid rehabilitation, replaces

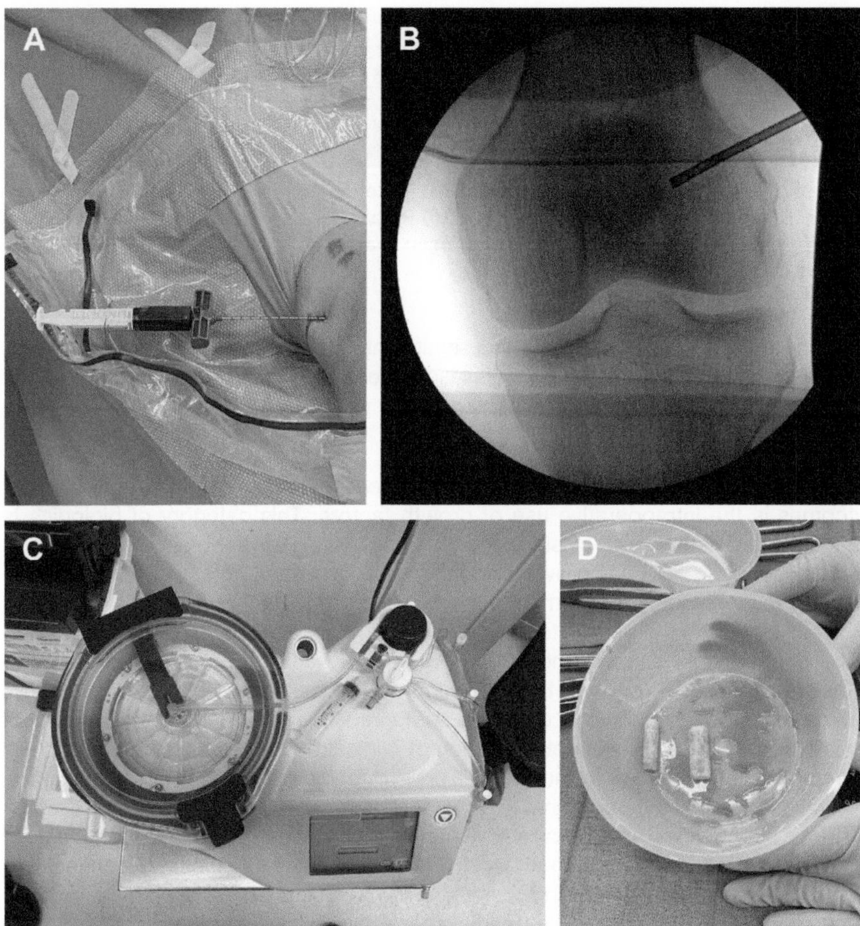

Fig. 1. (*A*) Showing BMAC, (*B*) Bone marrow aspiration from the distal femur (*B*–intraoperative fluoroscopy). (*C*) Centrifuging the bone marrow. (*D*) Allograft bone dowels soaked in BMAC. Arthrex Angel cPRP and Bone Marrow Processing System.

pathologic bone and the subchondral plate, provides immediate full-thickness mature hyaline cartilage tissue, and eliminates donor site morbidity.[10] However, the main drawback is the allograft nature, meaning the graft is predominantly osteoconductive and osteoinductive, rather than osteogenic. Additionally, allograft bone is thought to be incorporated by creeping substitution of native cells.[11] Thus, to provide additional biologic stimulus in the form of autologous hematopoietic-derived progenitor cells, as well as autologous growth factors, BMAC has been used clinically to augment OCA. From a technique standpoint, this is done by simply soaking the graft in BMAC (previously harvested and prepared) before implantation into the recipient site.[12] In laboratory studies, it has been shown that OCA plugs treated with BMAC are found to have increased osteogenic cell proliferation and osteogenic protein concentration than plugs treated with platelet-rich plasma (PRP).[13] Clinical results are currently not definitive, as the literature is limited to case series with conflicting results. Using cartilage transplantation-specific MRI scoring systems, addition of BMAC to OCA of the knee

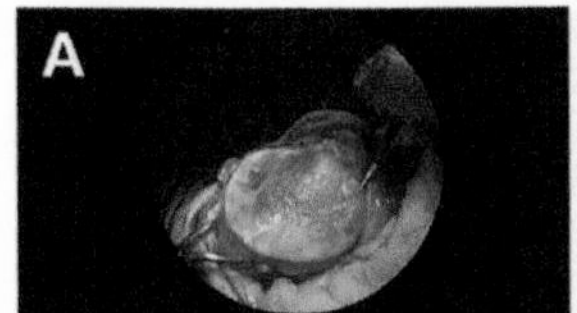

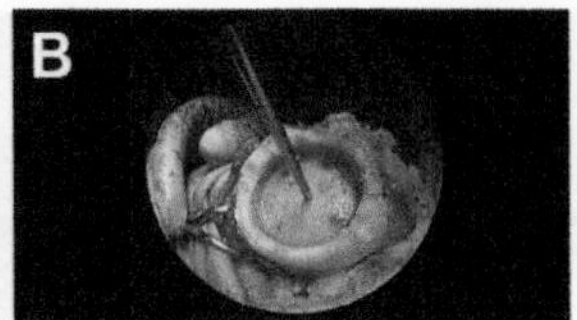

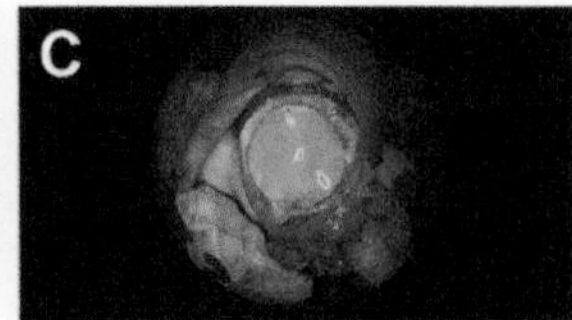

Fig. 2. Showing osteochondral allograft of the patella, augmented with BMAC. (*A*) Pan-patellar osteochondral lesion of the patella. (*B*) Preparation of the recipient site. (*C*) Placement of osteochondral allograft, which has been soaked with BMAC, previously harvested from the distal femur.

has generally been shown to have no significant added benefit in clinical or radiographic outcomes,[14,15] except potentially in larger condylar defects[16] (**Fig. 2**A, B).

FACTOR-BASED AUGMENTATION

Another strategy to harness or induce natural healing cascades to improve surgical outcomes is the intraoperative use of growth factors. This category of biologics is thought to stimulate healing by supplementing the healing environment by the addition of independent stand-alone growth factors, or bulk growth factors. Common applications of this technique, in the form of nonspecific growth factor augmentation are PRP and fibrin clots. PRP is thought to work by delivering platelet growth factors, adhesion proteins, and cytokines including PDGF, TGF, and vascular endothelial growth factor to diseased tissue.[17] Together this is thought to induce connective tissue synthesis and angiogenesis, which can expedite acute repair and stimulate the healing of chronic injuries. Historically, determination of clinical outcomes and utility has been hindered by heterogenous formulations. This is due to differences in kits, preparation protocols, and leukocyte content.[17]

PRP has been trialed as surgical augmentation across many pathologic conditions, of which rotator cuff repair has been subject to the most high-level studies.[18] It is considered by some to be of particular use in accelerating the healing process for high-use or high-demand populations based on an early prospective study that showed significantly improved patient reported outcomes and strength compared with standard repair at 3 months but not at later time points.[18] However, other studies and meta-analyses had mixed results with several finding no significant effect with PRP augmentation.[18] Recently, there has been renewed interest in the benefits of leukocyte poor PRP (LP-PRP). One recent meta-analysis of studies assessing LP-PRP and/or leukocyte rich PRP (LR-PRP) with a control found significant improvements in ret-ear rate, Constant, University of California, Los Angeles (UCLA), merican Shoulder and Elbow Surgeons (ASES), and visual analog scale (VAS) scores relative to control while LR-PRP was no different than control except for VAS. Although promising, there is a need for more high-quality studies including information on formulation, especially leukocyte concentration.

Fibrin clots are formed as a result of blood's natural clotting processes but can also be expedited by mechanical stirring.[19] Blood is typically extracted to form an exogenous clot, capturing the platelets and their payloads, and is then reinserted inside the knee. Typically, peripheral blood is used; however, there is some evidence that fibrin clots from bone marrow may possess greater levels of cytokines.[20] Application of these clots is thought to provide a scaffold, provide mitogenic factors, and even deliver cellular nutrition.[21] As platelets themselves are captured in the clot, it is thought to serve as a reservoir of factors that is released over time.[22] Although factors are not

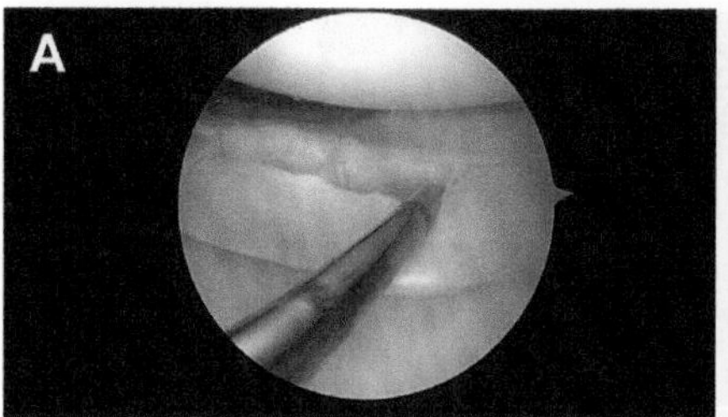

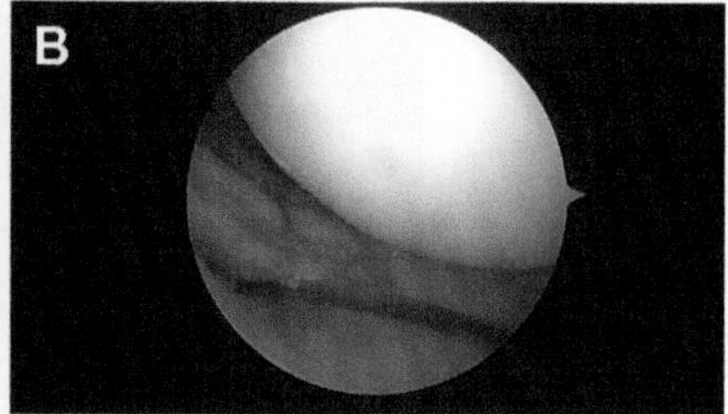

Fig. 3. Showing arthroscopic meniscus repair. (*A*) Vertical longitudinal tear is demonstrated with arthroscopic probe. (*B*) Repair sutures are placed to achieve compression across the tear. Depending on indications, patient factors, and surgeon preference, an isolated meniscus tear of this pattern could be amenable to biologic augmentation.

concentrated as they are in PRP, fibrin clots have benefits of structural support, higher platelet capture rate, and cost effectiveness as no machinery is required.[22] One cited downside is that delivery to the desired site of injury can be challenging.

One common application of fibrin clot augmentation is in meniscal repair. This has historically been used in repairs of less vascularized regions of the meniscus with evidence of fibrous connective tissue that developed into fibrocartilaginous tissue.[23] This has been applied to other tear patterns such as radial and even degenerative horizontal tears, often using inside-out technique.[19,24] A recent meta-analysis noted that multiple studies have shown positive results; however, many of these outcomes are somewhat obscured by concomitant ACL reconstruction, which releases factors during tunnel drilling.[25] The 2 remaining studies in the review assessing augmented meniscal repair in isolation showed an overall 70% to 75% success rate in horizontal tears but were not comparative studies[24,26] (**Fig. 3**A, B). On the horizon, fibrin may have utility as a delivery vehicle because it has been found to maintain mesenchymal stem cell viability in vitro.[21] There has also been work on addressing the difficulty with delivery by wrapping it in a polyester sheet.[27]

BIOMECHANICAL AUGMENTATION

Beyond cells and growth factors, biologic strategies in surgical augmentation also include structural augmentation using various forms of tissue scaffolds. This is most commonly done in tendon and ligament repair, with much of the recent literature focusing on structural augmentation in rotator cuff repair. Use of tissue patches consisting of autogenous, allogenic, xenogeneic, or synthetic materials has been described for the treatment of massive or irreparable rotator cuff tears. This is done in an onlay fashion (over top of the repair site), or in a bridging construct (with the patch serving as a standalone bridge between the retracted or deficient native tendon and the bony insertion).[28] Autograft options have largely been limited to long head biceps and fascia lata and may be associated with donor site morbidity. In the literature, xenograft, allograft, and synthetic patches have been shown to have good structural healing rates, ranging from 60% to 100%, albeit in small series.[28] In the recent literature, the most common graft has been acellular dermis, which is functionally a collagen matrix patch; results have been positive, with improvement in pain, function, strength, and motion, with good imaging integrity of repairs at up to 50 months postop.[29,30] In laboratory studies in animal models with more rigorous testing parameters, augmented rotator cuff repair with acellular dermal patch has been shown to produce a repair construct with similar biomechanical properties to native tendon by 12 weeks; additionally, on histological

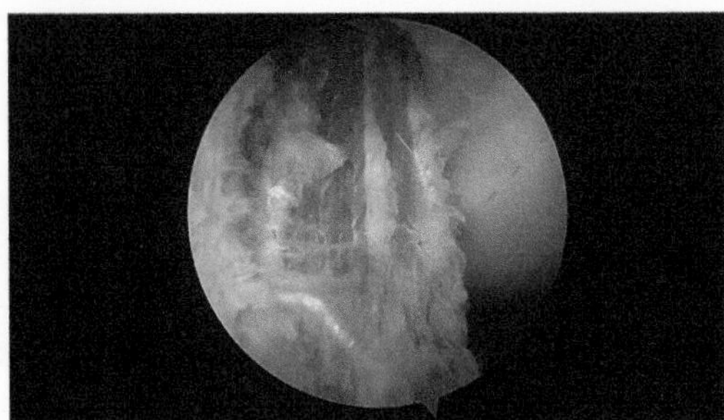

Fig. 4. Showing ACL Reconstruction with suture brace augmentation. A quadriceps autograft ACL reconstruction is shown, with suture tape augmentation as a mechanical checkrein. There are 2 separate suture tape strands that are tensioned separately of the ACL graft to avoid overtensioning.

analysis, there is similar appearance to native tendon with native tendon cell infiltration of the acellular patch.[30] Despite these positive findings, it has been shown that the mechanism of healing even with the use of patch augmentation is still through initial macrophage infiltration followed by fibrovascular scar formation.[31]

Although by definition not a biologic-based technique, there has been recent interest in use of suture tape for augmentation of soft tissue repair and reconstruction, for added time zero biomechanical strength.[32] Several areas in which this technique has been studied include augmented elbow ulnar collateral ligament (UCL) repair in the throwing athlete, and ligamentous repair or reconstruction in the knee.[33,34] In the setting of elbow UCL injury, the gold standard treatment of UCL reconstruction is associated with long rehabilitation periods, on average 12 to 18 months.[35] Recently an augmented repair technique has been popularized, in which the torn UCL is primarily repaired, and suture brace is placed for augmentation.[36] Biomechanical studies have shown promising results,[37–39] and clinical studies have shown good outcomes at short term with high rates of return to play and low failure rates, with a significantly accelerated rehabilitation of 6.7 months on average.[36] In the knee, suture tape augmentation has been described for various ligamentous reconstruction and repair techniques, including of the ACL[32,40] and medial collateral ligament (MCL).[41,42]

The suture tape serves as a rigid brace and checkrein for the repaired or reconstructed tissue because it has superior mechanical properties. Thus, when the repair/reconstruction is stretched to a certain point, the suture brace will take up tension and prevent further loading on the repair tissue. This avoids supraphysiologic loads on the healing tissue but allows full load-bearing by the repair tissue before this point at which the suture tape becomes taut. Concerns with this technique include possible overtensioning leading to stress shielding or inadequate physiologic loading to the repair tissue (as it is known that proper tissue healing does require a baseline level of physiologic loading),[43,44] overconstraint of the joint that is spanned leading to stiffness or chondral overload,[45,46] and local soft tissue reaction related to the nonabsorbable suture material.[47] Additionally, the long-term effects of suture tape augmentation are unknown (**Fig. 4**).

SUMMARY

In summary, orthobiologic use in the surgical setting is a promising frontier for improving on the inherent limitations of native tissue biology to reduce treatment failure rates and improve patient outcomes. Orthobiologics used in surgery fall broadly into 3 main categories: cell-based, factor-based, and biomechanical augmentation strategies. Cell-based therapies such as BMAC and adipose-derived mesenchymal progenitor cells have been used for augmentation of cartilage restoration and bony nonunion surgery. Factor-based augmentation has been described for augmentation of meniscus repair, and tendon and ligament repair. Biomechanical augmentation has gained popularity in rotator cuff repair, elbow UCL primary repair, and ligamentous reconstruction in the knee. The field of orthobiologics is still young, and many questions remain unanswered regarding exact therapeutic targets, mechanism of action, delivery method, patient-specific differences in autologous harvest yields, and off-target effects. Continued general patient awareness, clinician knowledge, and high-level clinical and basic science research will drive further understanding of orthobiologics.

CLINICS CARE POINTS

- Research on orthobiologics is still ongoing and many questions remain unanswered regarding delivery methods, patient specific differences, off-target effects, etc.
- The current literature is limited to case series with conflicting results, where some show benefits and others show none.
- BMAC used in cell-based augmentation has been shown to improve bony healing for fractures and nonunions, however, the current data is mainly preclinical and done in the setting of animal studies.
- Factor-based augmentations, such as PRP and fibrin clots, are used to accelerate the healing process in a cost-efficient manner by delivering platelet growth factors and other proteins and cells, however, there are mixed results with PRP, and delivery method complications with fibrin clots.
- Suture tapes used in biologic augmentation show good short-term benefits and high rates of return to play, however, long-term benefits are unknown.

CONFLICT OF INTEREST

All authors declare that they have no conflict of interest.

REFERENCES

1. Calcei JG, Rodeo SA. Orthobiologics for bone healing. Clin Sports Med 2019;38: 79–95.
2. Lin KM, Rodeo SA. Tendon and ligament healing. In: RA, editor. Orthopaedic basic science. 5th edition. Rosemont (IL): American Academy of Orthopaedic Surgeons; 2021. p. 433–44.
3. Galatz LM, Gerstenfeld L, Heber-Katz E, et al. Tendon regeneration and scar formation: the concept of scarless healing. J Orthop Res 2015;33:823–31.
4. Chahla J, Kennedy MI, Aman ZS, et al. Ortho-biologics for ligament repair and reconstruction. Clin Sports Med 2019;38:97–107.
5. Lopa S, Colombini A, Moretti M, et al. Injective mesenchymal stem cell-based treatments for knee osteoarthritis: from mechanisms of action to current clinical evidences. Knee Surg Sports Traumatol Arthrosc 2019;27:2003–20.
6. Lin K, VandenBerg J, Putnam SM, et al. Bone marrow aspirate concentrate with cancellous allograft versus iliac crest bone graft in the treatment of long bone nonunions. OTA Int 2019;2:e012.

7. Pittenger MF, Mackay AM, Beck SC, et al. Multilineage potential of adult human mesenchymal stem cells. Science 1999;284:143–7.
8. Liu XN, Yang CJ, Kim JE, et al. Enhanced tendon-to-bone healing of chronic rotator cuff tears by bone marrow aspirate concentrate in a rabbit model. Clin Orthop Surg 2018;10:99–110.
9. Lim JK, Hui J, Li L, et al. Enhancement of tendon graft osteointegration using mesenchymal stem cells in a rabbit model of anterior cruciate ligament reconstruction. Arthroscopy 2004;20:899–910.
10. Zouzias IC, Bugbee WD. Osteochondral allograft transplantation in the knee. Sports Med Arthrosc Rev 2016;24:79–84.
11. Burchardt H. The biology of bone graft repair. Clin Orthop Relat Res 1983;(174): 28–42.
12. Cook JL. Editorial commentary: bone marrow aspirate biologics for osteochondral allografts-because we can or because we should? Arthroscopy 2019;35: 2445–7.
13. Stoker AM, Baumann CA, Stannard JP, et al. Bone marrow aspirate concentrate versus platelet rich plasma to enhance osseous integration potential for osteochondral allografts. J Knee Surg 2018;31:314–20.
14. Wang D, Lin KM, Burge AJ, et al. Bone marrow aspirate concentrate does not improve osseous integration of osteochondral allografts for the treatment of chondral defects in the knee at 6 and 12 months: a comparative magnetic resonance imaging analysis. Am J Sports Med 2019;47:339–46.
15. Ackermann J, Mestriner AB, Shah N, et al. Effect of autogenous bone marrow aspirate treatment on magnetic resonance imaging integration of osteochondral allografts in the knee: a matched comparative imaging analysis. Arthroscopy 2019;35:2436–44.
16. Oladeji LO, Stannard JP, Cook CR, et al. Effects of autogenous bone marrow aspirate concentrate on radiographic integration of femoral condylar osteochondral allografts. Am J Sports Med 2017;45:2797–803.
17. Everts P, Onishi K, Jayaram P, et al. Platelet-rich plasma: new performance understandings and therapeutic considerations in 2020. Int J Mol Sci 2020;21(20): 7794.
18. Le ADK, Enweze L, DeBaun MR, et al. Current clinical recommendations for use of platelet-rich plasma. Curr Rev Musculoskelet Med 2018;11:624–34.
19. Chahla J, Kennedy NI, Geeslin AG, et al. Meniscal repair with fibrin clot augmentation. Arthrosc Tech 2017;6:e2065–9.
20. Hashimoto Y, Nishino K, Orita K, et al. Biochemical characteristics and clinical result of bone marrow-derived fibrin clot for repair of isolated meniscal injury in the avascular zone. Arthroscopy 2022;38:441–9.
21. Warth RJ, Shupe PG, Gao X, et al. Fibrin clots maintain the viability and proliferative capacity of human mesenchymal stem cells: an in vitro study. Clin Orthop Relat Res 2020;478:653–64.
22. Siegel KR, Clevenger TN, Clegg DO, et al. Adipose stem cells incorporated in fibrin clot modulate expression of growth factors. Arthroscopy 2018;34:581–91.
23. Arnoczky SP, Warren RF, Spivak JM. Meniscal repair using an exogenous fibrin clot. An experimental study in dogs. J Bone Joint Surg Am 1988;70:1209–17.
24. Nakayama H, Kanto R, Kambara S, et al. Successful treatment of degenerative medial meniscal tears in well-aligned knees with fibrin clot implantation. Knee Surg Sports Traumatol Arthrosc 2020;28:3466–73.

25. Zaffagnini S, Poggi A, Reale D, et al. Biologic augmentation reduces the failure rate of meniscal repair: a systematic review and meta-analysis. Orthop J Sports Med 2021;9. 2325967120981627.
26. Kamimura T, Kimura M. Meniscal repair of degenerative horizontal cleavage tears using fibrin clots: clinical and arthroscopic outcomes in 10 cases. Orthop J Sports Med 2014;2. 2325967114555678.
27. Yamanashi Y, Kato T, Akao M, et al. Meniscal repair using fibrin clots made from bone marrow blood wrapped in a polyglycolic acid sheet. Arthrosc Tech 2021;10: e2541–6.
28. Frank RM, Cvetanovich G, Savin D, et al. Superior capsular reconstruction: indications, techniques, and clinical outcomes. JBJS Rev 2018;6:e10.
29. Badhe SP, Lawrence TM, Smith FD, et al. An assessment of porcine dermal xenograft as an augmentation graft in the treatment of extensive rotator cuff tears. J Shoulder Elbow Surg 2008;17:35s-9s.
30. Neumann JA, Zgonis MH, Rickert KD, et al. Interposition dermal matrix xenografts: a successful alternative to traditional treatment of massive rotator cuff tears. Am J Sports Med 2017;45:1261–8.
31. Nicholson GP, Breur GJ, Van Sickle D, et al. Evaluation of a cross-linked acellular porcine dermal patch for rotator cuff repair augmentation in an ovine model. J Shoulder Elbow Surg 2007;16:S184–90.
32. EAM C, Huntington LS, Tulloch S. Suture tape augmentation of anterior cruciate ligament reconstruction increases biomechanical stability: a scoping review of biomechanical, animal, and clinical studies. Arthroscopy 2022;38:2073–89.
33. Wicks ED, Stack J, Rezaie N, et al. Biomechanical evaluation of suture tape internal brace reinforcement of soft tissue allografts for ACL reconstruction using a porcine model. Orthop J Sports Med 2022;10. 23259671221091252.
34. Waly AH, ElShafie HI, Morsy MG, et al. All-inside anterior cruciate ligament reconstruction with suture tape augmentation: button tie-over technique (BTOT). Arthrosc Tech 2021;10:e2559–70.
35. Carr JB 2nd, Camp CL, Dines JS. Elbow ulnar collateral ligament injuries: indications, management, and outcomes. Arthroscopy 2020;36:1221–2.
36. Dugas JR, Looze CA, Capogna B, et al. Ulnar collateral ligament repair with collagen-dipped fibertape augmentation in overhead-throwing athletes. Am J Sports Med 2019;47:1096–102.
37. Urch E, Limpisvasti O, ElAttrache NS, et al. Biomechanical evaluation of a modified internal brace construct for the treatment of ulnar collateral ligament injuries. Orthop J Sports Med 2019;7. 2325967119874135.
38. Roth TS, Beason DP, Clay TB, et al. The effect of ulnar collateral ligament repair with internal brace augmentation on articular contact mechanics: a cadaveric study. Orthop J Sports Med 2021;9. 23259671211001069.
39. Bodendorfer BM, Looney AM, Lipkin SL, et al. Biomechanical comparison of ulnar collateral ligament reconstruction with the docking technique versus repair with internal bracing. Am J Sports Med 2018;46:3495–501.
40. Heusdens CHW, Blockhuys K, Roelant E, et al. Suture tape augmentation ACL repair, stable knee, and favorable PROMs, but a re-rupture rate of 11% within 2 years. Knee Surg Sports Traumatol Arthrosc 2021;29:3706–14.
41. Black AK, Schlepp C, Zapf M, et al. Technique for arthroscopically assisted superficial and deep medial collateral ligament-meniscotibial ligament repair with internal brace augmentation. Arthrosc Tech 2018;7:e1215–9.

42. van Eck CF, Nakamura T, Price T, et al. Suture tape augmentation improves laxity of MCL repair in the ACL reconstructed knee. Knee Surg Sports Traumatol Arthrosc 2021;29:2545–52.
43. Lai VJ, Reynolds AW, Kindya M, et al. The use of suture augmentation for graft protection in acl reconstruction: a biomechanical study in porcine knees. Arthrosc Sports Med Rehabil 2021;3:e57–63.
44. Cook JL, Smith P, Stannard JP, et al. A canine arthroscopic anterior cruciate ligament reconstruction model for study of synthetic augmentation of tendon allografts. J Knee Surg 2017;30:704–11.
45. Hopper GP, Heusdens CHW, Dossche L, et al. Medial patellofemoral ligament repair with suture tape augmentation. Arthrosc Tech 2019;8:e1–5.
46. Mercer N, Kanakamedala A, Azam M, et al. Clinical outcomes after suture tape augmentation for ankle instability: a systematic review. Orthopaedic J Sports Med 2022;10. 232596712210957.
47. Esenyel C, Demirhan M, Kilicoglu O, et al. Evaluation of soft tissue reactions to three nonabsorbable suture materials in a rabbit model. Acta Orthop Traumatol Turc 2009;43:366–72.

Regulatory Considerations of Orthobiologic Procedures

Kudo Jang, MD[a,1], William A. Berrigan, MD[b,2,3], Ken Mautner, MD[a,c,*]

KEYWORDS

• PRP • MFAT • SVF • BMAC • Birth tissue products • FDA

KEY POINTS

- Platelet-rich plasma (PRP) is not considered a human cellular-based product (HCT/P) and is regulated as blood-derived product under 21 CFR 640.
- Bone marrow products that undergo minimal manipulation for homologous use and are not combined with another article are not considered an HCT/P; regulation is similar to PRP.
- Nano fat, fat grafts, and microfragmented adipose tissue that do not alter tissue micro-architecture are regulated as HCT/Ps and are under moderate regulation; they do not require premarket approval (PMA) by the FDA.
- Bone marrow aspirate concentrate that is altered beyond centrifugation and concentration and adipose-derived products that are enzymatically or mechanically digested are under strict regulation; they require PMA by the FDA
- Birth tissue products are not permitted for use for orthopedic purposes outside of research with an investigational new drug application.

INTRODUCTION

Regenerative medicine is a rapidly growing field of novel therapies used in the treatment of musculoskeletal conditions. Despite growing experience among providers and developing evidence, the field continues to be under researched. Even so, some research can be associated with inflated expectations of regenerative capabilities and the ability to treat unmet medical needs.[1–3] Although this has stimulated growth in legitimate and appropriate research discussion, the growing enthusiasm has also permitted more exuberant and at times inappropriate information for both providers and patients. This information can potentially harm patients while also

[a] Department of Physical Medicine and Rehabilitation, Emory University School of Medicine, Atlanta, GA, USA; [b] Department of Orthopaedics, University of California San Francisco, CA, USA; [c] Department of Orthopedics, Emory University School of Medicine, Atlanta, GA, USA
[1] Present address: 1441 Clifton Road, Atlanta, GA 30322.
[2] Present address: 1968 Hawks Lane, Atlanta, GA 30329.
[3] Present address: 1500 Owens Street; San Francisco, CA 94158
* Corresponding author. 1968 Hawks Lane, Atlanta, GA 30329.
E-mail address: kmautne@emory.edu
Twitter: @WBerriganMD (W.A.B.); @DrKenMautner (K.M.)

Phys Med Rehabil Clin N Am 34 (2023) 275–283
https://doi.org/10.1016/j.pmr.2022.08.016
1047-9651/23/

threatening research progress in the field, necessitating a stringent need for regulation.[4] These regulatory, ethical, scientific, and clinical concerns are the primary aim of this article .

The Necessity for Federal Regulation

The United States holds the largest number of stem cell clinics globally.[5] Hundreds of these clinics directly market unproven stem cell-related therapies to consumers. These unproven treatments without appropriate testing, manufacturing standards, and clinical supervision have several inherent risks.[1,6] Yet, despite these risks, the direct-to-consumer industry for these unproven stem cell clinics is growing, with marketing strategies targeting orthopedics/sports conditions, neurologic conditions, and cosmetic/antiaging/sexual conditions.[7]

Food and Drug Administration Regulations of Human Cells, Tissues, and Cellular-Based Products

Several regulations by the Food and Drug Administration (FDA) have been developed over time to enhance the discretion of these products and encourage the proper study of evidence-based treatments. In 1997 the FDA proposed a centralized plan for regulation, which eventually became the Title 21 Code of Federal Regulations Part 1271 (21 CFR 1271).[8,9] This policy, in use today, defined what is known as human cells, tissues, and cellular-based products (HCT/Ps).

The FDA defines HCT/Ps as "articles containing or consisting of human cells or tissues that are intended for implantation, transplantation, infusion, or transfer into a human recipient." All HCT/Ps must pass Part 1271. This parameter addresses the primary constraints of structural versus nonstructural tissue, minimal manipulation, the homologous purpose of the product, and its autologous versus allogeneic properties.

In defining minimal manipulation, the FDA separates structural tissue from nonstructural tissue. For structural tissue, this is defined as processing that does not alter the original relevant characteristics of the tissue relating to the tissue's utility for reconstruction, repair, or replacement. In nonstructural tissue, minimal manipulation is described as processing that does not alter the relevant biological characteristics of cells or tissues.[9] Examples of structural versus nonstructural tissues are displayed in **Table 1**.

Beyond minimal manipulation, it is necessary to determine the homologous use of the product. Homologous use is defined by the FDA as the repair, reconstruction, replacement, or supplementation of a recipient's cells or tissues with an HCT/P that performs the same basic function or functions in the recipient as in the donor (CFR 1271.3(c)).[9] This may include identical cells and tissues, or cells and tissues that are not identical but perform one or more of the same basic functions.[10] If the HCT/P performs multiple functions, the basic functions that the HCT/P is expected to perform in the recipient must be a basic function that the HCT/P performed in the donor. Basic functions should be understood and not require study to prove that it is basic to the donor.

Finally, the product must be deciphered as allogeneic or autologous. All allogeneic products intended for stem cell use fail regulation under 21 CFR.10. These products cannot have a systemic effect or be dependent on the metabolic activity of living cells for their primary function.

The FDA has sent warning letters for noncompliance with homologous use mandates and minimal manipulation rules to companies such as Liveyon, Genetech, R3, and Cord for Life, among others. Despite warning letters and enforcement actions, unproven stem cell clinics still exist that continue to market these interventions.[11]

Table 1
Examples of structural and nonstructural tissues

Structural Tissue	Nonstructural Tissue
Bone	Reproductive cells or tissues
Skin	Cord blood
Amniotic membrane	Amniotic fluid
Blood vessels	Bone marrow aspirate
Adipose tissue	Lymph nodes
Articular cartilage	Parathyroid glands
Nonarticular cartilage	Peripheral nerve
Tendons and ligaments	Pancreatic tissue

Tiers of Human Cells, Tissues, and Cellular-Based Products Regulation

HCT/Ps are regulated in tiers based on the degree of perceived risk to public health. The tier-based approach is addressed in the "tissue rules" under the communicable disease authority of the Public Health Service (PHS) Act (42 US .C. 264). These regulations define those HCT/Ps that do not require premarket approval (PMA) and registration, manufacturing, and reporting steps that must be taken to prevent the introduction, transmission, and spread of communicable diseases. The PHS Act is the authority on which the FDA has relied for CFR Part 1271.[12]

There are two primary tiers of regulation that address minimally invasive orthopedic procedures in the PHS Act, Sections 351 and 361. Those HCT/Ps under Section 361 do not require PMA by the FDA. To qualify as an HCT/P that is regulated under Section 361, the tissue product must meet all three criteria defined in CFR 1271.10. This includes a tissue product that has a homologous purpose, autologous usage, and minimal manipulation of tissue. HCT/Ps that do not meet these criteria fall under the regulation of Section 351 of the PHS Act. These products are regulated as a drug, device, or biologic product that requires PMA.[13] To obtain PMA, a product must meet an additional level of regulation. New drugs require an investigational new drug (IND) approval and must comply with good manufacturing practice regulations.

There are cases where a biologic or establishment may qualify for an exception to criteria defined in part 1271. These exceptions are in CFR 1271.15(b), which states "you are not required to comply with the requirements of this Part if you are an establishment that removes HCT/Ps from an individual and implants such HCT/Ps into the same individual during the same surgical procedure." For this to apply, the HCT/P still must be autologous, implanted in the same surgical procedure, and the HCT/P must remain in its original form, that is, with minimal manipulation of tissue. Cell isolation, expansion, activation, or enzymatic digestion do not fall under this category and are not allowed.[13]

DISCUSSION

Regenerative Medicine and Orthobiologics

The conservative management for various orthopedic injuries, such as tendinopathy, ligamentous injuries, and osteoarthritis, has evolved with orthobiologics. Most of the biologics used within the clinical settings are autologous and include platelet-rich plasma (PRP), bone marrow aspirate (BMA), and adipose-derived stem cells (ASCs). Other allogeneic sources, however, have also been trialed and include birth tissue products such as the umbilical cord, placental tissue, and amniotic fluid.[13] These products are used in purported antiinflammatory usage but are unsure about their ability to regenerate poorly healing tissues such as articular cartilage, tendons, and ligaments.[14] The regulations related to these individualized biologics vary and specific considerations should be considered when implementing them into common practice based on FDA HCT/P regulations.

Platelet-rich plasma

PRP is a biologic product defined as a portion of the plasma fraction of autologous blood with an elevated platelet concentration above the baseline to the concentration of 1,000,000 platelets per microliter.[15] The product is obtained from the blood of patients and is processed through a method of centrifugation. The FDA's definition of PRP stipulates that preparation requires a single, uninterrupted venipuncture to be centrifuged within hours of collection.[9] This definition constitutes PRP as a blood-derived product that is regulated under 21 CFR 640 and does not fall under the definition of an HCT/P per the 21 CFR 1271.[9]

There is substantial variability in PRP preparations, conceivably due to differences in patients' daily platelet levels, procurement methods, concentration mechanisms, and other exogenous factors.[14] Many of these may originate from specific device differences. PRP is regulated through the device that is used to manufacture it, and these devices have been brought to market via the 510(k) pathway.[16–18] The 510k pathway clears products that are substantially equivalent to an already cleared predicate device.[19] For PRP, the device is a platelet and plasma separator that produces the PRP. Through this pathway, PRP receives FDA clearance to be used in a variety of orthopedic conditions. Clearance, however, is not synonymous with FDA approval and PRP for musculoskeletal conditions is considered "offlabel" use.[16]

Bone marrow aspirate

Bone marrow-based stem cell therapies emerged as a promising biologic tool due to the presence of pluripotent mesenchymal stem cells (MSCs) and growth factors. These cells via paracrine and autocrine pathways decrease cell apoptosis and inflammation, activate cell proliferation and differentiation, and induce angiogenesis.[20,21] The aspiration of bone marrow is most often taken from the iliac crest, and aspirate volume depends on the processing system and the goal of treatment. The BMA can then be concentrated into BMA concentrate (BMAC) to result in a product with a higher concentration of nucleated bone marrow cells compared with BMA.[13,20] This concentrated product is subject to FDA regulation.

Autologous bone marrow products are not considered HCT/Ps if they undergo only minimal manipulation, are for homologous use, and are not combined with another article (except water, crystalloids, sterilizing agent, preserving agent, or storage agent). Bone marrow is considered a nonstructural tissue and the relevant biological characteristics cannot be altered to be considered minimally manipulated. This includes the differentiation and activation state, proliferation potential, and metabolic activity. If a manufacturer performs cell selection on a mobilized peripheral blood apheresis product to obtain a higher concentration of hematopoietic/progenitor cells for transplantation, the product is considered minimally manipulated and is not regulated under the 21 CFR 1271 as an HCT/P. By this, the concentrated peripheral blood stem/progenitor cells are not altered with regard to their relevant biological characteristics to repopulate the bone marrow.[12] It should be noted that the injection of BMAC for orthopedic indications is considered offlabel use.[13]

In contrast to BMAC products that have only undergone minimal manipulation and are intended for homologous use, bone marrow that has been altered beyond centrifugation and concentration is more tightly regulated. The FDA is clear that isolating and expanding cells after bone marrow aspiration is not within minimal manipulation. Any cell expansion is controlled within the jurisdiction as a 351 Product (drug or biologic product) requiring PMA.[9,13]

Adipose tissue-derived products

ASC therapies for orthopedic conditions have come to the forefront of biological treatments given promising preclinical and clinical data from animal and human studies.[22–25] Adipose tissue is rich in MSCs, and its extraction has an excellent safety profile with easy accessibility and a self-replenishing abundance.[26,27] To extract adipose, the tissue is aspirated via tumescent liposuction either from the abdomen, hip, thigh, or infrapatellar fat pad. It can then be processed by a few different methods. In one method, the fat either undergoes mechanical emulsification or enzymatic digestion to obtain a liquefied heterogeneous suspension of a multitude of cells, referred to as stromal vascular fraction (SVF). The alternative is for the fat to be progressively reduced in size, eliminating residue and blood elements, via rinsing, resizing, and reshaping the fat without digestive enzymes. This occurs with microfragmented adipose tissue (MFAT), nano fat, or with a fat graft/fat transfer.[13,28,29] Each adipose-derived tissue product is subject to different regulations by the FDA.[13,28]

SVF involves processing by enzymatic digestion and/or isolation of cellular components. Owing to the processing required for the preparation of the ASCs in SVF, the use of SVF-derived stem cell injections does not qualify as minimally manipulated tissue. Therefore, it is regulated as a 351 Product (strict regulation and oversight as a drug, device, or biological product for patient use and marketing).[13] MFAT, nano fat, and fat grafts/fat transfers, in contrast, may be evaluated separately given the mechanism of action. Specifically, if these treatments and devices only process fat through steps of rinsing, sizing, cleansing, or shaping the tissue to facilitate removal of debris, the cell and tissue microarchitecture are preserved as "such HCT/P" and are considered minimally manipulated.[30,31] MFAT, nano fat, and fat grafts/transfers, when used in this manner, are minimally manipulated, autologous, and used within a single procedure. These devices have also been cleared by the FDA for homologous use as cushioning and support for other tissues. They are not, however, indicated to treat orthopedic and musculoskeletal conditions at this time. Still, they do qualify for the same surgical procedure exemption under CFR 1271.15(b) and with that, clinical application off label may be permitted with proper discussion and informed consent from the patient. Any adipose-derived products beyond this, including SVF, require PMA and the use of an IND.

Birth tissue products

In theory, birth tissue products, such as umbilical and amniotic cells, are a potent source of MSCs with high proliferative capacity and expansion potential. The cells contain antiinflammatory cytokines such as interleukin (IL)-1RA and IL-10 in addition to factors that upregulate anabolic pathways such as epidermal growth factor, fibroblast growth factor, platelet-derived growth factor, and vascular endothelial growth factor.[32,33] The cells and fluid also upregulate tissue inhibitors of metalloproteinase, which can halt the progression of certain disease processes[34,35] and contain hyaluronic acid and proteoglycans for lubrication and reduction of shear forces.[36,37] It should be noted that on delivery and injection of the cells per the manufacturer's suggestions, there are no actual live cellular products.[38]

There are limited data suggestive of effective and positive outcomes for orthopedics sports indications.[13,39] The FDA regulates these products under the umbrella of an HCT/P. Under this regulation, the lyophilization and packaging of amniotic membrane tissue as particles is considered more than minimal manipulation as it alters the original relevant characteristics of the HCT/P.[40] The original relevant characteristics, in this case, would be considered the integration of the amniotic membrane as a barrier, generally including the tissue's physical integrity, tensile strength, and elasticity. The use of MSCs from birth tissue products is not accepted by the FDA.

In 2017, the FDA outlined a framework for the regulation of regenerative medicine products and outlined the intent to exercise enforcement discretion until November 2020 for certain regenerative medicine products. This was regarding the IND and PMA requirements to give manufacturers time to determine what requirements apply and effectively engage with the FDA. During the period of enforcement discretion, products, mostly related to birth tissue products, were allowed to be used in the clinic setting to demonstrate safety and efficacy. The period of enforcement discretion was extended until May 2021. After this time, many amniotic fluid and membrane injectables were withdrawn from the market due to noncompliance with the FDA regulations for minimal manipulation and the failure to properly investigate the product or obtain an IND.[41] Several companies engaged with the FDA and regenerative medicine advanced therapy designations were obtained with ongoing studies for a few of these products. None have been approved for any orthopedic use and at this time they cannot be used in the clinic setting unless they are a part of a research trial with an IND from the FDA.

Future directions

Clinicians who use orthobiologics need to be aware of the shifting environment. The FDA regulations and enforcement have responded to the growth of unproven stem cell clinics and placed multiple regulations on products, with the hope that it will allow the field to grow safely and effectively. These regulations are always subject to change, and it is prudent to be cognizant of current protocols and recommendations for clinical practice. There exists a need to navigate the clinical environment with a standard of care and best practice statement that mirrors the current regulations by the FDA. This recommendation statement should define specific nomenclature, laws, and licensure limitations. The American Medical Society of Sports Medicine has addressed this gap with its most recent statement on the responsible use of regenerative medicine and orthobiologics in sports medicine.[42] This comprehensive position statement aids in moving clinicians and regulatory bodies. Through this, future research is encouraged to establish protocols for the field that may develop into the standard of care for practitioners.

SUMMARY

Many fraudulent stem cell clinics market unproven treatments, which consumers and physicians need to be aware of. The best way to address these ethical, legal, and scientific issues is to understand the current landscape of orthobiologics and be aware of the current FDA guidelines. It is only through this understanding that legitimate research can be performed to continue to advance the field.

CLINICS CARE POINTS

- The Food and Drug Administration (FDA) regulates minimally manipulated fat transfers, stromal vascular fraction (SVF), and birth tissue products under the Title 21 Code of Federal Regulations Part 1271. This specifically defines human cells, tissues, or cellular or tissue-based products (HCT/Ps).

- HCT/Ps must define whether a product is structural or nonstructural, minimally manipulated, used for a homologous purpose, and whether it is autologous or allogenic.
- Autologous platelet-rich plasma and bone marrow aspirate concentrate with minimal manipulation are not considered an HCT/P and are regulated as blood-derived products under 21 CFR 640.
- Bone Marrow Concentrate that undergoes alteration beyond centrifugation and concentration is considered more than minimal manipulation, which would be regulated as a 351-product requiring premarket approval (PMA).
- SVF is regulated as a 351 product and cannot be used outside of an IND, as enzymatic or mechanical digestion is considered beyond minimal manipulation.
- Nano fat, fat grafts, and micro-fragmented adipose tissue that do not alter tissue microarchitecture are regulated as HCT/Ps and are under moderate regulation; they do not require PMA by the FDA.
- All mesenchymal stem cells from birth tissue products are now classified as a 351 product requiring PMA and currently should not be used in clinics outside of the company's IND.
- Physicians can use any legally available product off label, according to their clinical judgment, but the marketing materials can only reflect onlabel claims.

DISCLOSURE

K. Mautner is a speaker and consultant for Lipogems.

REFERENCES

1. Bauer G, Elsallab M, Abou-El-Enein M. Concise Review: A Comprehensive Analysis of Reported Adverse Events in Patients Receiving Unproven Stem Cell-Based Interventions. Stem Cells Transl Med 2018;7(9):676–85.
2. Murdoch CE, Scott CT. Stem cell tourism and the power of hope. Am J Bioeth 2010;10(5):16–23.
3. Caulfield T, Sipp D, Murry CE, et al. SCIENTIFIC COMMUNITY. Confronting stem cell hype. Science 2016;352(6287):776–7.
4. Shapiro SA, Finnoff JT, Awan TM, et al. Highlights from the American Medical Society for Sports Medicine position statement on responsible use of regenerative medicine and orthobiologics in sports medicine. Br J Sports Med 2022;56(3):121–2.
5. Berger I, Ahmad A, Bansal A, et al. Global Distribution of Businesses Marketing Stem Cell-Based Interventions. Cell Stem Cell 2016;19(2):158–62.
6. Arango-Rodriguez ML, Ezquer F, Ezquer M, et al. Could cancer and infection be adverse effects of mesenchymal stromal cell therapy? World J Stem Cells 2015;7(2):408–17.
7. Turner L, Knoepfler P. Selling Stem Cells in the USA: Assessing the Direct-to-Consumer Industry. Cell Stem Cell 2016;19(2):154–7.
8. Research USDoHaHSFaDACfBEa. Guidance for Industry: Regulation of Human Cells, Tissues, and Cellular and Tissue-Based Products (HCT/Ps) Small Entity Compliance Guide. 2007.
9. Title 21 Code of Federal Regulations Part 1271 Human Cells, Tissues, and Cellular and Tissue-Based Products.
10. Establishment registration and listing for manufacturers of human cellular and tissue-based products–FDA. Proposed rule. Fed Regist 1998;63(93):26744–55.

11. Sipp D. Direct-to-consumer stem cell marketing and regulatory responses. Stem Cells Transl Med 2013;2(9):638–40.
12. US Department of Health and Human Services FaDA. Regulatory Considerations for Human Cells, Tissues, and Cellular and Tissue-Based Products: Minimal Manipulation and Homologous Use. https://www.fda.gov/media/109176/download#:~:text=4%20Examples%20of%20HCT%2FPs,semen%20or%20other%20reproductive%20tissue. [Accessed 10 March 2022].
13. Fang WH, Vangsness CT Jr. Food and Drug Administration's Position on Commonly Injected Biologic Materials in Orthopaedic Surgery. Am J Sports Med 2021;49(12):3414–21.
14. Huebner K, Frank RM, Getgood A. Ortho-Biologics for Osteoarthritis. Clin Sports Med 2019;38(1):123–41.
15. Marx RE. Platelet-rich plasma (PRP): what is PRP and what is not PRP? Implant Dent 2001;10(4):225–8.
16. Beitzel K, Allen D, Apostolakos J, et al. US definitions, current use, and FDA stance on use of platelet-rich plasma in sports medicine. J Knee Surg 2015;28(1):29–34.
17. Arshi A, Petrigliano FA, Williams RJ, et al. Stem Cell Treatment for Knee Articular Cartilage Defects and Osteoarthritis. Curr Rev Musculoskelet Med 2020;13(1):20–7.
18. Jones IA, Togashi RC, Thomas Vangsness C Jr. The Economics and Regulation of PRP in the Evolving Field of Orthopedic Biologics. Curr Rev Musculoskelet Med 2018;11(4):558–65.
19. Sweet BV, Schwemm AK, Parsons DM. Review of the processes for FDA oversight of drugs, medical devices, and combination products. J Manag Care Pharm 2011;17(1):40–50.
20. Kim GB, Seo M-S, Park WT, et al. Bone Marrow Aspirate Concentrate: Its Uses in Osteoarthritis. Int J Mol Sci 2020;21(9):3224.
21. Veronesi F, Giavaresi G, Tschon M, et al. Clinical use of bone marrow, bone marrow concentrate, and expanded bone marrow mesenchymal stem cells in cartilage disease. Stem Cells Dev 2013;22(2):181–92.
22. Heidari N, Borg TM, Olgiati S, et al. Microfragmented Adipose Tissue Injection (MFAT) May Be a Solution to the Rationing of Total Knee Replacement: A Prospective, Gender-Bias Mitigated, Reproducible Analysis at Two Years. Stem Cells Int 2021;2021:9921015.
23. Heidari N, Noorani A, Slevin M, et al. Patient-Centered Outcomes of Microfragmented Adipose Tissue Treatments of Knee Osteoarthritis: An Observational, Intention-to-Treat Study at Twelve Months. Stem Cells Int 2020;2020:8881405.
24. Ude CC, Sulaiman SB, Min-Hwei N, et al. Cartilage regeneration by chondrogenic induced adult stem cells in osteoarthritic sheep model. PLoS One 2014;9(6):e98770.
25. Guercio A, Di Marco P, Casella S, et al. Production of canine mesenchymal stem cells from adipose tissue and their application in dogs with chronic osteoarthritis of the humeroradial joints. Cell Biol Int 2012;36(2):189–94.
26. Bacakova L, Zarubova J, Travnickova M, et al. Stem cells: their source, potency and use in regenerative therapies with focus on adipose-derived stem cells - a review. Biotechnol Adv 2018;36(4):1111–26.
27. Jurgens WJ, Oedayrajsingh-Varma MJ, Helder MN, et al. Effect of tissue-harvesting site on yield of stem cells derived from adipose tissue: implications for cell-based therapies. Cell Tissue Res 2008;332(3):415–26.

28. Oedayrajsingh-Varma MJ, van Ham SM, Knippenberg M, et al. Adipose tissue-derived mesenchymal stem cell yield and growth characteristics are affected by the tissue-harvesting procedure. Cytotherapy 2006;8(2):166–77.
29. Desando G, Bartolotti I, Martini L, et al. Regenerative Features of Adipose Tissue for Osteoarthritis Treatment in a Rabbit Model: Enzymatic Digestion Versus Mechanical Disruption. Int J Mol Sci 2019;20(11):2636.
30. Malanga GA, Bemanian S. Microfragmented adipose injections in the treatment of knee osteoarthritis. J Clin Orthop Trauma 2019;10(1):46–8.
31. FDA Office of Communication O, (OCOD) aD. Same Surgical Procedure Exception under 21 CFR 1271.15(b): Questions and Answers Regarding the Scope of the Exception. Accessed May 2022.
32. Heikkinen J, Mottonen M, Pulkki K, et al. Cytokine levels in midtrimester amniotic fluid in normal pregnancy and in the prediction of pre-eclampsia. Scand J Immunol 2001;53(3):310–4.
33. Chow SS, Craig ME, Jones CA, et al. Differences in amniotic fluid and maternal serum cytokine levels in early midtrimester women without evidence of infection. Cytokine 2008;44(1):78–84.
34. Bennett NT, Schultz GS. Growth factors and wound healing: biochemical properties of growth factors and their receptors. Am J Surg 1993;165(6):728–37.
35. Korenovsky YV, Remneva OV. [Reference ranges of matrix metalloproteinase-1, -2, -9 and tissue inhibitor of matrix metalloproteinases-1 concentrations in amniotic fluid in physiological pregnancy]. Biomed Khim 2016;62(1):96–8.
36. Meinert M, Eriksen GV, Petersen AC, et al. Proteoglycans and hyaluronan in human fetal membranes. Am J Obstet Gynecol 2001;184(4):679–85.
37. Lee TY, Schafer IA. Glycosaminoglycan composition of human amniotic fluid. Biochim Biophys Acta 1974;354(2):264–74.
38. Panero AJ, Hirahara AM, Andersen WJ, et al. Are Amniotic Fluid Products Stem Cell Therapies? A Study of Amniotic Fluid Preparations for Mesenchymal Stem Cells With Bone Marrow Comparison. Am J Sports Med 2019;47(5):1230–5.
39. Dresser R. Ethical issues in embryonic stem cell research. JAMA 2001;285(11):1439–40.
40. Regulatory Considerations for Human Cells, Tissues, and Cellular and Tissue-Based Products: Minimal Manipulation and Homologous Use (2020).
41. FDA. FDA Extends Enforcement Discretion Policy for Certain Regenerative Medicine Products. Available at: https://www.fda.gov/news-events/press-announcements/fda-extends-enforcement-discretion-policy-certain-regenerative-medicine-products. Accessed April 4, 2022.
42. Finnoff JT, Awan TM, Borg-Stein J, et al. American Medical Society for Sports Medicine Position Statement: Principles for the Responsible Use of Regenerative Medicine in Sports Medicine. Clin J Sport Med 2021;31(6):530–41.

Orthobiologic Standardization and Clinical Outcome Measurement

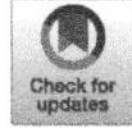

Joshua Martin, MD[a,*], Gerard Malanga, MD[b]

KEYWORDS

- Standardization • PRP • MFAT

KEY POINTS

- Controversy regarding the use of platelet-rich plasma (PRP) and other orthobiologics is largely secondary to a lack of standardization and quality control.
- The PLRA system (platelets, leukocytes, red blood cells, and activation) should be considered to quantify PRP products.
- Bone marrow aspirate concentrate should have similar components quantified (nucleated cells, leukocytes, red blood cells).
- Tracking outcomes with high-quality data are essential for the acceptance and advancement of orthobiologics

INTRODUCTION

It is well established in modern westernized medicine that for a drug to work, one must have both the correct drug as well as the correct dose. The wrong substance or chemical composition, and the intervention reasonably would not have an effect. A dose too low for the desired biologic effect, and the intervention would be considered not much different than a placebo. For medications that are produced by pharmaceuticals, with a relatively straightforward composition and structure, there is a long history of standardization, regulation, and ensuring that outcomes of the well-described intervention are supported by clinical evidence. Orthobiologics, especially those derived from an individual's own blood or cells, provide unique challenges for standardization. There is inherent variability in the cell counts and cellular compositions between individuals. In addition, products harvested, processed, and injected during one clinic visit are often not tested for quality control. To make matters more difficult, concentrations of various orthobiologic products used certainly matters, and as of this writing there are no accepted field-wide standards of the ideal orthobiologic composition. To address these

[a] Washington, DC, USA; [b] Department of Physical Medicine & Rehabilitation, Rutgers School of Medicine, New Jersey Regenerative Institute, 197 Ridgedale Avenue, Suite 210, Cedar Knolls, NJ 07927, USA

* Corresponding author. 8402 Donnybrook Drive, Chevy Chase, MD 20815.
E-mail address: joshuaericmartin@gmail.com

Phys Med Rehabil Clin N Am 34 (2023) 285–290
https://doi.org/10.1016/j.pmr.2022.08.017
1047-9651/23/© 2022 Published by Elsevier Inc.

needs there have been numerous calls for the standardization of various orthobiologics.[1–3] This article further addresses the history of and rationale for standardization, current orthobiologic best practices, as well as clinical outcome measurement.

HISTORY

There is a long history of standardization and regulation of drugs in the United States, which provides insights into potential pathways for orthobiologics to find their own appropriate pathway. As early as 1820, physicians met to establish the U.S. Pharmacopia, an independent, nongovernmental, nonprofit organization, that sets quality, purity, and strength standards called monographs for drugs in the United States[4,5]. Subsequently in 1905 the American Medical Association initiated a voluntary program, of drug approval that would last until 1955. To earn the right to advertise therapeutic claims in the Journal of the American Medical Association (JAMA) and related journals companies had to submit evidence for review by the AMA's Council on Pharmacy and Chemistry as well as outside experts. Shortly thereafter in 1906 congress passed the Food and Drugs Act, prohibiting interstate commerce in misbranded and adultered food, drinks, and drugs. The purview of the US Food and Drug Administration (FDA) was widened in 1938 with the Federal Food, Drug, and Cosmetic Act requiring drugs to be shown to be safe before marketing, and in 1962 the Kefauver-Harris Drug amendments for the first time required drug manufacturers to prove the effectiveness of their products before marketing them.[4] At this time the US Pharmacopia still independently sets monograph standards, which are then enforced by the FDA.

As per orthobiologics in the United States, in 2005 the FDA proposed and in 2005 implemented a tiered, risk-based approach to the regulation of human cells, tissues, and cellular-based products, which has been updated several times to establish safety regulations in how these products are acquired, manipulated, and used.[6] These regulations heavily focus on what is not allowed, with safety as the primary focus. As there is currently no recognized orthobiologic counterpart to US pharmacopeia, standards about what *should be* included in orthobiologics for efficacy is extremely limited. At this time platelet-rich plasma (PRP) is the only human blood, cell, or tissue product for which there is FDA guidance, specifying that there must be a minimum platelet concentration of 250,000 platelets per microliter.[7] There is no FDA guidance regarding red blood cell concentration or leukocyte concentration, which do matter, and the 250,000 platelets/uL may be below what is desired.

BACKGROUND: NEED FOR STANDARDIZATION

There is a pressing need for the standardization of orthobiologics, considering the cellular components, concentrations, and methods of injections may vary wildly, currently without significant standards of care. There is a growing body of evidence that these factors matter significantly for patient outcomes, yet there is no accepted the guidance of minimum standards for most of these interventions. In regard to PRP, commercially available PRP systems vary widely in platelet concentration, with some systems not actually concentrating platelets at all.[8,9] Many clinicians do not use cell counts to confirm they are getting a true PRP product, which is problematic because platelet concentration affects tenocyte behavior[10] and leukocyte concentration affects pain outcomes in joints such as knee osteoarthritis.[11] Parameters to consider include not only platelet and white blood cell concentrations, but also the presence or absence of red blood cells, which are thought to be detrimental due to free radical damage from heme components, activation status of the platelets, as well as volume of PRP injected as the total dose of any medicine is volume x concentration.

Table 1
PLRA system

	Criteria	Measurement	Comments
P	Platelet count	Volume in mL AND cells/μL	Total dose = volume × concentration
L	Leukocyte content	Percentage (%) of cells	If white cells are present the percentage of neutrophils should also be reported
R	Red blood cell content	Percentage (%) of cells	This measurement should ideally be as low as possible, <1%
A	Activation	Method should be reported	

In order to determine the best parameters for orthobiologic treatment it is imperative that these basic characteristics are quantified for all future studies. It also creates confusion and muddies the knowledge regarding orthobiologics when otherwise great studies are hampered by poor products. Top tier journals such as JAMA have been publishing papers where there is no description regarding the "PRP" product used,[12] and in many cases the quantified "PRP" product does not actually have an increased concentration of PRP, as defined by 2x at the very minimum.[13] Negative results should be expected from the use of poor products, and subsequent meta-analyses would also appear equivocal noting a vast variety of results. Until there is standardization and quality control the mainstream medical community may reasonably look upon various orthobiologics with incredulity.

DISCUSSION

Best Practices for Standardization

Various classification systems have been proposed for the use of PRP in orthobiologic use. At a bare minimum the proposed PLRA classification should be considered, which does include the pertinent cellular components that are thought the affect outcomes for injection.[3] The PLRA system includes **Table 1**:

A similar system may be also used for bone marrow concentrate, except nucleated cells and colony-forming unit-fibroblast (CFU-F) cells are desired rather than platelets, and the product typically is not activated. CFU-F cells are a subset of nucleated cells that are multipotent. CFU-F populations are not homogeneous but rather contain a hierarchy of progenitors including multipotential skeletal stem stems, which constitute from one-tenth to one-third of all CFU-F cells.[14] CFU-F cells are counted by plating and growing colonies of cells, so numbers may not be available in real-time for injections. Yet, CFU-F is of importance for quality control to ensure technique of bone marrow aspirate concentrate aspiration and concentration has been satisfactory, especially considering that whole blood does contain nucleated cells. It should be noted that CFU-F cells are rather sparse, roughly 1 out of every 30,000 cells in the iliac crest.[15] In addition, the number of colonies formed per unit of marrow cells plated, or colony-forming efficiency (CFE) does decrease with age.[14] Cell viability is another marker that is more readily measured than CFU-F and is affected by technique. For bone marrow concentrate in clinical use, volume of total injection, total nucleated cells (cells/μL), and red blood cell content (%) should be recorded. Cell viability and CFU-F may play an important role in quality control as well.

In terms of desired concentrations, for PRP, the platelet count should be high, as below 2x is much less likely to provide significant benefit. Early research and clinical data have suggested the desired platelet concentration may be age dependent, with Chris Centeno's group noting that in lab data young adults show healing at 2–3x baseline, but higher concentrations are recommended for more advanced ages, with recommendations for middle age 5–7x (35–45), older individuals 10 to 14x, and the elderly 20 × .[16] Studies regarding leukocyte concentration for various applications (tendon vs joint) are ongoing and should be recorded. Monocytes are thought to interact differently than neutrophils in the healing response, so if a leukocyte-rich product is used these components should be quantified. Red blood cell concentration should be as low as possible, as the heme components produce free radicals which may damage tendon and cartilage cells. In bone marrow aspirate concentrate it is also desirable to reduce red blood cells as much as possible, and research is ongoing about the ideal amount of nucleated cells and CFU-F cells.

MFAT (microfragmented adipose tissue) typically is thick and opaque, and in a clinical setting does not lend itself well to cell counting. Nevertheless, total amount of MFAT and system used to process the MFAT should be recorded. There are ongoing studies regarding obtaining stromal vascular fraction (SVF) from adipose, and once injections of these more pure cellular components become allowable by the FDA in the United States similar counts may be obtained. This would include nucleated cell concentration, leukocytes, red blood cells, and volume injected.

Another consideration for standardization for regenerative injections is consistent and accurate technique for injection. Considering that the mechanisms of action for regenerative injections are thought to modulate local tissue processes, placing the injectate in the right area is critical. There is increased accuracy of injection of even large joints such as knees with ultrasound guidance,[17] and for joints fluoroscopy may be another consideration. For tendon injury typically the target for PRP is the location of tendon with greatest tendinopathy, which may be visualized under ultrasound.

Best practices for outcome measurement

In the use of orthobiologics, and musculoskeletal medicine in general, patient-reported outcomes are essential to improving care. The goal is typically to improve pain, function, and quality of life, which are typically patient-reported. There are numerous validated standardized questionnaires to capture these outcomes, such as the numeral pain scale (NPS) for pain and functional outcomes such as the Knee Osteoarthritis Outcome Score (KOOS) and Western Ontario and McMaster Universities Osteoarthritis Index (WOMAC) for knee osteoarthritis. When tracking outcomes it is important to include these pain and function scores, which these typically track. To optimize data, it is important to enroll as many patients as possible, as well as follow-up data over time for more longitudinal data. When consenting patients for their procedures it is also appropriate to obtain consent for tracking their outcomes, and then contact may be maintained for longitudinal outcomes via email or phone calls, especially if they do not follow-up during desired post-injection time points.

Even though double-blinded placebo-controlled studies are often considered the gold standard for clinical data, if these were the only studies available most potential data would be lost. There is great value in following outcomes from clinical practice, and various other treatments, such as steroid or hyaluronic acid for knee osteoarthritis, may still be compared with the orthobiologic injection. Often orthobiologics are used in chronic conditions where there has been little to no pain or functional relief for years, so a demonstrable benefit above baseline is also of clinical significance.

SUMMARY

There is ongoing controversy about the effectiveness of orthobiologics, with the lack of standardization, quality control, and outcome measurement contributing to this confusion. There are several classification systems that exist, such as the PLRA system for PRP, to address the issue of standardization, but the systems have not yet had widespread use. By adopting a standard and tracking outcomes, just as US pharmacopeia and the FDA did years ago for drug development, the orthobiologic field may advance and overcome much of the uncertainty in terms of safety and efficacy. In order to have the best patient outcomes it is imperative to know exactly what and how much we are injecting of any particular product, and to ensure we keep up with the quality of these injections.

CLINICS CARE POINTS

- Orthobiologic injections should be under ultrasound guidance to ensure the correct target tissue receives the desired product
- Clinicians should use products that have shown the capability to deliver a quality product. For platelet-rich plasma (PRP): adequate platelets, reduced neutrophils and elimination of red blood cells (RBCs).
- Practices should engage in quality control, where there are routine measurements to ensure the desired product is in fact produced. This should be performed for each technician, as technical skill handling commercial devices may make a difference in final product

For PRP injections we recommend the following:

- Record the platelet concentration, leukocyte concentration (%), RBC concentration (%), and volume injected. Activation, if used, should be immediately before injection
- Platelet concentration should target at least 2x blood concentration in young adults, and higher in older individuals. RBCs should be kept to close to zero.

For Bone Marrow aspirate injections we recommend the following:

- Record the total nucleated cell count, RBC concentration (%), percent viability, and volume injected. When possible colony-forming unit-fibroblast has use for validating aspiration and concentration technique.

For Microfragmented Adipose tissue injections we recommend the following:

- Record the amount of MFAT injected. At this time it is difficult to get cell counts from a dense lipophilic product

For Outcome measurement we recommend:

- Log which body part(s) are injected, including underlying diagnosis
- Include parameters about each injection as described above
- Log any adverse responses
- Log regenerative procedures with relevant outcome scores (ie, numeral pain scale and Knee Osteoarthritis Outcome Score) in a database that includes relevant time frame follow-up (3 months, 6 months, 1 year, 2 year+)

DISCLOSURE

The authors have nothing to disclose.

REFERENCES

1. Chahla J, Cinque ME, et al. A Call for Standardization in Platelet-Rich Plasma Preparation Protocols and Composition Reporting. The J Bone Joint Surg 2017; 99(20):1769–79. https://doi.org/10.2106/JBJS.16.01374.

2. Fadadu PP, Mazzola AJ, Hunter CW, et al. Review of concentration yields in commercially available platelet-rich plasma (PRP) systems: a call for PRP standardization. Reg Anesth Pain Med 2019;44:652–9.
3. Mautner K, Malanga GA, Smith J, et al. A Call for a Standard Classification System for Future Biologic Research: The Rationale for New PRP Nomenclature. PM R The J Inj Funct Rehabil 2015;7(4 Suppl):S53–9.
4. The History of Drug Regulation. U.S. Food and Drug Administration. Available at: https://www.fda.gov/media/109482/download. Accessed February 6, 2022.
5. Kozlowski S. CDER Conversation: Ensuring That Standardization Does Not Impede Biological Product Innovation. In: FDA.gov. 2019. Available at: https://www.fda.gov/drugs/news-events-human-drugs/cder-conversation-ensuring-standardization-does-not-impede-biological-product-innovation/. Accessed February 6, 2022.
6. Regulatory Considerations for Human Cells, Tissues, and Cellular and Tissue-Based Products: Minimal Manipulation and Homologous Use. Food and Drug Administration Center for Biologics Evaluation and Research. Available at: https://www.fda.gov/media/109176/download. Accessed February 6, 2022.
7. CFR- Code of Federal Regulatioms Title 21. Food and Drug Administration Department of Health and Human Services. Subchapter F- Biologics. Available at: https://www.accessdata.fda.gov/scripts/cdrh/cfdocs/cfcfr/CFRSearch.cfm?fr=640.34. Accessed February 6, 2022.
8. Fadadu PP, Anthony JM, Hunter CW, Davis TT. Review of Concentration Yields in Commercially Available Platelet-Rich Plasma (PRP) Systems: A Call for PRP Standardization. Reg Anesth Pain Med 2019. https://doi.org/10.1136/rapm-2018-100356.
9. Carr BJ, Canapp SO, Mason DR, et al. Canine Platelet-Rich Plasma Systems: A Prospective Analysis. Front Vet Sci 2015;2:73.
10. Giusti Ilaria, D'Ascenzo Sandra, Mancò Annalisa, et al. Platelet Concentration in Platelet-Rich Plasma Affects Tenocyte Behavior in Vitro. Biomed Res Int 2014; 2014:630870.
11. Riboh JC, Saltzman BM, Lisa Fortier Adam B Yanke, et al. Effect of Leukocyte Concentration on the Efficacy of Platelet-Rich Plasma in the Treatment of Knee Osteoarthritis. Am J Sports Med 2016;44(3):792–800.
12. Kearney RS, Ji C, Warwick J, et al. Effect of Platelet Rich plasma injection versus Sham injection on Tendon Dysfunction Patients with Chronic Midportion Achilles tendinopathy: A Randomized Clinical Trial. JAMA 2021;326(2):137–44.
13. Bennell KL, Paterson KL, Metcalf BR, et al. Effect of Intra-Articular Platelet-Rich Plasma vs Placebo Injection on Pain and Medial Tibial Cartilage Volume in Patients With Knee Osteoarthritis: The RESTORE Randomized Clinical Trial. JAMA: The J Am Med Assoc 2021;326(20):2021–30.
14. Kuznetsov SA, Mankani MH, Bianco P, et al. Enumeration of the Colony-Forming Units-Fibroblast from Mouse and Human Bone Marrow in Normal and Pathological Conditions. Stem Cell Res 2009;2(1):83–94.
15. Hernigou Ph, Poignard A, Beaujean F, et al. Percutaneous Autologous Bone-Marrow Grafting for Nonunions. Influence of the Number and Concentration of Progenitor Cells." The J Bone Joint Surg Am Volume 2005;87(7):1430–7.
16. Berger DR, Centeno CJ, Steinmetz NJ. Platelet lysates from aged donors promote human tenocyte proliferation and migration in a concentration-dependent manner. Bone Joint Res 2019;8(1):32–40.
17. Fang WH, Chen XT, Vangsness CT. Ultrasound-Guided Knee Injections Are More Accurate Than Blind Injections: A Systematic Review of Randomized Controlled Trials. Arthrosc Sports Med Rehabil 2021;3(4):e1177–87.

Regional Anesthesia for Orthobiologic Procedures

Michael Khadavi, MD[a,*], Danielle Rehor, BS[b,1], Alex Roney, BS[c], Luga Podesta, MD[d,e], David R. Smith, MD[f]

KEYWORDS

- Peripheral nerve block • Regional anesthesia • Orthobiologics • Stem cell
- Regenerative medicine • Platelet-rich plasma

KEY POINTS

- Peripheral nerve blocks (PNB) can lessen procedural pain and eliminate the known detrimental effects of local anesthetics on orthobiologic target tissues.
- Knowledge of the risks of PNBs and prevention strategies can minimize their occurrence.
- PNBs should only be performed on an awake and communicative patient, with ultrasound-guidance, small volumes (2–3 mL) at multiple perineural locations, with the lowest possible local anesthetic dose.
- Bupivacaine carries the greatest risk of systemic toxicity.

INTRODUCTION

Orthobiologics is a growing field with a rapidly growing evidence base and frequency of use. These procedures are often performed on an outpatient basis. Many of these procedures, such as into a tendon or bone, may be challenging due to injection discomfort and consequent patient movement without some form of anesthesia. Although both intravenous (IV) sedation and target site local anesthetic (LA) injection are commonly used, their use is not without risk of complication or adverse effects. In the case of LA use into or around the target tissue, all commercially available LAs

[a] Kansas City Orthopedic Alliance, 4504 West 139th Street, Leawood, KS 66224, USA; [b] University of Kansas School of Medicine, 3901 Rainbow Boulevard, Kansas City, KS 66160, USA; [c] Liberty University College of Osteopathic Medicine, 600 Barrington Way, Lynchburg, VA 24502, USA; [d] Regenerative Sports Medicine, Bluetail Medical Group Naples, 1875 Veterans Park Drive, Suite 2201, Naples, FL 34109, USA; [e] Podesta Orthopedic and Sports Medicine Institute, 1875 Veterans Park Drive, Suite 2201, Naples, FL 34109, USA; [f] Division of Anaesthesia, Queens University, Astra Fellow in Regional Anesthesia, Virginia Mason Clinic, Interventional Pain Medicine, Kingston Orthopaedic Pain Institute, 800 John Marks Avenue, Kingston, Ontario K7K 0J7, Canada
[1] Present address: 8532 West 109th Terrace, Overland Park, KS 66210.
* Corresponding author. 10777 Nall Avenue, Suite 300, Overland Park, KS 66211.
E-mail address: mjkhadavi@gmail.com

Phys Med Rehabil Clin N Am 34 (2023) 291–309
https://doi.org/10.1016/j.pmr.2022.08.018
pmr.theclinics.com

have negative effects on tenocytes, chondrocytes, and platelets, with ropivacaine the least and bupivacaine the most harmful to these tissues.[1–6] Similarly, many providers use IV sedation, which comes with a host of mild complications such as nausea, vomiting, flu-like symptoms, hypotension, dysesthesia, and headache.[7–9] Life-threatening risks include airway obstruction, cardiac arrhythmias, pulmonary embolus, and aspiration.[9–13] Furthermore, heavily sedated patients can become disoriented and agitated, which can further challenge the procedure.

These situations can be avoided by blocking the sensory nerve supply to our orthobiologic target at a site some distance away from the treatment area, via a peripheral nerve block (PNB). Nerve blocks, also termed regional anesthesia, have been used since the late 1800s[14] and were in fact preferred due to the morbidity and mortality of general anesthesia in that period. More recently, they have been used with great success in a wide range of surgeries, including both large and small orthopedic surgeries.[12,15–19] When used for perioperative pain control, PNBs are associated with dramatic decreases in complications,[17] even compared with neuraxial nerve blocks.[20]

The literature is robust and formal educational curricula are well established for PNB techniques in many orthopedic surgical procedures; however, any mention of regional blockade before an orthobiologic injection is exceedingly rare in the literature. Yet, anesthetic goals for orthobiologic procedures differ from those in surgery. A complete block of both sensory and motor fibers is necessary in surgical settings; however, a sensory-only block is not only sufficient but also preferred in orthobiologic settings. In addition, a less than complete, "imperfect" block will often suffice.

These procedures have the potential to simultaneously minimize procedural pain and eliminate LAs detrimental effects on target tissues. Furthermore, limiting patient movement and anxiety while allowing for a more rapid procedure reduces the risk of infection and other complications.[21–24] In our experience, PNBs may allow even intraosseous injections to be performed in a clinic setting without the risks and adverse effects of heavy IV sedation.

While many orthobiologic providers are already performing PNBs on some occasions, most subspecialists who perform these treatments—such as physiatrists, primary care sports medicine physicians, and orthopedic surgeons—receive no formal training in PNB techniques and risks.

This article aims to summarize the basic concepts of regional anesthetic usage as pertains to orthobiologics, including the risks of PNBs, strategies to minimize these risks, and specific PNB techniques for several commonly performed orthobiologic procedures.

Risks and Precautions of Peripheral Nerve Blocks for Orthobiologic Procedures

It is the authors' belief that the enhanced efficacy, safety, and comfort provided by PNBs outweigh the inherent risks for many intratendinous and intraosseous orthobiologic procedures; however, an understanding of these risks and strategies toward their prevention is necessary to enhance PNB safety. These risks can be separated into two main categories: local anesthetic systemic toxicity (LAST) and target nerve damage from either LA chemical toxicity or physical injury from the needle and injection.

LAST is usually the result of LA toxicity to the central nervous system (CNS) or heart but can also cause hematologic, allergic, and local tissue reactions. It typically manifests within 5 minutes of injection but can appear several hours after anesthetic administration; the former associated with intravascular injection and the latter with slower uptake of LA from the soft tissues where they have been deposited. Strategies to mitigate both situations are discussed below.[25] CNS symptoms include confusion, metallic taste, dizziness, tinnitus, circumoral numbness, muscle twitching, seizure, loss of consciousness, coma, respiratory depression, and death. Cardiovascular symptoms include hypertension, tachycardia, bradycardia, arrhythmias, and asystole. However, the estimated 40% of patients with LAST present atypically. The incidence of LAST has been estimated at 3 in 10,000 PNBs,[26,27] and half are caused by non-anesthesia providers. Although self-limiting symptoms are common, the overall mortality rate of LAST is between 4% and 10%.[25]

The risk of LA systemic absorption in PNBs is lower than for plexus blocks, especially in the neck,[27] but higher than the subcutaneous and musculoskeletal injections that physiatrists are most experienced with, because of:

- Higher volumes of LA
- The highly vascularized anatomy that is more prone to indirect absorption or unintentional intravascular injection[25,28]

Low muscle mass rather than low total body weight is a risk factor for LAST, as systemically circulating LAs get stored in muscle. The use of epinephrine with LA in PNBs can both decrease intravascular uptake and serve as an intravascular marker but carries additional risks that may not be outweighed by the benefits.[29] Other risk factors for LAST include the high and low extremes of age and comorbidities, particularly heart and liver disease but also kidney disease and diabetes mellitus.[25–27] Ultrasound-guidance reduces LAST by 65%.[25,30,31]

Among LAs, bupivacaine poses the greatest risk of LAST, compared with lidocaine or ropivacaine.[11,32] Its uniquely high cardiac toxicity leads to more cardiac arrest and thus carries the highest morbidity and mortality in LAST among LAs.[27,33] However, American Society of Regional Anesthesia and Pain Medicine (ASRA)'s advisory panel on LAST opines that ropivacaine may have similar toxicity to bupivacaine.[27] Higher LA dose is a risk factor for LAST; however, a few cases have been reported with relatively low LA doses, as small as 0.31 mg/kg.[25] Because miscalculation of maximum LA dose is a common reason for overdose and LAST,[34] maximum volumes corresponding to maximum doses of recommended LAs in PNBs are presented in **Table 1** for three

Table 1
Concentration and maximum doses of lidocaine and ropivacaine

	Concentration (mg/mL)	Max Dose (mg/kg)	Max Volume per kg (mL/kg)	Max LA Volume (mL) for 50 kg Person (110lb)	Max LA Volume (mL) for 70 kg Person (154lb)	Max LA Volume (mL) for 85 kg Person (187lb)
Lidocaine 1%	10	5	0.5	25	35	42.5
Lidocaine 2%	20	5	0.25	12.5	17.5	21.25
Lidocaine 1% c Epi	10	7	0.7	35	49	59.5
Lidocaine 2% c Epi	20	7	0.35	17.5	24.5	29.75
Ropivacaine 0.5%	5	3	0.6	30	42	51
Ropivacaine 0.2%	2	3	1.5	75	105	127.5

$$Max\ Volume\ per\ kg\ IBM = \frac{Max\ Dose\ (\frac{mg}{kg})}{Concentration\ (\frac{mg}{ml})}$$

Max, maximum; c, with; Epi, epinephrine.

*Max doses and volumes must be calculated using ideal body weight and not total body weight.

sample lean body weights.[34,35] However, the risk of systemic toxicity increases continuously with escalating dose, rather than with a sudden increase once the maximum dose is reached. No more than the lowest possible LA dose should be used.[25,27,35]

If signs or symptoms of LAST occur, quick recognition and treatment are crucial for patient outcomes, beginning with immediate cessation of LA injection once any cardiovascular or mental status change is noticed. Treatment continues with respiratory and cardiac support, administration of 100% oxygen, benzodiazepines for seizures, and IV access to allow treatment with lipid emulsion therapy which acts as a "sink" for LAs.[25,26,36,37] Pharmacology, indications, and dosing of lipid emulsion therapy are outside the scope of this article.

A common procedural complication with often similar presentation to LAST is the vasovagal reaction. This presents as dizziness, light-headedness, weakness, nausea, sweating, or syncope and is known to occur in 1% to 8% of outpatient injections.[38,39] In a sitting position, venous blood will pool in the legs and diminish the body's ability to augment preload to the heart when cardiac output drops because of the bradycardia seen in vasovagal reactions.[40,41] Moreover, when possible, it is recommended to avoid performing painful injections in a sitting position. If a vasovagal response occurs, treatment begins with halting the procedure, placing the patient's legs above their heart (Trendelenburg position), and applying a cold compress on their forehead. Oxygen, IV fluids, and vasoactive medications may be needed in the rare, severe case.[42] Atropine and ephedrine can be used to support heart rate, blood pressure, and cardiac output as described in advanced cardiovascular life support (ACLS) guidelines.[42]

Local risks of PNBs include toxicity from the LA to the target nerve and mechanical trauma to the nerve from intraneural penetration or injection. These can present as motor or sensory deficits and pain in the sensory distribution of that peripheral nerve. Although transient deficits lasting up to 2 weeks occur in 8% to 15% of PNBs, incidence of long-lasting nerve injury is 2 to 4 per 10,000 PNBs.[28]

This can be prevented by retracting and repositioning the needle if pain or paresthesia occurs during the injection, a situation that can only occur if the patient is awake. Furthermore, it is important that the physician instruct the patient before the injection on the importance of reporting paresthesia and how to recognize them before performing the block, and again just before starting. We suggest a statement such as "when I get near the nerve, you may feel a "zing" down the arm. Please tell me if you experience this and I will reposition my needle and it will go away." Then, when injecting around the nerve, it is helpful to ask, "are you having any discomfort right now? Any uncomfortable sensations going down the arm?" Anxiolytic medications may be considered as long as the patient is still able to effectively communicate.

An indirect risk from some PNBs is injury that can occur secondary to the expected, temporary weakness after a block.[43,44] These injuries may be prevented by proper warning before the procedure and precautions such as arm slings for upper extremity weakness and crutches or an ankle boot for lower extremity weakness.

Contraindications to PNBs include an inability to cooperate with the injection, preexisting neurologic deficit, active local or systemic infection, and obesity obscuring optimal ultrasonographic visualization. Coagulopathy, anticoagulants, and heart and liver disease represent relative contraindications to PNBs.[12,27]

Last, an "incomplete block" is not uncommon and should be counseled. Several common reasons for this include inability of the LA to diffuse into the deeper nerve fibers, insufficient time for the block to take effect, and target innervation by nerves additional to those blocked. The latter scenario may knowingly occur in cases in which a portion of innervation is intentionally left unblocked because of challenges in blocking the remaining innervation branches. However, nerve anomalies are common and may explain some fraction of these incomplete nerve blockade phenomena.[45] In these scenarios, consideration may be given to injecting a few milliliters of ropivacaine around the target structure, with an even smaller volume into the target structure itself. PNB success rates are improved when expected onset time of the LA is observed.[46]

Clinics key points

- Major PNB risks include local nerve damage and local anesthetic systemic toxicity (LAST).
- LAST most often presents with CNS and cardiac signs and symptoms, but atypical presentations are common.
- The risk of LAST increases with lower muscle mass, higher local anesthetic (LA) doses, and comorbidities.
- Bupivacaine is the LA with the highest risk of LAST.
- LA maximum doses should be calculated and confirmed; however, the lowest possible LA dose should be used.
- An awake patient allows for early recognition of intraneural needle placement and LAST symptoms.
- Brace and support the limb for weakness resulting from the PNB.

General Nerve Block Techniques

As the local anatomy and volume of LA for PNBs may be unfamiliar to even the most experienced ultrasound-guided proceduralist, the aforementioned risks and several unique techniques must be considered. When first learning PNB techniques, more superficial PNBs and those not part of a vascular plexus may be ideal—such as the suprascapular nerve (SSN), tibial nerve (TN) at the ankle, or radial nerve. These procedures should only be performed by a skilled ultrasound proceduralist.

Ultrasound guidance improves the success rate[47–50] and safety[25,30,31] and decreases the required volume of LA in PNBs;[51] however, these risks are not completely eliminated. A brief anatomic scan with particular attention to nearby nerve branches and vessels is essential to prevent inadvertent puncture or intravascular injection. A "straight-line view" setup (**Fig. 1**) with the provider, body part, and ultrasound monitor in a line is recommended to enhance provider comfort and accuracy. On approaching the target nerve, aspiration followed by a "test" injection of a small volume of 1 mL LA may be injected just before reaching the nerve. If no "halo" occurs, advancing farther with another test dose is recommended.[27] Multiple small-volume LA perineural injections in different locations around the nerve will reduce the risk of concomitant intravascular uptake. We suggest a volume of 2 to 3 mL and no more than 5 mL of LA in one needle position to create a "halo" about the nerve before the needle is repositioned and another small volume is injected. Even if a "halo" occurs around the nerve, inadvertent or concomitant intravascular injection is possible. Each injection should be slow, without resistance, and with a "halo" flow pattern. If any of these do not occur, immediate repositioning is necessary to prevent injection into an unintended structure.

Although optimal LA concentration and dose for orthobiologic procedures have not been studied, the surgical anesthesiology literature suggests that low volumes may often be sufficient, with volumes as low as 0.11 mL/mm^2 nerve cross-sectional area advocated.[52] Surgical literature suggests that at the same total dose, a lower injected volume of higher concentration provides more complete block than the converse.[53–56] There is also evidence that at the same total LA dose, higher injected volumes may result in greater systemic absorption and thus greater potential of LAST. In any case, the lowest possible LA dose should always be used.[25,27]

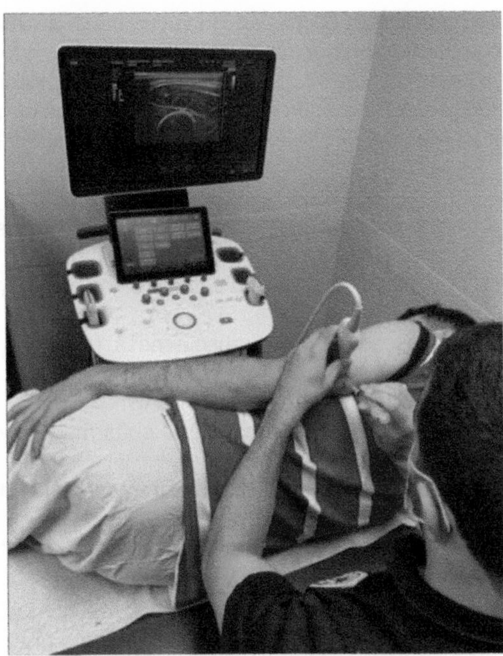

Fig. 1. Physician, patient, and ultrasound oriented in a "straight line view," allowing the physician a comfortable position with an easy view back and forth between the ultrasound monitor and injection site.

Further education and training through guidelines, publications, and organizations such as the ASRA and the New York School of Regional Anesthesia are recommended.

Clinics key points

- Always use a "straight line view" when possible.
- Multiple small-volume LA injections about the nerve with "halo" visualization may reduce the risk of inadvertent intravascular injection of a large volume of LA.
- Further and continuing training on PNBs is suggested.

COMMON NERVE BLOCK TECHNIQUES

Peripheral Nerve Block for Plantar Fascia Orthobiologic Procedures

The plantar fascia is innervated by the TN.[57,58] Although both the anatomic innervation of the plantar fascia and technique for TN block at the ankle have been studied,[12,47,59,60] PNBs specifically for plantar fascia procedures have not been described. At the ankle, the TN is also termed the posterior TN and divides into three branches to innervate the skin and intrinsic muscles of the plantar foot via the medial plantar nerve, lateral plantar nerve, and medial calcaneal nerve. Owing to this distal location, a TN block at or just above the ankle may result in paresthesia and weakness in just this distal distribution, with ankle plantarflexion and dorsiflexion strength maintained.

Technique: TN block at the ankle
Indication: Plantar fascia intratendinous procedures
Positioning: Side-lying, facing away with affected leg down and nearest to physician
Suggested Needle: 1 ½ inch, 22 or 25-gauge

Needle Approach: Posterior to anterior, in-plane
LA volume: 3 to 5 mL

The TN has a significant anatomic variation in the number and location of its branches[61] and blocking 10 cm proximal to the tarsal tunnel will assure that all branches are adequately blocked. With the patient in side-lying position with the affected leg on bottom, the ultrasound probe is placed in an axial position over the posteromedial ankle to identify the medial ankle tendons (**Fig. 2**). The TN will be visualized just deep and posterior to the vasculature and anterior to the flexor hallucis longus tendon. From here, the probe is translated proximally by 10 cm. Needle entry is just medial to the Achilles tendon toward the TN.

Peripheral nerve block for achilles tendon orthobiologic procedures

The Achilles tendon is innervated by the TN and sural nerves, the latter originating from the common peroneal nerve (CPN) and TN.[62] Blockade of the TN and CPN just past their bifurcation in the popliteal fossa provides superior anesthesia compared with blocking the sciatic nerve before this bifurcation[63] and is thus our preferred PNB technique for Achilles and other ankle procedures.[64] Subsequent weakness in plantarflexion and dorsiflexion is anticipated,[58] and a well-fitting orthopedic boot is necessary after this block to avoid tripping and falls.

Technique: TN and CPN blocks at the knee (“popliteal block”)
Indication: Achilles intratendinous procedures; intraosseous injection of distal tibia and talus
Positioning: Prone, treatment leg away from physician
Suggested Needle: 2 ½ or 3 ½ inch, 22 or 25-gauge Quincke
Needle Approach: Medial to lateral, in-plane
LA Volume: 5 to 10 mL for TN; 5 mL for CPN

With the patient in prone and the US probe in axial position over the posterior knee, the sciatic nerve and its TN and CPN branches can be traced from proximal to distal or distal to proximal. The popliteal artery and its branches should be identified without and with color Doppler. The block location is found by moving the transducer until just past the bifurcation of TN and CPN (**Fig. 3**). A medial approach avoids

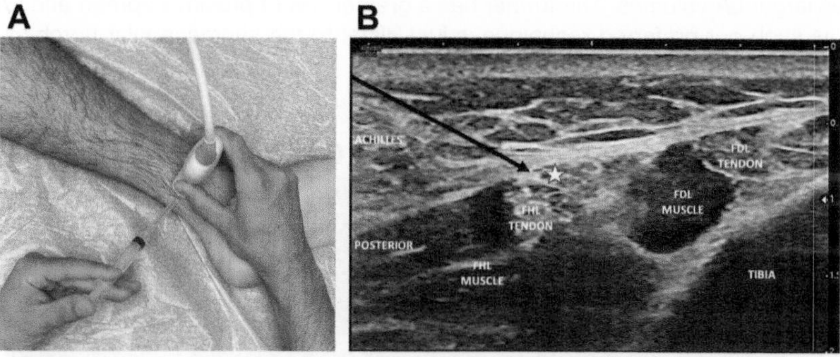

Fig. 2. (*A*) Probe positioning for tibial nerve block at the ankle with (*B*) corresponding US image of an in-plane tibial nerve block in short axis to the nerve. FDL Muscle, flexor digitorum longus muscle; FDL Tendon, flexor digitorum longus tendon; FHL Muscle, flexor hallucis longus muscle; FHL Tendon, flexor hallucis longus tendon; US, ultrasound; ☆ = tibial nerve, → = needle path.

unintentional puncture of the more superficial CPN. With meticulous, small-volume injection technique, the perineural injection about the TN is performed, followed by the CPN. Two separate needle entrance sites will sometimes be required depending on patient-specific anatomy.

Peripheral nerve block for rotator cuff interventions

Although interscalene blocks remain the gold standard for shoulder surgery regional anesthesia, this block is riskier than PNBs, with an expected phrenic nerve blockade and significant risks of respiratory distress[15,65] and LAST.[26,27] Fortunately, two of the most commonly diseased rotator cuff tendons, the supraspinatus, and infraspinatus[66] are innervated by the SSN, which may be targeted with a simple and less risky SSN block.

SSN blocks are widely studied and clinically used in the treatment of scapular fractures, various shoulder pathologies such as frozen shoulder, rotator cuff tendinopathy, glenohumeral arthritis, shoulder dislocations,[67–71] radiofrequency neurotomy,[72] and surgical and postsurgical regional anesthesia.[16] The SSN is a mixed sensory and motor nerve that branches from the superior trunk of the brachial plexus, travels toward the scapula and through the suprascapular notch to the supraspinatus fossa to provide innervation to the supraspinatus via its first branch, then the acromioclavicular joint, subacromial bursa, and then the infraspinatus and 70% of the glenohumeral capsule.[73] It is important to be aware that an SSN block will not anesthetize the subscapularis, teres minor, or long head biceps tendons.

Technique: SSN block
Indication: Supraspinatus and infraspinatus intratendinous procedures
Positioning: Sitting, facing away from physician
Suggested Needle: 2 ½ or 3 ½ inch Quincke, 22 or 25-gauge
Needle Approach: Inferomedial to superolateral, in-plane
LA Volume: 5 to 10 mL

Several SSN block techniques have been described, each with differing risks, ease of performance, and completeness of SSN blockade,[67,74–77] including direct SSN blockade proximal to the suprascapular notch from an anterior approach as it courses deep to the omohyoid and indirect blocks in which the nerve is not visualized and requires larger LA volumes. The former has a greater risk of proximal spread and LAST and as such our preferred technique is just distal to the suprascapular notch at the lateral floor of the supraspinatus fossa.

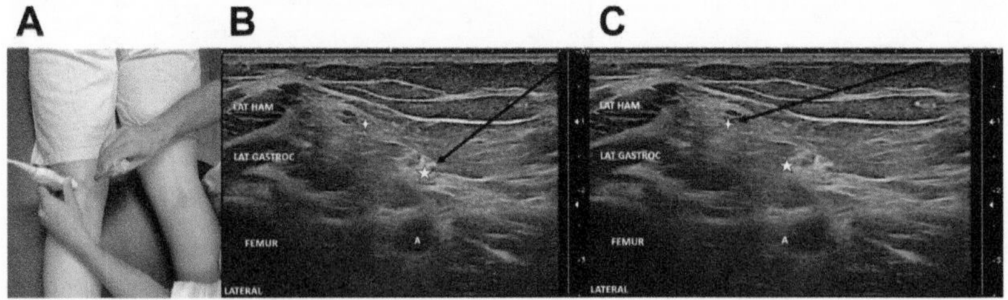

Fig. 3. (*A*) Probe positioning for popliteal block with corresponding US image of an in-plane tibial nerve (*B*) and common peroneal nerve (*C*) injection, both in short axis to the nerves. A, popliteal artery; Lat Gastroc, lateral gastrocnemius; Lat Ham, lateral hamstrings; ☆ = tibial nerve; ✧ = common peroneal nerve; → = needle path.

This block may be performed with the patient sitting upright (**Fig. 4**). Shoulder adduction and forward flexion may assist by bringing the nerve into a more superficial position. Scanning the lateral supraspinatus fossa will find the suprascapular notch on its anterior border with the SSN and artery running deep and in a posterolateral direction in a shallow canal known as the suprascapular canal. In our experience, color Doppler often misses the small accompanying artery, but the nerve can most easily be found just as it exits anteriorly from the suprascapular notch. With the US probe placed short axis to the SSN and artery, the needle is directed from an inferomedial approach, in-plane through the overlying trapezius, supraspinatus, and finally the supraspinatus fascia overlying the suprascapular canal. In some larger patients, the suprascapular canal is difficult to visualize, and the needle may be directed beneath the supraspinatus fascia in the lateral suprascapular fossa without direct nerve visualization.[78]

Before the SSN block, the patient should be advised of anticipated rotator cuff weakness. If a sling is given, we suggest the range of motion exercises such as pendulums and wall crawls to reduce the risk of immobility-associated adhesive capsulitis.

Peripheral Nerve Block for Elbow Common Extensor Tendon Procedures

Regional anesthesia literature describes proximal interscalene and axillary plexus blocks[17–19,79] for most elbow surgery regional anesthesia; however, these blocks are associated with higher respiratory and systemic risks.[80] Thus, PNB of the radial nerve may be considered.

Although the proximal tendon of the extensor carpi radialis brevis is the most relevant in lateral epicondylitis, blockade of the entire common extensor tendon is necessary for optimal anesthesia. Variations commonly occur in nerve branching patterns to the components of the wrist extensors, including branching directly from the radial nerve, the posterior antebrachial cutaneous nerve, the posterior interosseous nerve, and even the radial sensory nerve in over 20% of individuals.[81–83] Therefore, to maximize efficacy of this blockade, the authors suggest blocking the radial nerve proximal to branching of the posterior antebrachial cutaneous nerve at the intermuscular septum of the arm. Consequent wrist drop and lateral forearm and thumb numbness should be explained beforehand and a wrist splint may be considered.

Technique Description: Radial nerve block
Indication: Elbow common extensor intratendinous procedures
Positioning: Side-lying with affected arm on top, facing away from the physician
Suggested Needle: 1 ½ inch, 22 or 25-gauge
Needle Approach: Posterior to anterior, in-plane
LA Volume: 5 to 10 mL

With the patient side-lying, facing away from the physician and with the affected arm on top (**Fig. 5**), the radial nerve may be found either from proximal to distal, posterolateral along the spiral groove. In an axial plane, the nerve will be visualized coursing the intermuscular septum between the triceps brachii and brachialis after which the posterior antebrachial cutaneous nerve diverges. Just proximal to this location, the block is performed. Either an anterior or posterior approach may be performed, and the latter is our preference.

Peripheral Nerve Blocks for Medial Knee Intraosseous Procedures

The innervation of the boney and capsular anatomy of the knee is complex, with over a dozen nerve branches that originate from the CPN, TN, sciatic nerve, femoral nerve, and obturator nerves.[84,85] Furthermore, several common variant innervation patterns have been described.[85] No studies have yet been aimed at regional anesthesia

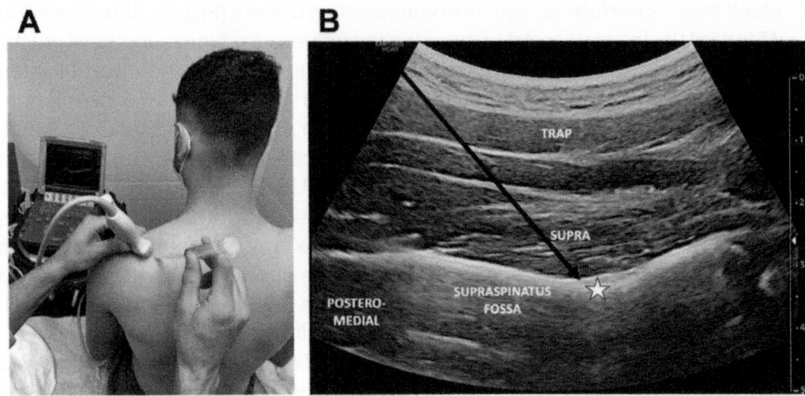

Fig. 4. (*A*) Probe positioning for a suprascapular block within the supraspinatus fossa with (*B*) corresponding US image of an in-plane suprascapular nerve injection, short axis to the nerve. Supra, supraspinatus; Trap, trapezius; fx1 = suprascapular nerve; → = needle path.

techniques specifically for intraosseous injections of the knee; however, the extensive innervation anatomy of the knee has been studied over the past 80 years.[86] More recently, knee innervation pattern literature has focused on regional anesthesia techniques for knee surgeries[87–90] and for knee radiofrequency neurotomy procedures.[85,91]

Within the medial knee, the medial femoral condyle and capsule are most commonly innervated by the:

- Nerve to the vastus medialis (NVM)—a branch of the femoral nerve
- Superior medial geniculate nerve (SMGN)—an articular branch of the TN (ABTN)
- Posterior division of the obturator nerve (PON), and the medial tibial plateau is innervated primarily by the:
- Inferior medial geniculate nerve (IMGN)—a branch off the anastomosis of the ABTN and the PON
- Infrapatellar branch of the saphenous nerve (SN)

Historically, a femoral nerve block was used for postoperative pain management after knee surgeries; however, the immediate postoperative period was challenged by quadriceps weakness[87,88] and incomplete postoperative analgesia for more extensive surgeries such as total knee arthroplasty.[89] Adductor canal block (ACB) has become popular and widely used for major knee surgery with the advantage of motor sparing due to the lack of blockade of several components of the quadriceps muscle.[87]

The adductor canal begins at the apex of the femoral triangle and ends at the adductor hiatus, just posterior to the sartorius and carries the SN and NVM. The NVM enters the adductor canal at the apex of the femoral triangle and then exits the adductor canal and courses medially and parallel to it midway down the thigh, separated by aponeurosis. The NVM has been found to provide more afferent innervation than previously thought to the medial knee. Therefore, for maximal medial knee blockade, an ACB should be performed midway or just proximal to midway down the thigh to include the NVM.

The other nerves to the medial knee are the SMGN, IMGN, and PON. While not always necessary, these nerves can be blocked simultaneously as they course posteriorly through the popliteal plexus of Rudinger, via the IPACK (Interspace between the Popliteal Artery and Capsule of the Knee) block.[89,90] However, for anyone not

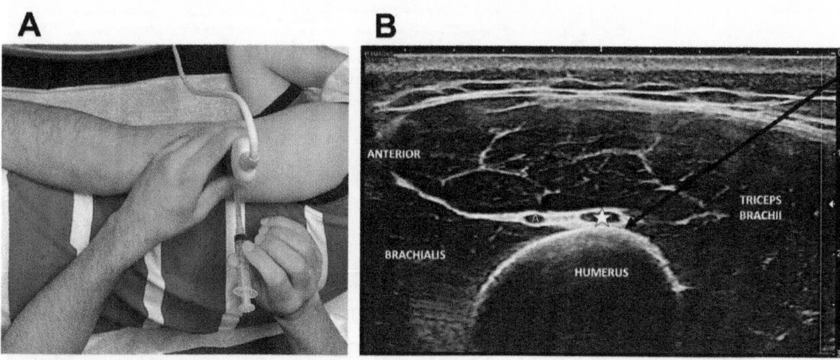

Fig. 5. (*A*) Probe positioning for radial nerve block just proximal to its passing through the intermuscular septum with (*B*) corresponding US image of an in-plane injection in short axis to the radial nerve. A, radial artery; fx1 = radial nerve; → = needle path.

highly experienced in PNBs who desires blockade beyond the ACB, we suggest SMGN and IMGN blocks.

It is important to be aware that the lateral knee remains sensate as the NVM, nerve to the vastus lateralis, superior lateral geniculate nerve, inferior lateral geniculate nerve, and recurrent fibular nerve are spared. However, as osteoarthritis effecting primarily the medial compartment is very common, these PNBs for the medial knee remain highly useful in clinical orthobiologics practice.

Technique: ACB
Indication: Intraosseous injection to the medial femoral condyle and medial tibial plateau of the knee, medial meniscus, and medial collateral ligament injection
Positioning: Supine, treatment leg toward physician, slight external rotation (frog-leg)
Suggested Needle: 2 ½ or 3 ½ inch, 22 or 25 gauge Quincke
Needle Approach: Anterolateral to posteromedial, in-plane
LA Volume: 10 mL

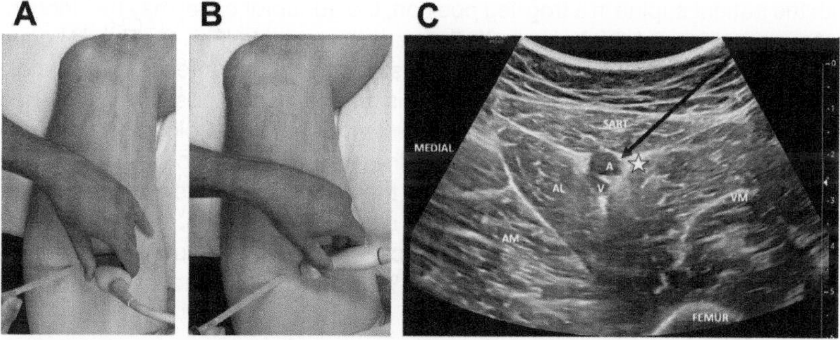

Fig. 6. (*A*) Initial probe positioning at mid-thigh with subsequent "move away and look back" positioning (*B*) for an adductor canal block. (*C*) Corresponding US image of an in-plane injection of the adductor canal in short axis. Note the sartorius overlying the adductor canal at this level. A, femoral artery; AL, adductor longus; AM, adductor magnus; Sart, sartorius; V, femoral vein; VM, vastus medialis; fx1 = nerves; → = needle path.

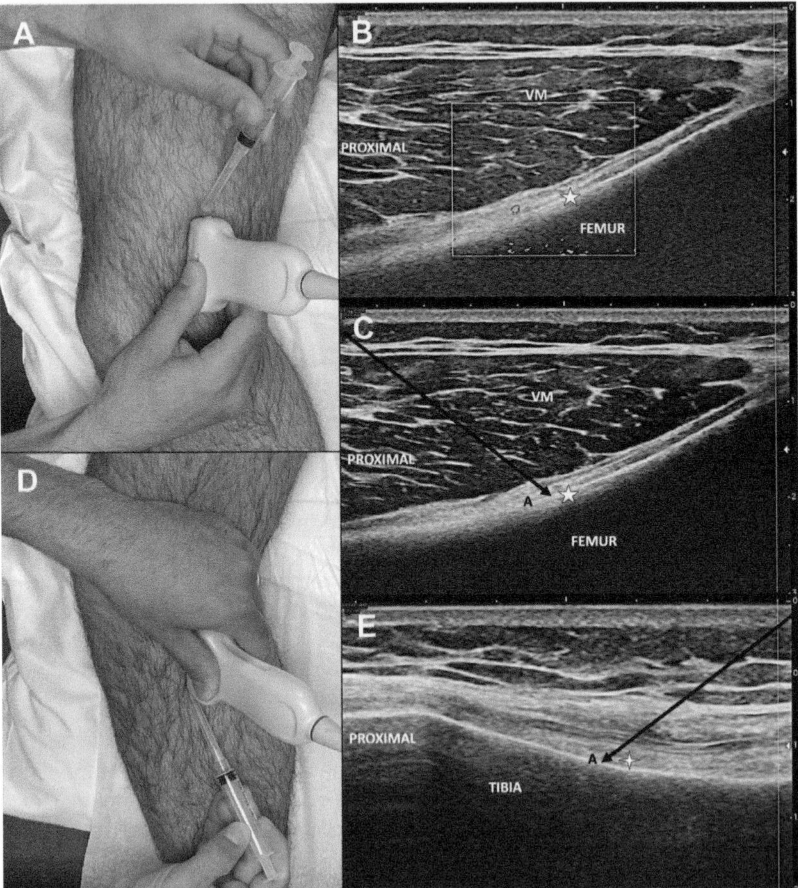

Fig. 7. (*A*) Probe position for SMGN injection. Color Doppler (*B*) may assistance in identifying the artery followed by an in-plane injection of the SMGN (*C*). Probe position (*D*) and in-plane injection of the IMGN. A, geniculate arteries; VM, vastus medialis; fx1 in (*B*) and (*C*); superior medial geniculate nerves; fx2 in (*E*); inferior medial geniculate nerves; → = needle path.

With the patient supine in a frog-leg position, the adductor canal may be identified at or just proximal to mid-thigh, beneath the sartorius muscle (**Fig. 6**). The SN courses just anterior to the femoral artery. After skin sterilization, the anterior to posterior, in-plane needle approach begins in short axis to the canal, positioning the needle deep to the sartorius and just anterior to the femoral artery. Color Doppler may aid in avoiding small vascular branches, such as the descending geniculate artery. Moving the transducer away from you while pressing the distal edge of the transducer into the skin will create a shallower angle and better needle visualization. This technique can be remembered as "move away and look back." Mild transient quadriceps weakness is possible as the NVM is responsible for 8% of the motor function of this muscle group.[89]

Technique: SMGN and IMGN blocks
Indication: Intraosseous injection to the medial femoral condyle and medial tibial plateau of the knee, medial meniscus, and medial collateral ligament injection
Positioning: Supine, treatment leg toward physician, external rotation (frog-leg)

Suggested Needle: 1 ½ or 2 ½ inch, 25-gauge
Needle Approach: Proximal to distal (SMGN), distal to proximal (IMGN), both in-plane
LA Volume: 2 to 5 mL for each nerve

In the same supine, frog-leg position, the ultrasound probe is placed in a coronal plane along the distal medial thigh at the medial femoral epicondyle. Deep to the vastus medialis, the small SMGN and accompanying vasculature will be visualized as they course anteriorly along the boney surface at the flair of the epicondyle. Color Doppler may be helpful to visualize the accompanying artery (**Fig. 7**). An in-plane approach is used, in short axis to the nerve and from distal to proximal until periosteum is reached.

The ultrasound probe is then moved to the medial tibia plateau, and in a coronal plane at the base of the flair of the medial tibial plateau, the small IMGN is found next to its vasculature, hugging the periosteum. As this nerve also courses from posterior to anterior, the nerve should be blocked in its most posterior location. In short axis to the nerve, a long-axis injection approach is taken from distal to proximal.

CLINICS CARE POINTS

- For a tibial nerve block at the ankle, find the nerve in the tarsal tunnel and track it proximally. The posterior tibial artery is another useful landmark as they travel together in a neurovascular bundle.
- For a popliteal block, the common peroneal nerve (CPN) is easy to find at the fibular head, and as you move proximally it is just medial to the short head of the biceps femoris. After finding the CPN, track it proximally to find the tibial nerve as they bifurcate from the sciatic nerve.
- The supraspinatus fossa is deep with the suprascapular nerve (SSN) at its lateral floor. SSN is easiest to find anteriorly as it exits the suprascapular notch, then travels posterolaterally. A 22 gauge is often easier to guide than a 25 gauge for this block.
- The radial nerve should be blocked in the posterior compartment before it passes the intermuscular septum for common extensor tendon procedures. Find the nerve against the posterolateral mid-humerus and track it proximally until it is away from the shaft of the humerus for a good site for blockade.
- Adductor canal block will include the nerve to the vastus medialis if performed just proximal to mid-thigh, where the femoral artery is directly under the sartorius: "Move away and look back" for better needle visualization (see **Fig. 6**).

SUMMARY AND FINAL RECOMMENDATIONS

The goal of the orthobiologic physician is to provide safe, effective, and minimally painful procedures. In the right setting, PNBs may facilitate all of these goals. An understanding of local and systemic risks of PNBs and LAs such as LAST will improve their safety. We suggest performing PNBs with:

- An awake and communicative patient
- Ultrasound-guidance
- Small volumes (2–3 mL) at multiple perineural locations around a nerve
- The lowest possible LA dose
- Constant monitoring for local and systemic symptoms during injection
- Lidocaine or ropivacaine and not bupivacaine

A well-performed PNB may provide excellent procedural comfort while eliminating complications from IV sedation and locally injected LA in the target tissue. Further studies comparing PNBs with locally injected LA and IV sedation on orthobiologic outcomes, procedural pain levels, and safety are necessary. We also suggest further study on minimum necessary LA doses for PNBs when used for orthobiologic procedures and on PNB techniques for other common orthobiologic procedures.

DISCLOSURE

M. Khadavi: Consultant for Arthrex. L. Podesta: Editor, Biologic Orthopedic Journal. D.R. Smith: Consultant for Gulf Coast Biologics, Fort Myers, FL.

REFERENCES

1. Durant TJ, Dwyer CR, McCarthy MB, et al. Protective Nature of Platelet-Rich Plasma Against Chondrocyte Death When Combined With Corticosteroids or Local Anesthetics. Am J Sports Med 2017;45(1):218–25.
2. Dregalla RC, Uribe Y, Bodor M. Effect of local anesthetics on platelet physiology and function. J Orthop Res 2021;39(12):2744–54.
3. Bedi A, Trinh TQ, Olszewski AM, et al. Nonbiologic Injections in Sports Medicine. JBJS Rev 2020;8(2):e0052.
4. Piper SL, Laron D, Manzano G, et al. A comparison of lidocaine, ropivacaine and dexamethasone toxicity on bovine tenocytes in culture. J Bone Joint Surg Br. 2012;94(6):856–62.
5. Zhang AZ, Ficklscherer A, Gülecyüz MF, et al. Cell Toxicity in Fibroblasts, Tenocytes, and Human Mesenchymal Stem Cells-A Comparison of Necrosis and Apoptosis-Inducing Ability in Ropivacaine, Bupivacaine, and Triamcinolone [published correction appears in Arthroscopy. 2021 Apr;37(4):1357]. Arthroscopy 2017;33(4):840–8.
6. Jayaram P, Kennedy DJ, Yeh P, et al. Chondrotoxic Effects of Local Anesthetics on Human Knee Articular Cartilage: A Systematic Review. PM R 2019;11(4): 379–400.
7. Schaufele MK, Marín DR, Tate JL, et al. Adverse events of conscious sedation in ambulatory spine procedures. Spine J 2011;11(12):1093–100.
8. American Society of Anesthesiologists Task Force on Sedation and Analgesia by Non-Anesthesiologists. Practice guidelines for sedation and analgesia by non-anesthesiologists. Anesthesiology 2002;96(4):1004–17.
9. Arepally A, Oechsle D, Kirkwood S, et al. Safety of conscious sedation in interventional radiology. Cardiovasc Intervent Radiol 2001;24(3):185–90.
10. Liu SS, YaDeau JT, Shaw PM, et al. Incidence of unintentional intraneural injection and postoperative neurological complications with ultrasound-guided interscalene and supraclavicular nerve blocks. Anaesthesia 2011;66(3):168–74.
11. Clarkson CW, Hondeghem LM. Mechanism for bupivacaine depression of cardiac conduction: fast block of sodium channels during the action potential with slow recovery from block during diastole. Anesthesiology 1985;62(4):396–405.
12. Wiederhold BD, Garmon EH, Peterson E, et al. Nerve Block Anesthesia. In: StatPearls. Treasure Island (FL): StatPearls Publishing; 2022.
13. Bellolio MF, Gilani WI, Barrionuevo P, et al. Incidence of Adverse Events in Adults Undergoing Procedural Sedation in the Emergency Department: A Systematic Review and Meta-analysis. Acad Emerg Med 2016;23(2):119–34.

14. Mian A, Chaudhry I, Huang R, et al. Brachial plexus anesthesia: A review of the relevant anatomy, complications, and anatomical variations. Clin Anat 2014;27(2): 210–21.
15. Divella M, Vetrugno L, Orso D, et al. Which regional anesthesia technique is the best for arthroscopic shoulder surgery in terms of postoperative outcomes? A comprehensive literature review. Eur Rev Med Pharmacol Sci 2021;25(2):985–98.
16. Ritchie ED, Tong D, Chung F, et al. Suprascapular nerve block for postoperative pain relief in arthroscopic shoulder surgery: a new modality? Anesth Analg 1997; 84(6):1306–12.
17. Cunningham DJ, LaRose MA, Zhang GX, et al. Regional anesthesia reduces inpatient and outpatient perioperative opioid demand in periarticular elbow surgery. J Shoulder Elbow Surg 2022;31(2):e48–57.
18. Lin E, Choi J, Hadzic A. Peripheral nerve blocks for outpatient surgery: evidence-based indications. Curr Opin Anaesthesiol 2013;26(4):467–74.
19. Gadsden JC, Tsai T, Iwata T, et al. Low interscalene block provides reliable anesthesia for surgery at or about the elbow. J Clin Anesth 2009;21(2):98–102.
20. Memtsoudis SG, Cozowicz C, Bekeris J, et al. Peripheral nerve block anesthesia/analgesia for patients undergoing primary hip and knee arthroplasty: recommendations from the International Consensus on Anesthesia-Related Outcomes after Surgery (ICAROS) group based on a systematic review and meta-analysis of current literature. Reg Anesth Pain Med 2021;46(11):971–85.
21. Gibbons C, Bruce J, Carpenter J, et al. Identification of risk factors by systematic review and development of risk-adjusted models for surgical site infection. Health Technol Assess 2011;15(30). 1-iv.
22. Korol E, Johnston K, Waser N, et al. A systematic review of risk factors associated with surgical site infections among surgical patients. PLoS One 2013;8(12): e83743.
23. Cheng H, Chen BP, Soleas IM, et al. Prolonged Operative Duration Increases Risk of Surgical Site Infections: A Systematic Review. Surg Infect (Larchmt) 2017; 18(6):722–35.
24. Schneider B, Kennedy DJ, Casey E, et al. Trainee involvement in transforaminal epidural steroid injections associated with increased incidence of vasovagal reactions. PM R 2014;6(10):914–9.
25. Gitman M, Barrington MJ. Local Anesthetic Systemic Toxicity: A Review of Recent Case Reports and Registries. Reg Anesth Pain Med 2018;43(2):124–30.
26. Macfarlane AJR, Gitman M, Bornstein KJ, et al. Updates in our understanding of local anaesthetic systemic toxicity: a narrative review. Anaesthesia 2021; 76(Suppl 1):27–39.
27. Neal JM, Barrington MJ, Fettiplace MR, et al. The Third American Society of Regional Anesthesia and Pain Medicine Practice Advisory on Local Anesthetic Systemic Toxicity: Executive Summary 2017. Reg Anesth Pain Med 2018;43(2): 113–23.
28. Helander EM, Kaye AJ, Eng MR, et al. Regional Nerve Blocks-Best Practice Strategies for Reduction in Complications and Comprehensive Review. Curr Pain Headache Rep 2019;23(6):43.
29. Brummett CM, Williams BA. Additives to local anesthetics for peripheral nerve blockade. Int Anesthesiol Clin 2011;49(4):104–16.
30. Lirk P, Hollmann MW, Strichartz G. The Science of Local Anesthesia: Basic Research, Clinical Application, and Future Directions. Anesth Analg 2018; 126(4):1381–92.

31. Barrington MJ, Uda Y. Did ultrasound fulfill the promise of safety in regional anesthesia? Curr Opin Anaesthesiol 2018;31(5):649–55.
32. Neal JM, Bernards CM, Butterworth JF 4th, et al. ASRA practice advisory on local anesthetic systemic toxicity. Reg Anesth Pain Med 2010;35(2):152–61.
33. Mazoit JX. Arrêt cardiaque et anesthésiques locaux [Cardiac arrest and local anaesthetics]. Presse Med 2013;42(3):280–6. French.
34. Williams DJ, Walker JD. A nomogram for calculating the maximum dose of local anaesthetic. Anaesthesia 2014;69(8):847–53.
35. El-Boghdadly K, Pawa A, Chin KJ. Local anesthetic systemic toxicity: current perspectives. Local Reg Anesth 2018;11:35–44.
36. Wadlund DL. Local Anesthetic Systemic Toxicity. AORN J 2017;106(5):367–77.
37. Neal JM, Neal EJ, Weinberg GL. American Society of Regional Anesthesia and Pain Medicine Local Anesthetic Systemic Toxicity checklist: 2020 version. Reg Anesth Pain Med 2021;46(1):81–2.
38. Kennedy DJ, Schneider B, Casey E, et al. Vasovagal rates in flouroscopically guided interventional procedures: a study of over 8,000 injections. Pain Med 2013;14(12):1854–9.
39. Al-Assam H, Azzopardi C, McGarry S, et al. Vasovagal reactions in ultrasound guided musculoskeletal injections: A study of 2,462 procedures. J Clin Orthop Trauma 2021;24:101706.
40. Rapp SE, Pavlin DJ, Nessly ML, et al. Effect of patient position on the incidence of vasovagal response to venous cannulation. Arch Intern Med 1993;153(14): 1698–704.
41. Akella K, Olshansky B, Lakkireddy D, et al. Pacing Therapies for Vasovagal Syncope. J Atr Fibrillation 2020;13(1):2406.
42. Vidri R, Emerick T, Alter B, et al. Managing Vasovagal Reactions in the Outpatient Pain Clinic Setting: A Review for Pain Medicine Physicians Not Trained in Anesthesiology. Pain Med 2022;23(6):1189–93.
43. Finn DM, Agarwal RR, Ilfeld BM, et al. Fall Risk Associated with Continuous Peripheral Nerve Blocks Following Knee and Hip Arthroplasty. Medsurg Nurs 2016;25(1):25–49.
44. Muraskin SI, Conrad B, Zheng N, et al. Falls associated with lower-extremity-nerve blocks: a pilot investigation of mechanisms. Reg Anesth Pain Med 2007; 32(1):67–72.
45. Feigl GC, Schmid M, Zahn PK, et al. The posterior femoral cutaneous nerve contributes significantly to sensory innervation of the lower leg: an anatomical investigation. Br J Anaesth 2020;124(3):308–13.
46. Chadha M, Si S, Bhatt D, et al. The Comparison of Two Different Volumes of 0.5% Ropivacaine in Ultrasound-Guided Supraclavicular Brachial Plexus Block Onset and Duration of Analgesia for Upper Limb Surgery: A Randomized Controlled Study. Anesth Essays Res 2020;14(1):87–91.
47. Redborg KE, Antonakakis JG, Beach ML, et al. Ultrasound improves the success rate of a tibial nerve block at the ankle. Reg Anesth Pain Med 2009;34(3):256–60.
48. Chin KJ, Wong NW, Macfarlane AJ, et al. Ultrasound-guided versus anatomic landmark-guided ankle blocks: a 6-year retrospective review. Reg Anesth Pain Med 2011;36(6):611–8.
49. Liu SS, Ngeow J, John RS. Evidence basis for ultrasound-guided block characteristics: onset, quality, and duration. Reg Anesth Pain Med 2010;35(2 Suppl): S26–35.
50. Salinas FV. Evidence Basis for Ultrasound Guidance for Lower-Extremity Peripheral Nerve Block: Update 2016. Reg Anesth Pain Med 2016;41(2):261–74.

51. Munirama S, McLeod G. A systematic review and meta-analysis of ultrasound versus electrical stimulation for peripheral nerve location and blockade. Anaesthesia 2015;70(9):1084–91.
52. Eichenberger U, Stöckli S, Marhofer P, et al. Minimal local anesthetic volume for peripheral nerve block: a new ultrasound-guided, nerve dimension-based method. Reg Anesth Pain Med 2009;34(3):242–6.
53. Nakamura T, Popitz-Bergez F, Birknes J, et al. The critical role of concentration for lidocaine block of peripheral nerve in vivo: studies of function and drug uptake in the rat. Anesthesiology 2003;99(5):1189–97.
54. Taboada Muñiz M, Rodríguez J, Bermúdez M, et al. Low volume and high concentration of local anesthetic is more efficacious than high volume and low concentration in Labat's sciatic nerve block: a prospective, randomized comparison. Anesth Analg 2008;107(6):2085–8.
55. O'Donnell BD, Iohom G. An estimation of the minimum effective anesthetic volume of 2% lidocaine in ultrasound-guided axillary brachial plexus block. Anesthesiology 2009;111(1):25–9.
56. Fredrickson MJ, Abeysekera A, White R. Randomized study of the effect of local anesthetic volume and concentration on the duration of peripheral nerve blockade. Reg Anesth Pain Med 2012;37(5):495–501.
57. Bourne M, Talkad A, Anatomy VM, et al. Foot fascia. In: StatPearls. Treasure Isl (FL): StatPearls Publishing; 2021.
58. Standring S. Gray's anatomy. 41tst ed. Edinburgh: Elsevier Churchill Livingstone; 2016.
59. Benimeli-Fenollar M, Montiel-Company JM, Almerich-Silla JM, et al. Tibial Nerve Block: Supramalleolar or Retromalleolar Approach? A Randomized Trial in 110 Participants. Int J Environ Res Public Health 2020;17(11):3860.
60. Shah A, Morris S, Alexander B, et al. Landmark Technique vs Ultrasound-Guided Approach for Posterior Tibial Nerve Block in Cadaver Models. Indian J Orthop 2020;54(1):38–42.
61. Bareither DJ, Genau JM, Massaro JC. Variation in the division of the tibial nerve: application to nerve blocks. J Foot Surg 1990;29(6):581–3.
62. O'Brien M. The anatomy of the Achilles tendon. Foot Ankle Clin 2005;10(2): 225–38.
63. Eldegwy MH, Ibrahim SM, Hanora S, et al. Ultrasound-guided sciatic politeal nerve block: a comparison of separate tibial and common peroneal nerve injections versus injecting proximal to the bifurcation. Middle East J Anaesthesiol 2015;23(2):171–6.
64. Nakagawa A, Miyake R, Naito Y. Masui. Ultrasound-guided sciatic nerve block in the popliteal fossa for the postoperative pain control after Achilles tendon repair 2012;61(5):546–8.
65. Herrick MD, Liu H, Davis M, et al. Regional anesthesia decreases complications and resource utilization in shoulder arthroplasty patients. Acta Anaesthesiol Scand 2018;62(4):540–7.
66. Freygant M, Dziurzyńska-Białek E, Guz W, et al. Magnetic resonance imaging of rotator cuff tears in shoulder impingement syndrome. Pol J Radiol 2014;79:391–7.
67. Dahan TH, Fortin L, Pelletier M, et al. Double blind randomized clinical trial examining the efficacy of bupivacaine suprascapular nerve blocks in frozen shoulder. J Rheumatol 2000;27(6):1464–9.
68. Lewis RN. The use of combined suprascapular and circumflex (articular branches) nerve blocks in the management of chronic arthritis of the shoulder joint. Eur J Anaesthesiol 1999;16(1):37–41.

69. Gleeson AP, Graham CA, Jones I, et al. Comparison of intra-articular lignocaine and a suprascapular nerve block for acute anterior shoulder dislocation. Injury 1997;28(2):141–2.
70. Breen TW, Haigh JD. Continuous suprascapular nerve block for analgesia of scapular fracture. Can J Anaesth 1990;37(7):786–8.
71. Schneider-Kolsky ME, Pike J, Connell DA. CT-guided suprascapular nerve blocks: a pilot study. Skeletal Radiol 2004;33(5):277–82.
72. Shah RV, Racz GB. Pulsed mode radiofrequency lesioning of the suprascapular nerve for the treatment of chronic shoulder pain. Pain Physician 2003;6(4):503–6.
73. Basta M, Sanganeria T, Varacallo M. Anatomy, shoulder and upper limb, suprascapular nerve. In: StatPearls. Treasure Island (FL): StatPearls Publishing; 2021.
74. Parris WC. Suprascapular nerve block: a safer technique. Anesthesiology 1990; 72(3):580–1.
75. Dangoisse MJ, Wilson DJ, Glynn CJ. MRI and clinical study of an easy and safe technique of suprascapular nerve blockade. Acta Anaesthesiol Belg 1994;45(2): 49–54.
76. Gado K, Emery P. Modified suprascapular nerve block with bupivacaine alone effectively controls chronic shoulder pain in patients with rheumatoid arthritis. Ann Rheum Dis 1993;52(3):215–8.
77. Laumonerie P, Blasco L, Tibbo ME, et al. Distal suprascapular nerve block-do it yourself: cadaveric feasibility study. J Shoulder Elbow Surg 2019;28(7):1291–7.
78. Schoenherr JW, Flynn DN, Doyal A. Suprascapular Nerve Block. In: StatPearls. Treasure Island (FL): StatPearls Publishing; 2022.
79. Hacıbeyoğlu G, Kocadağ G, Özkan A, et al. Brachial plexus block for elbow surgery in a patient with spinal muscular atrophy. J Clin Anesth 2021;72:110275.
80. Zhai WW, Wang XD, Li M, et al. A study on diaphragm function after interscalene brachial plexus block using a fixed dose of ropivacaine with different concentrations. Zhonghua Yi Xue Za Zhi 2016;96(28):2229–33.
81. al-Qattan MM. The nerve supply to extensor carpi radialis brevis. J Anat 1996; 188(Pt 1):249–50.
82. Cho H, Lee HY, Gil YC, et al. Topographical anatomy of the radial nerve and its muscular branches related to surface landmarks. Clin Anat 2013;26(7):862–9.
83. Jeon A, Kim YG, Kwon SO, et al. Relationship between the Branching Patterns of the Radial Nerve and Supinator Muscle. Biomed Res Int 2021;2021:8691114.
84. Tran J, Peng PWH, Chan VWS, et al. Overview of Innervation of Knee Joint. Phys Med Rehabil Clin N Am 2021;32(4):767–78.
85. Roberts SL, Stout A, Dreyfuss P. Review of Knee Joint Innervation: Implications for Diagnostic Blocks and Radiofrequency Ablation. Pain Med 2020;21(5): 922–38.
86. GARDNER E. The innervation of the knee joint. Anat Rec 1948;101(1):109–30.
87. Jaeger P, Nielsen ZJ, Henningsen MH, et al. Adductor canal block versus femoral nerve block and quadriceps strength: a randomized, double-blind, placebo-controlled, crossover study in healthy volunteers. Anesthesiology 2013;118(2): 409–15.
88. Charous MT, Madison SJ, Suresh PJ, et al. Continuous femoral nerve blocks: varying local anesthetic delivery method (bolus versus basal) to minimize quadriceps motor block while maintaining sensory block. Anesthesiology 2011;115(4): 774–81.
89. Johnston DF, Sondekoppam RV, Uppal V, et al. Hybrid Blocks for Total Knee Arthroplasty: A Technical Description. Clin J Pain 2018;34(3):222–30.

90. Sankineani SR, Reddy ARC, Eachempati KK, et al. Comparison of adductor canal block and IPACK block (interspace between the popliteal artery and the capsule of the posterior knee) with adductor canal block alone after total knee arthroplasty: a prospective control trial on pain and knee function in immediate postoperative period. Eur J Orthop Surg Traumatol 2018;28(7):1391–5.
91. Tran J, Peng PWH, Lam K, et al. Anatomical Study of the Innervation of Anterior Knee Joint Capsule: Implication for Image-Guided Intervention. Reg Anesth Pain Med 2018;43(4):407–14.

Printed and bound by CPI Group (UK) Ltd, Croydon, CR0 4YY

03/10/2024

01040476-0011